METASTASIS
Clinical and Experimental Aspects

Proceedings of the EORTC Metastasis Group International Conference
on Clinical and Experimental Aspects of Metastasis, London, April 21-23,
1980

edited by

K. HELLMANN
Imperial Cancer Research Fund
London, England

P. HILGARD
Bristol-Myers International
Brussels, Belgium

S. ECCLES
Institute of Cancer Research
Sutton, Surrey, England

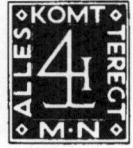

1980

SPRINGER-SCIENCE+BUSINESS MEDIA, B.V.

ISBN 978-94-009-8927-6   ISBN 978-94-009-8925-2 (eBook)
DOI 10.1007/978-94-009-8925-2

DEVELOPMENTS IN ONCOLOGY

VOLUME 4

Previously published in this series:

1. F.J. Cleton and J.W.I.M. Simons, eds., Genetic Origins of Tumor Cells
   ISBN 90-247-2272-1
2. J. Aisner and P. Chang, eds., Cancer Treatment Research
   ISBN 90-247-2358-2
3. B.W. Ongerboer de Visser, D.A. Bosch and W.M.H. van Woerkom-Eykenboom, eds.,
   Neuro-Oncology: Clinical and Experimental Aspects
   ISBN 90-247-2421-X

Series ISBN: 90-247-2338-8

METASTASIS

PREFACE

The Metastasis Group of the European Organization for Research on Treatment of Cancer (EORTC) held an International Meeting at the Royal Institution in London on April 21st-23rd, 1980. The subject was "Clinical and Experimental Aspects of Metastasis" and these Proceedings are the record of that Meeting.

Almost all of those who presented a paper or a poster have written up their contributions as chapters of the Proceedings and we have made no distinction here between posters and oral communications. The Organizers and Editors owe a considerable debt of gratitude to all the contributors who without exception presented the results of their work in a clear and concise manner that did much to reveal the essence of the complex problems central to current thinking on metastasis. Moreover most manuscripts arrived well within the deadline - a circumstance which in our experience is unusual.

Of the large audience who attended the Meeting many had come from the far distant corners of the World and to them as well as to the presenters of papers the Organizers wish to express their deep appreciation.

The Organizers would also like to express their indebtedness to the organizations whose financial contribution made this EORTC Metastasis Group Meeting possible and a list of them follows.

The keen interest which was shown in the Meeting has led many to ask about future meetings and these it is hoped can be arranged before long, though the framework within which this will take place remains to be settled.

for the EORTC Metastasis Group

K. Hellmann, Chairman

P. Hilgard, co-Chairman

S. Eccles

ACKNOWLEDGEMENTS

The Organizing Committee, which consisted of:

J. Castro, London
S. Eccles, Sutton
K. Hellmann, London
P. Hilgard, Brussels
F. Spreafico, Milano

thanks the following for their generous support of the EORTC Metastasis Conference

Abbott Laboratories Ltd.
Bayer Pharma-Forschungszentrum
Boehringer Ingelheim Ltd.
Boots Co. Ltd.
Bristol-Myers International
Cancer Research Campaign
Dome Laboratories
Eli Lilly & Co. Ltd.
Glaxo Holdings
Imperial Cancer Research Fund
I.C.I. Ltd.
Lederle Laboratories Ltd.
Monsanto Company
Montedison Pharmaceuticals Ltd.
Roche Products Ltd.
Wellcome Foundation Ltd.

They would also like to thank all the staff of the Cancer Chemotherapy Department, Imperial Cancer Research Fund who helped at the Meeting and whose unstinting efforts made this occasion run as smoothly as it did.

They would particularly like to thank Mrs. Jean Hartley who not only organized the secretariat, but who also collated all the papers of the Proceedings and retyped many of them. Thanks are also due to Ms. Stephanie Jibson whose valiant efforts resulted in the exhaustive Index of this book.

CONTENTS

X

CONTENTS

CONTENTS

CONTENTS

CONTENTS

CONTENTS

CONTENTS

CONTENTS

CONTENTS

CONTENTS

CONTRIBUTORS

Ikuo Abe,
Dept. of Oncology,
The Research Inst. for
    Tuberculosis & Cancer,
Tohoku University,
Sendai, Japan.

K. Adams,
Dept. of Radiotherapy
    Research,
Inst. of Cancer Research,
Sutton, Surrey, UK

J.E. Agnew,
The Royal Free Hospital &
    School of Medicine,
London, NW3 2QG, UK

H. Alani,
Royal Free Hospital,
London, NW3 2QG, UK

Giulio Alessandri,
Istituto di Ricerche
    Farmacologiche "Mario Negri",
Via Eritrea, 62, 20157 Milan,
Italy.

Magne Alpsten,
Dept. of Surgery I,
Sahlgrenska Sjukhuset,
Göteborg, Sweden.

J. Ammon,
Chefarzt der Abteilung
    für Radiologie der Med.
    Fakultät der TH Aachen,
Goethestrasse 27-29,
D-5100 Aachen,
West Germany.

R. Arnould,
Institut Jules Bordet,
1000 Brussels,
Rue Heger-Bordet 1,
Belgium.

Mitsuo Asamura,
Dept. of Clinical Cancer
    Chemotherapy,
The Research Inst. for
    Tuberculosis & Cancer,
Tohoku University, Sendai,
Japan.

G. Atassi,
Institut Jules Bordet,
1000 Brussels,
Rue-Heger Bordet, 1,
Brussèls

S. Bajwa,
University of Southern
    California School of
    Medicine,
Los Angeles, California, 90033,
USA

I. Basic,
Dept. of Animal Physiology,
University of Zagreb,
Zagreb,
Yugoslavia

A. Baxter,
Depts. of Oncology and
    Pathology,
University of Glasgow,
Glasgow,
Scotland, UK

D.J. Beard,
Depts. of Human Metabolism
    & Clinical Biochemistry,
University of Sheffield
    Medical School,
Sheffield, UK

A.C. Begg,
Gray Laboratory,
Mount Vernon Hospital,
Northwood,
Middlesex, UK

CONTRIBUTORS

Germana de Bellis Vitti,
Laboratory for Haemostasis
  & Thrombosis Research,
Istituto di Ricerche
  Farmacologiche "Mario Negri",
Via Eritrea 62, 20157 Milan,
Italy.

H.J. Bengelsdorff,
Research Laboratories of
  Behringwerke AG,
3550 Marburg/Lahn, FRG

C. Bignell,
Radiobiological Institute TNO,
151 Lange Kleiweg, Rijswijk,
Netherlands.

G.D. Birkmayer,
Inst. für Zellbiologie,
München,
West Germany

Bernt Boeryd,
Dept. of Pathology,
University of Linköping,
Sweden

E. Bogenmann,
Swiss Inst. for Experimental
  Cancer Research,
1066 Epalinges,
Switzerland.

J.L. Boublil,
Centre Antoine Lacassagne,
36 Av. Voie Romaine,
Nice, France.

K. Bosslet,
Inst. für Immunologie und
  Genetik am Deutschen
  Krebsforschungszentrum
Heidelberg, FRG

Julie Boston
Marie Curie Memorial
  Foundation, Oxted,
Surrey, UK

N. Bowley,
Royal Postgraduate Medical
  School,
London, UK

F. Calabresi,
"Regina Elena" Inst. for
  Cancer Research,
Rome,
Italy.

S.K. Calderwood,
Cancer Unit,
Royal Victoria Infirmary,
Newcastle upon Tyne,
UK

K.C. Calman,
Department of Pathology,
University of Glasgow,
Glasgow,
Scotland, UK

M. Caputo,
"Regina Elena" Cancer Inst.,
Rome,
Italy.

J.E. Castro,
Royal Postgraduate Medical
  School,
Hammersmith Hospital,
London, W12, UK

R.L. Carter,
Institute for Cancer Research,
Fulham Road,
London, SW3 6JB, UK

P. Cassell,
Wexham Park Hospital,
Slough,
Berks, UK

CONTRIBUTORS

S.A. Cederholm-Williams,
Dept. of Haematology,
John Radcliffe Hospital,
Oxford, UK

J. Coel,
Institut Jules Bordet,
1000 Brussels,
Belgium.

Mario Colucci,
Laboratory for Haemostasis and
   Thrombosis Research,
Istituto "Mario Negri",
Milan,
Italy.

A. Corsi,
"Regina Elena" Cancer Inst.,
Rome,
Italy.

G.T. Craig,
Dept. of Oral Pathology,
University of Sheffield,
Sheffield, UK

R. Cuman,
Istituto di Farmacologia,
Universita di Trieste,
Trieste, Italy.

Federica Delaini,
Laboratory for Haemostasis nad
   Thrombosis Research,
Istituto "Mario Negri",
Milan,
Italy.

H. Denck,
Institut für Krebsforschung
   der Universität Wien,
1090 Wien,
Austria

K.P. Dingemans,
Laboratory for Pathological
   Anatomy,
University of Amsterdam,
The Netherlands

B. Dixon,
Dept. of Radiotherapy,
University of Leeds,
Leeds, UK

J.A. van Dongen,
Dept. of Surgery,
The Netherlands Cancer Inst.,
Amsterdam,
The Netherlands.

Maria B. Donati,
Laboratory for Haemostasis
   & Thrombosis Research,
Istituto "Mario Negri",
Milan,
Italy.

D.L. Douglas,
Depts. of Human Metabolism
   and Clinical Biochemistry,
University of Sheffield
   Medical School,
Sheffield, UK

S.A. Eccles,
Institute of Cancer Research,
Sutton,
Surrey, UK

Jan Eldh,
Dept. of Plastic Surgery,
University of Göteborg,
Sweden

S. Elgebaly,
University of Connecticut,
Farmington,
Connecticut 06032, USA

CONTRIBUTORS

D. Eljuga,
Central Institute for Tumors
  and Allied Diseases,
Zagreb,
Yugoslavia.

H. Ellis,
Department of Surgery,
Westminster Hospital Medical
  School,
London, SW1, UK

M. Endo,
2nd Dept. of Pathology,
Fukushima Medical College,
Fukushima 960,
Japan.

M. Evans,
Cancer Chemotherapy Dept.,
Imperial Cancer Research Fund,
London, WC2, UK

I. Florentin,
I.C.I.G.,
94800 Villejuif,
France.

M. Frick,
Institut fur Zellforschung,
Deutsches Krebsforschungszentrum,
Heidelberg,
West Germany.

C.S.B. Galasko,
Dept. of Orthopaedic Surgery,
University of Manchester,
Hope Hospital,
Salford, UK.

Silvio Garattini,
Istituto "Mario Negri",
Milan, Italy.

S. Garbisa,
Nat. Inst. for Dental Research,
National Cancer Institute,
Bethesda, MD 20205,
USA

Raffaella Giavazzi,
Istituto "Mario Negri",
Milan,
Italy.

J. Gilbert,
Northwick Park Hospital,
Harrow, Middlesex,
UK

T. Giraldi,
Istituto di Farmacologia,
Universita di Trieste,
Trieste,
Italy.

J.P. Giroud,
Fac. Med. Cochin Port Royal,
76574 Paris Cedex,
France.

A. Goldin,
Division of Cancer Treatment,
National Cancer Institute,
Bethesda, Maryland,
USA

C. Greco,
"Regina Elena" Inst. for
  Cancer Research,
Rome,
Italy.

J. Griffiths,
Royal Marsden Hospital,
London, SW3, UK

CONTRIBUTORS

D. Guy,
Cancer Research Unit,   ,
Dept. of Clinical Biochemistry,
Royal Victoria Infirmary,
Newcastle upon Tyne, UK

P. Hanson,
Institut Jules Bordet,
1000 Brussels,
Belgium,

S.E. Heckford,
Division of Tumour Immunology,
Inst. of Cancer Research,
Sutton, Surrey, UK

K. Hellmann,
Cancer Chemotherapy Department,
Imperial Cancer Research Fund,
London, WC2, UK.

C.N. Hensby,
Hammersmith Hospital & Royal
  Postgraduate Med. School,
London, W12, UK

H.B. Hewitt,
King's College Hospital
  Medical School,
London, SE5, UK

Yuhji Higuchi,
Third Dept. of Internal Medicine,
University of Tokushima,
Japan.

P. Hilgard,
Bristol-Myers International,
185 Chaussee de la Hulpe,
B1170 Brussels,
Belgium.

C.J. Hillyard,
Royal Postgraduate Medical
  School,
Hammersmith Hospital,
London, W12, UK

P. van Hoorde,
Dept. of Radiotherapy &
  Nuclear Medicine,
University Hospital,
B-9000 Ghent,
Belgium

Katsuyoshi Hori,
Department of Oncology,
The Research Institute for
  Tuberculosis & Cancer,
Tohoku University,
Sendai, Japan.

Kou M. Hwang,
University of Southern
  California School of
  Medicine,
Los Angeles, California,90033,
USA

M. Ishihara,
Research Institute,
Daiichi Pharmaceutical Co.,
Tokyo, Japan.

Lars Ivarsson,
Dept. of Surgery 1,
Sahlgrenska Sjukhuset,
Göteborg,
Sweden

A. Iwakawa,
Dept. of Pathology,
Faculty of Medicine,
Kyushu University,
Fukuoka, Japan.

CONTRIBUTORS

P.D.E. Jones,
Department of Surgery,
Royal Postgraduate Medical School,
London, W12, UK

Kazuo Kagawa,
Third Department of Internal
  Medicine,
The University of Tokushima
  School of Medicine,
Tokushima, Japan.

Ryunosuke Kanamuru,
Department of Clinical Cancer
  Chemotherapy,
The Research Inst. for
  Tuberculosis & Cancer,
Tohoku University, Sendai,
Japan.

J.A. Kanis,
Depts. of Human Metabolism &
  Clinical Biochemistry,
University of Sheffield Medical
  School,
Sheffield, UK

K. Karrer,
Institut für Krebsforschung der
  Universität Wien,
1090 Wien,
Austria

J.H. Karstens
Chefarzt der Abteilung für
  Radiologie der Med.Fakultät
  der TH Aachen,
Goethestrasse 27-29,
D5100 Aachen,
West Germany

T. Kawaguchi,
2nd Dept. of Pathology,
Fukushima Medical College,
Fukushima 960, Japan.

J.A. Kellen,
Dept. of Clinical Biochemistry
University of Toronto,
Toronto, Ontario,
Canada

O. Khan,
Hammersmith Hospital and
  Royal Postgraduate Med.
  School,
London, W12, UK

Untae Kim,
Roswell Park Memorial Inst.,
Buffalo,
New York, 14263, USA

M. Kinjo,
Dept. of Pathology,
Faculty of Medicine,
Kyushu University, Fukuoka,
Japan.

S. Kohga,
Dept. of Pathology,
Faculty of Medicine,
Kyushu University, Fukuoka,
Japan.

Kenichi Kohno,
Department of Surgery,
Akita University School
  of Medicine,
Akita 010, Japan.

CONTRIBUTORS

A. Kolin,
Department of Clinical Bio-
    chemistry,
University of Toronto,
Toronto, Ontario,
Canada.

L. Kreel,
Northwick Park Hospital,
Harrow,
Middlesex, UK

R. Kurrle,
Research Laboratories of
    Behringwerke AG,
3550 Marburg/L hn,
FRG

Eve Lacey,
Dept. of Orthopaedic Surgery,
University of Manchester,
Hope Hospital,
Salford, UK

M.S. Lakshmi,
Cancer Research Unit,
University of Newcastle upon
    Tyne,
Royal Victoria Infirmary,
Newcastle upon Tyne, UK

C.M. Lalanne,
Centre Antoine Lacassagne,
36 Av. Voie Romaine,
Nice, France.

L. Lassiani
Istituto di Farmacologia,
Università di Trieste,
Trieste,
Italy.

A.L. Latner,
Cancer Research Unit,
Dept. of Clinical Biochemistry
    and Metabolic Medicine,
Royal Victoria Infirmary,
Newcastle upon Tyne, UK

A.E. Lee,
Imperial Cancer Research
    Fund,
London, WC2, UK

R.K. Lees,
Ludwig Institute for
    Cancer Research,
1066 Epalinges,
Switzerland.

F. Legros,
Institut Jules Bordet,
1000 Brussels,
Belgium

S. Legros,
Institut Jules Bordet,
1000 Brussels,
Belgium.

F.J. Lejeune,
Institut Jules Bordet,
1000 Brussels,
Belgium

C. Leuchtenberger,
Institute of Pathology,
Lausanne,
Switzerland.

A. Libert,
Institut Jules Bordet,
1000 Brussels,
Belgium

CONTRIBUTORS

L. Liotta,
Nat. Inst. for Dental Research,
National Cancer Institute,
Bethesda, MD 20205,
USA.

A. Liteanu,
Institut Jules Bordet,
1000 Brussels,
Belgium.

Julia Lockwood,
Marie Curie Memorial Foundation,
Oxted,
Surrey

J. Lovett,
Department of Surgery,
University of Connecticut,
Farmington, Connecticut,06032,
USA.

J. Lundy,
Department of Pathology,
University of Connecticut,
Farmington, Connecticut,06032,
USA

B. Maat,
Radiobiological Inst. TNO,
151 Lange Kleiweg,
Rijswijk,
The Netherlands.

I. MacIntyre,
Royal Postgraduate Medical
   School,
Hammersmith Hospital,
London, W12, UK

M. Magudia,
Marie Curie Memorial Foundation,
Oxted, Surrey,
UK

A. Malcolm,
Department of Pathology,
University of Glasgow,
Glasgow,
Scotland, UK

B. Malenica,
Central Inst. for Tumors
   and Allied Diseases,
Zagreb,
Yugoslavia

A. Malkin
Department of Surgery,
University of Toronto,
Toronto,
Ontario, Canada

Alberto Mantovani,
Istituto di Ricerche
   Farmacologiche "Mario Negri",
Milan,
Italy.

Francis S. Markland,
Dept. of Biochemistry &
   Cancer Center,
University of Southern
   California School of Medicine
Los Angeles, Calif. 90033,
USA

M. Mareel,
Dept. of Radiotherapy & Nuclear
   Medicine,
Universith Hospital,
B-9000 Ghent,
Belgium.

R. Masse,
C.E.A.-I.P.S.N., Toxicol.
   Exptl. Lab,
92542 Montrouge Cedex,
France

CONTRIBUTORS

R.T. Mathie,
Department of Surgery,
Royal Postgraduate Medical School,
Hammersmith Hospital,
London, W12, UK

S. Matzku,
German Cancer Research Center,
Institute of Nuclear Medicine,
Heidelberg, FRG

A. Mayer,
Institut für Zellforschung,
Deutsches Krebsforschungszentrum,
Heidelberg,
West Germany.

C. Meyvisch,
Laboratory of Experimental
  Cancerology,
University Hospital,
B-9000 Ghent,
Belgium.

G. Milano,
Centre Antoine Lacassagne,
36 Av. Voie Romaine,
Nice, France.

L. Milas,
Department of Experimental
  Radiotherapy,
The University of Texas System
  Cancer Center,
M.D. Anderson Hospital & Tumor
  Institute, Houston, Texas,
USA.

K.J. Miller,
Imperial Cancer Research Fund,
Lincoln's Inn Fields,
London, WC2, UK

Youko Mimata,
Department of Clinical Cancer
  Chemotherapy,
The Research Inst. for
  Tuberculosis & Cancer,
Tohoku University, Sendai,
Japan.

Karen M. Miner,
Departments of Developmental
  and Cell Biology & Physiology,
College of Medicine,
University of California,
Irvine, Calif. 92717,
USA

H.D. Mitcheson,
Hammersmith Hospital & Royal
  Postgraduate Medical School,
London, W.12, UK

J.H. Mulder,
Dept. of Internal Medicine,
Rotterdam Radiotherapeutic
  Inst., Rotterdam,
The Netherlands.

J.C. Murray,
Nat. Inst. for Dental Research,
National Cancer Institute,
Bethesda, MD20205,
USA

CONTRIBUTORS

K. Nakamura,
2nd Department of Pathology,
Fukushima Medical College,
Fukushima 960,
Japan.

N. Namer,
Centre Antoine Lacassagne,
36 Av. Voie Romaine,
Nice,
France.

F.E. Neal,
Dept. of Radiotherapy &
   Oncology,
Weston Park Hospital,
Sheffield, UK.

Anthony Neri,
Depts. of Developmental & Cell
   Biology & Physiology,
College of Medicine,
University of California,
Irvine,
California 72717, USA

Adele Nicolas,
Royal Postgraduate Medical
   School,
Hammersmith Hospital,
London, W12, UK

Garth L. Nicolson,
Department of Tumor Biology,
University of Texas System Cancer
   Center,
M.D. Anderson Hospital & Tumor Inst.
Houston, Texas 77030, USA

C. Nisi,
Istituto di Farmacologia,
Università di Trieste,
Trieste,
Italy

D. Nolibe,
C.E.A.-I.P.S.N.,
Toxicol. Exptl. Lab.,
92542 Montrouge Cedex,
France.

A. Nuchowicz,
Institut Jules Bordet,
1000 Brussels,
Belgium.

H. Ogawa,
Research Institute,
Daiichi Pharmaceutical Co.,
Tokyo,
Japan.

Siegfried Öhl,
Innere Universitätsklinik und
   Poliklinik (Tumorforschung)
Westdeutsches Tumorzentrum,
Essen,
West Germany

L.N. Owen,
Dept. of Clinical Veterinary
   Medicine,
Madingley Road,
Cambridge, UK

L. Ozzello,
Inst. of Pathology,
Lausanne,
Switzerland.

L. Pang,
Imperial Cancer Research
   Fund,
Lincoln's Inn Fields,
London, WC2, UK

CONTRIBUTORS

S.P. Parbhoo,
Academic Department of Surgery,
Royal Free Hospital,
London, NW3 2QG, UK

B. Patkos,
University of Southern
  California School of Med.,
Los Angeles,
California 90033, USA

J.H. Peacock,
Department of Radiotherapy Research,
Institute of Cancer Research,
Sutton, Surrey, UK

M. Pelletier,
Fac. Med. Cochin Port
  Royal 75674,
Paris Cedex,
France.

Hans-Inge Peterson,
Laboratory of Bioreology,
Dept. of Surgery I,
Sahlgrenska Univ. Hospital,
Göteborg, Sweden

Lars-Erik Peterson,
Dept. of Statistics,
University of Göteborg,
Sweden.

Adreina Poggi,
Laboratory for Haemostasis
  & Thrombosis Research,
Istituto "Mario Negri",
Milan,
Italy.

Morris Pollard,
Lobund Laboratory,
University of Notre Dame,
Notre Dame, Indiana 46556,
USA

F.E. Preston,
Dept. of Haematology,
University of Sheffield
  Med. School,
Sheffield, UK

N. Pridun,
Institut für Krebsforschung
  der Universität Wien,
1090 Wien,
Austria

L.M. van Putten,
Radiobiological Inst. TNO,
Rijswijk,
The Netherlands

L. Reading,
Depts. of Developmental and
  Cell Biology & Physiology,
College of Medicine,
Univ. of California, Irvine,
California, 92717,
USA

Parker Roberts,
University of Connecticut
  Health Center,
Farmington, Connecticut, 06032,
USA

L.A. Rogers,
Imperial Cancer Research
  Fund,
Lincoln's Inn Fields,
London, WC2, UK

E. Roos,
Division of Cell Biology,
The Netherlands Cancer Inst.,
Amsterdam,
The Netherlands.

CONTRIBUTORS

Stella Rushton,
Dept. of Orthopaedic Surgery,
Univ. of Manchester,
Hope Hospital, Salford,
UK

R.G.G. Russell,
Dept. of Radiotherapy &
  Oncology,
Weston Park Hospital,
Sheffield, UK

A. Sacchi,
"Regina Elena" Cancer Inst.,
Rome,
Italy.

Peter L. Salk,
Salk Institute,
San Diego, Calif. 92138,
USA

A. Salsbury,
Brompton Hospital,
Fulham Road,
London, SW3, UK

A.W. Samuel,
Dept. of Orthopaedic Surgery,
University of Manchester,
Hope Hospital, Salford,
UK

Sachiko Saito,
Dept. of Oncology,
The Research Inst. for Tuber-
  culosis & Cancer,
Tohoku University,
Sendai, Japan.

Haruo Sato,
Dept. of Oncology,
The Research Inst. for Tuber-
  culosis & Cancer,
Tohoku University,
Sendai, Japan.

Haruhiko Sato, Kazuaki Sato &
  Yoshihiro Sato,
Dept. of Clinical Cancer Chemo-
  therapy,
The Research Inst. for Tuber-
  culosis & Cancer, Tohoku
  University,
Sendai, Japan.

Hiroshi Satoh,
Sasaki Institute,
Tokyo,
Japan.

G. Sava,
Istituto di Farmacologia,
Università di Trieste,
Trieste,
Italy

V. Schirrmacher,
Inst. für Immunologie und
  Genetik am Deutschen
  Krebsforschungszentrum,
Heidelberg,
West Germany

A.B. Schleich,
Inst. für Zellforschung,
Deutsches Krebsforschungszentru
Heidelberg,
West Germany.

G. Schmidt,
Innere Universitätsklinik und
  Poliklinik,
Westdeutsches Tumorzentrum,
Essen,
West Germany

M. Schneider,
Centre Antoine Lacassagne,
36 Av. Voie Romaine,
Nice,
France.

CONTRIBUTORS

Friedrich Schüning,
Innere Universitätsklinik und
  Poliklinik,
Westdeutsches Tumorzentrum,
Essen,
West Germany

H.H. Sedlacek,
Research Laboratories of
  Behringwerke AG,
Marburg/Lahn,
West Germany

F.R. Seiler,
Research Laboratories of
  Behringwerke AG,
Marburg/Lahn,
West Germany

Nicola Semeraro,
Dept. of Microbiology,
Med. School, University
  of Bari,
Bari, Italy.

S.A. Shah,
Cancer Unit,
Royal Victoria Infirmary,
Newcastle upon Tyne,
UK

G.V. Sherbet,
Cancer Research Unit,
University of Newcastle
  upon Tyne,
Royal Victoria Infirmary,
Newcastle upon Tyne, UK

Jennifer Shewell,
Dept. of Radiobiology,
Medical College of St.
  Bartholomew's Hospital,
London, EC2. UK

A.C. Simpson,
Cancer Unit,
Royal Victoria Infirmary,
Newcastle upon Tyne, UK

Gabor Skolnik,
Dept. of Surgery I,
Sahlgrenska Sjukhuset,
Göteborg, Sweden.

K.A. Smith,
Gray Laboratory,
Mount Vernon Hospital,
Northwood,
Middlesex, UK

B. Sordat,
Swiss Inst. for Experimental
  Cancer Research
1066 Epalinges,
Switzerland.

H. Speakman,
Dept. of Radiotherapy,
University of Leeds,
Leeds, UK

Federico Spreafico,
Istituto "Mario Negri",
Milan,
Italy.

T.C. Stephens,
Dept. of Radiotherapy Research,
Inst. of Cancer Research,
Sutton, Surrey, UK

B.A. Stoll,
Department of Radiotherapy,
Royal Free Hospital,
London, NW3 2QG, UK

CONTRIBUTORS

Anders Sundbeck,
Laboratory of Biorheology,
Dept. of Surgery I,
Sahlgrenska University Hospital,
Göteborg,
Sweden.

Maroh Suzuki,
Dept. of Oncology,
The Research Inst. for Tuber-
culosis & Cancer,
Tohoku University,
Sendai, Japan.

N. Suzuki,
Department of Experimental
Radiotherapy,
The University of Texas System
Cancer Center,
M.D. Anderson Hospital & Tumor
Institute,
Houston, Texas, 77030,
USA

Toshio Takahashi,
Department of Surgery,
School of Medicine,
Akito University,
Japan.

I.C. Talbot,
Department of Pathology,
School of Medicine,
Leicester, UK

K. Tanaka & N. Tanaka,
Dept. of Pathology,
Faculty of Medicine,
Kyushu University,
Fukuoka, Japan

J.A. Teodorczyk-Injeyan,
Dept. of Clinical Biochemistry,
University of Toronto,
Toronto, Ontario,
Canada.

G. Terres,
Dept. of Physiology,
Tufts University School of
Medicine,
Boston, USA

R. Tchao,
Institut für Zellforschung,
Deutsches Krebsforschungszentrum,
Heidelberg,
West Germany

N. van Tieghem,
Institut Jules Bordet,
1000 Brussels,
Belgium.

M.J. Tisdale,
Dept. of Biochemistry,
St. Thomas's Hospital Medical
School,
London, SE1 7EH, UK

S. Tobai,
2nd Dept. of Pathology,
Fukushima Medical College,
Fukushima 960, Japan.

Eiro Tsubura,
3rd Dept. of Internal Medicine,
The University of Tokushima
Medical School,
Tokushima, Japan.

CONTRIBUTORS

G.A. Turner,
Cancer Research Unit,
Dept. of Clinical Biochemistry
   & Metabolic Medicine,
Royal Victoria Infirmary,
Newcastle upon Tyne, UK

J. Varani,
Dept. of Surgery,
University of Connecticut,
Farmington,
Connecticut 06032,
USA.

A. Vercammen-Grandjean,
Institut Jules Bordet,
1000 Brussels,
Belgium.

A. Verhest,
Institut Jules Bordet,
1000 Brussels,
Belgium.

M. Viot,
Centre Antoine Lacassagne,
36 Av. Voie Romaine,
Nice, France.

J.F. Watkins,
Dept. of Medical Microbiology,
Welsh National School of Med.,
Heath Park,
Cardiff, UK

H. White,
Royal Marsden Hospital,
London, SW3 6JJ, UK

D.C. Williams,
Marie Curie Memorial Foundation,
Oxted, Surrey, UK

G. Williams,
Hammersmith Hospital & Royal
   Postgraduate Medical School,
London, W12, UK

M. Williams,
Dept. of Experimental Radio-
   therapy,
The Univ. of Texas System
   Cancer Center,
M.D. Anderson Hospital & Tumor
   Institute,
Houston, Texas, 77030,
USA

N. Willmott,
Dept. of Oncology,
University of Glasgow,
Glasgow,
Scotland, UK

H.R. Withers,
Dept. of Experimental Radio-
   therapy,
The Univ. of Texas System
   Cancer Center,
M.D. Anderson Hospital &
   Tumor Institute,
Houston, Texas, 77030,
USA

M.A. van den Bergh Weerman,
Laboratory for Pathological
   Anatomy,
University of Amsterdam,
Amsterdam,
The Netherlands.

Toshiharu Yamaguchi,
Department of Surgery,
Akita University School
   of Medicine,
Akita 010, Japan.

XXXIV

CONTRIBUTORS

Toshiaki Yamamoto,
3rd Dept. of Internal Medicine,
The University of Tokushima
   Medical School,
Tokushima, Japan.

Takashi Yamashita,
3rd Dept. of Internal Medicine,
The University of Tokushima
   Medical School,
Tokushima, Japan.

Ganesa Yogeeswaran,
Salk Institute,
San Diego,
California 92138,
USA

M. Zöller,
German Cancer Research Center,
Institute of Nuclear Medicine,
Heidelberg,
West Germany.

G. Zupi,
"Regina Elena" Cancer Institute,
Rome,
Italy.

ADDENDUM

O. Bertermann, T. Mischkowsky
   and H. Krebs,
Department of Surgery,
University of Heidelberg,
West Germany.

J. Stjernswärd,
Ludwig Inst. for Cancer
   Research,
Bern, Switzerland.

THE SIGNIFICANCE OF METASTASES TO THE SURGEON

H. Ellis

I am honoured, as a surgeon, to open this important
Symposium on Clinical and Experimental Aspects of Metastasis.
It is my duty to set the scene for our discussion over the next
three days.

Metastases are the enemy of the cancer surgeon.   Even the
most horrendous primary cancer can usually be controlled either
by surgical excision, which may sometimes have to be of heroic
proportions, or by radiotherapy.   However, it is the secondary
deposits and not the primary tumour itself which usually
defeat the surgeon and kill his patient.

Until recently, the classical concept of tumour spread
envisaged an orderly march of local growth proceeding to
lymphatic spread and then to widespread dissemination and
eventually the death of the patient.   This view led to the
development of radical cancer surgery which was designed to
ablate the primary tumour and its lymphatic drainage in the
hope that dissemination would thus be prevented.   A century ago
the radical mastectomy operation was developed by Halsted with
this in mind, and this was followed rapidly by the evolution of
block dissection of the neck by Crile, the abdomino-perineal
excision of the rectum by Miles and the other classical cancer
operations.   For a time surgeons seemed to vie with each other
to produce bigger and better operations and any attempt at a
more conservative approach was considered as little short of
criminal.

However, in recent years a more critical evaluation of our
patients has led to the concept that there are two major groups
of malignant tumours.   The first category are those which are
locally invasive with late dissemination.   Here radical surgery
pays off and long-term survivals can be anticipated.   The
second category are those where micro-metastases are already
present at the time of initial presentation and so surgery, no
matter how radical, cannot possibly preserve the patient.

At present the status of the regional lymph nodes is the
best prognostic marker but it is far from accurate.   For
example, we know that about 90% of women with lymph node negative

breast cancer will survive for five years or more after adequate local therapy to the breast - but what of the 10% that relapse? Similarly, we know that 60% of patients with extensive lymph node involvement in this disease will be dead within five years - but what of the 40% that remain well?

What we clinicians urgently need are better markers for tumour prognosis; these may be histological, histochemical, biochemical or hormonal, alone or in combination. Once we have an effective marker for a particular tumour we can decide whether to use adequate local therapy alone in good prognosis cases, even though this might have to be very radical indeed, or to use some form of adjuvant therapy in those cases where we know that the prognosis is very grave.

There are many unsolved questions facing the surgeon dealing with his cancer patients to-day - I hope that some at least may be answered in this Symposium.

THE SPREAD OF RECTAL CANCER INTO VEINS AND THE MECHANISM OF DISTANT EMBOLISM

I.C. Talbot

INTRODUCTION

Since metastatic disease is the principal factor which determines the outcome in rectal cancer, occurring in 32% of cases (Dionne, 1965) and, as Willis (1930) states, distant metastases are generally the result of spread of tumour by the blood stream it is, perhaps, surprising that the relationship between local invasion of rectal veins and the development of blood-borne distant metastases has not hitherto been well defined.

MATERIALS AND METHODS

These are described in detail elsewhere (Talbot, 1980 and Talbot et al, 1980 (b)). A series of 703 cases of carcinoma of rectum were examined at St. Mark's Hospital, London, over a 7 year period. Surgically excised specimens were carefully dissected, using a technique devised by Bussey and Morson. Only those cases in which there was definite evidence of tumour spread into veins were classed as showing venous invasion; cases with possible or doubtful venous invasion were placed, together with those in which venous spread was not observed, in the "not demonstrated" category. Venous invasion was quantitated according to its extent; spread into sub-mucosal or intramuscular veins only was classed as "intramural" venous spread, whereas invasion of veins in the peri-rectal adipose tissue was classed as "extramural". The invaded veins were divided into 2 categories; those with only thin-walls in which smooth muscle was inconspicuous and those with thick-walls and a well developed muscular coat. Other histological features related to carcinomatous invasion of veins were noted; aneurysmal distention of veins, particularly by mucinous carcinoma, necrosis of tumour within veins, peri-venous inflammation with damage to the vein wall and replacement by granulation tissue and fibrous tissue, formation of a mantle of proliferated endothelial cells covering the tip of intravenous tumour, permeation of capillary channels in vein walls and direct contact between naked tumour cells and venous blood were all noted. These features are illustrated and described more fully by Talbot et al (1980 (b)). Careful follow-up of the patients revealed whether they were alive or dead 5 years after operation and, with reasonable certainty, whether metastatic tumour was present in the liver or elsewhere. 5 year survival rates were determined only on those patients who recovered from the immediate post-operative period (4 weeks) and were corrected to compensate for death from all causes in the national age-matched population.

RESULTS

Invasion of veins was found by histological examination in 52% of cases (Table 1.2.1.). Extramural veins were invaded in 36% of the whole series (Table 1.2.1.).

TABLE 1.2.1.

VENOUS INVASION	NUMBER	%
NOT DEMONSTRATED	338	48.1
PRESENT { Intramural 111 Extramural 254 }	365	51.9
TOTAL	703	100.0

The corrected 5 year survival rate when venous invasion was present was only 43%, but was as high as 73% when venous spread was not demonstrated (Table 1.2.2.). The survival rate of the smaller number of cases in which only intramural veins were involved was almost 2 in 3 (not very significantly different from cases in which venous invasion was not demonstrated), but when extramural veins were invaded the corrected 5 year survival rate was only 33%.

TABLE 1.2.2.

VENOUS INVASION	OPERATION SURVIVORS	5 YEAR SURVIVORS	CORRECTED 5 YEAR SURVIVAL RATE (%)
NOT DEMONSTRATED	328	206	73
PRESENT { Intramural Extramural	{ 108 248 } 356	{ 61 69 } 130	{ 66 33 } 43

These survival differences are related to the occurrence of liver and other distant metastases (Table 1.2.3.). 40% of cases with extramural venous spread developed liver metastases, whereas liver deposits developed in 23% of cases with invasion limited to intramural veins and in only 14% of cases in which spread into veins was not demonstrated.

TABLE 1.2.3.

VENOUS INVASION	NUMBER OF CASES	LIVER METASTASES	
		NUMBER	%
NOT DEMONSTRATED	338	48	14.2
INTRAMURAL	111	26	23.4
EXTRAMURAL	254	102	40.2
WHOLE SERIES	703	176	25.0

Table 1.2.4. shows that there is a more specific relationship between venous invasion and the development of metastases when the size (thickness of wall) of the invaded veins is taken into account.

TABLE 1.2.4.

VENOUS INVASION	NUMBER OF CASES	NUMBER WITH DISTANT METASTASES	%	PROBABILITY cf. "not demonstrated"
INTRAMURAL	111	33	29.7	$<0.1,>0.05$
EXTRAMURAL Thin-walled	161	63	39.1	<0.001
EXTRAMURAL Thin-walled	93	63	67.7	<0.001
NOT DEMONSTRATED	338	74	21.9	-

Taking cases with invasion of extramural veins, in which the 5 year survival rate was 33%, involvement of thin-walled veins is associated with a survival rate of 41%, but only 51 of 91 patients with spread into thick-walled extramural veins survived for 5 years (Table 1.2.5.)

TABLE 1.2.5.

INVADED EXTRAMURAL VEINS	OPERATION SURVIVORS	5 YEAR SURVIVORS	CORRECTED 5 YEAR SURVIVAL RATE (%)
Thin-walled	157	54	41
Thick-walled	91	15	19

Analysis of the other histological features of venous invasion was confined to those cases with spread into extramural veins. Aneurysmal distention of invaded extramural veins was seen in 106 out of 248 cases (Table 1.2.6.). The 5 year survival rate was 41% in these cases.

TABLE 1.2.6.

ANEURYSMAL DISTENSION OF INVADED EXTRAMURAL VEIN	OPERATION SURVIVORS	5 YEAR SURVIVORS	CORRECTED % SURVIVAL
Not seen	142	33	27
Present	106	36	41 (P<0.02)

Necrosis of intravenous tumour was observed in 75 cases (Table 1.2.7.)
However, there was no significant difference in the survival rate of cases with
such necrosis and those in which it was not observed.

TABLE 1.2.7.

NECROSIS IN EXTRAMURAL INTRAVASCULAR GROWTH	OPERATION SURVIVORS	5 YEAR SURVIVORS	CORRECTED % SURVIVAL
NOT SEEN	173	53	36
PRESENT	75	16	25 (0.2>P>0.1)

The relationship between inflammatory damage to the walls of invaded
extramural veins and survival is shown in Table 1.2.8. This shows that only 5
out of 53 patients survived for 5 years when the vein wall was intact. When the
vein wall was partially damaged the corrected 5 year survival rate was nearly
30% and when the wall was destroyed the survival rate was 57%, similar to that
of the series as a whole.

TABLE 1.2.8.

STATE OF EXTRAMURAL VEIN WALL	OPERATION SURVIVORS	5 YEAR SURVIVORS	CORRECTED % SURVIVAL
INTACT	51	5	11
DAMAGED	126	31	29
DESTROYED	69	33	57

A mantle of proliferated endothelial cells covering the tip of the tumour in
extramural veins was present in 60 cases (Table 1.2.9.) and was associated with
a high 5 year survival rate (53%), a highly significant result.

TABLE 1.2.9 .

ENDOTHELIAL CELL MANTLE	OPERATION SURVIVORS	5 YEAR SURVIVORS	CORRECTED % SURVIVAL
NOT SEEN	188	42	26
PRESENT	60	27	53 (P<0.001)

Spread of carcinoma cells apparently in capillary channels in vein walls with
or without permeation of the lumen was present in 24 cases (Table 1.2.10.)
Only one of these patients survived 5 years.

TABLE 1.2.10.

PERMEATION OF CAPILLARIES VEIN WALL	OPERATION SURVIVORS	5 YEAR SURVIVORS	CORRECTED % SURVIVAL
NOT SEEN	30	68	36.1
PRESENT	24	1	4.9 (P<0.01)

Direct contact between naked tumour cells and extramural venous blood was observed in 17 cases (Table 1.2.11.). Only 2 of these survived for 5 years.

TABLE 1.2.11.

BLOOD IN INVADED EXTRAMURAL VEIN	OPERATION SURVIVORS	5 YEAR SURVIVORS	CORRECTED % SURVIVAL
NOT IN CONTACT WITH GROWTH	231	67	32.8
IN CONTACT WITH GROWTH	17	2	14.6 (P<0.2)

DISCUSSION

As a result of these observations we can build up a picture of the way tumour and veins interact (Fig. 1.).

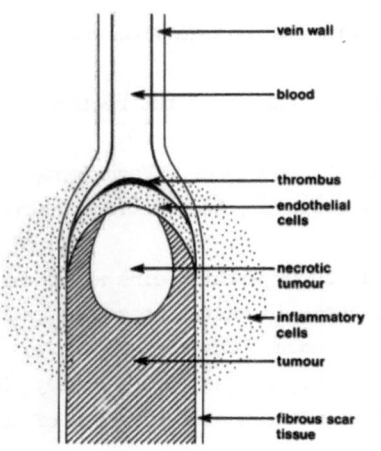

Fig. 1. Diagram of venous invasion and the host tissue reaction.

The inflammatory reaction in response to necrosis of the intravascular tumour results in damage to the vein wall, with consequent inhibition of malignant embolism, in accord with Willis's theory that a muscular element in the vein wall is important in dissemination of tumour by the blood stream. The following hypotheses are therefore suggested:

1. The inflammatory reaction to intravenous tumour necrosis results in inhibition of malignant embolism by endothelial proliferation and fibrous scarring of vein wall.

2. Invasion of veins by rectal cancer is invariably present, but is not detected in some cases when veins are destroyed.

3. The latter cases are unlikely to develop metastases.

4. Malignant emboli develop when vein walls are not severely damaged.

These results are not intended to be taken in isolation for epidemiological surveys or clinical trials. The inter-relationship between venous invasion and the Dukes stage and the histological grade of malignancy and correlation with survival rates, documented elsewhere (Talbot et al 1980, (a) and (b)) indicate that only by taking account of both the Dukes stage and the quantity of venous invasion can the most precise prediction of prognosis of patients with rectal cancer be arrived at.

ACKNOWLEDGEMENTS
This work was carried out with the generous support of Dr. B.C. Morson, the staff of St. Mark's Hospital, London and the Cancer Research Campaign.

REFERENCES
Dionne, L. 1965. Pattern of blood-borne metastasis from carcinoma of rectum. Cancer New York 18: 775-781.

Dukes, C.E. 1932. The classification of cancer of the rectum. J. Path. Bact. 35: 1489-94.

Nie, N.H., Hull, C.H., Jenkins, J.G., Steinbrenner, K and Bent, D.H. 1975. Statistical package for the social sciences, 2nd edition. McGraw Hill, New York and London.

Talbot, I.C. 1980. Spread of rectal cancer within veins and mechanisms of malignant embolism; in "Recent advances in gastrointestinal pathology", R. Wright (Editor), W.G. Saunders, London. Chapter 22.

Talbot, I.C., Ritchie, S., Leighton, M.H., Hughes, A.O., Bussey, H.J.R. and Morson, B.C. 1980a. The clinical significance of invasion of veins by rectal cancer. Brit. J. Surg., in press.

Talbot, I.C., Ritchie, S., Leighton, M., Hughes, A.O., Bussey, H.J.R. and Morson, B.C. 1980b. Invasion of veins by carcinoma of rectum. Method of detection, histological features and significance. Histopathology, in press.

Willis, R.A. 1930. The importance of venous invasion in the development of metastatic tumours in the liver. J. Path. Bact. 33: 849-861.

SQUAMOUS CARCINOMAS OF THE HEAD AND NECK: PATTERNS AND MECHANISMS OF LOCAL INVASION AND METASTASIS

R.L. Carter

Although the different anatomical sites of primary squamous carcinomas of the head and neck are important determinants in their spread, the overall pattern of growth and dissemination of this group of tumours is similar. The dominant features are local infiltration and metastasis to regional lymph nodes (Carter and Pittam, 1980). Clinically apparent metastases at distant sites are uncommon except in patients with carcinomas of the nasopharynx.

LOCAL SPREAD

The extent of local spread is often underestimated clinically because of the tendency of these tumours to invade beneath intact overlying mucosa. Infiltration of connective tissues, lymphatics and blood vessels is well known and two less familiar aspects of local invasion will be considered here: spread into perineural spaces and direct infiltration of bone.

Perineural spread

The perineural spaces, once erroneously regarded as lymphatics, form an important route of dissemination for squamous carcinomas of the head and neck (Carter et al., 1979). Perineural spread is found in over 25% of all major surgical resections and is occasionally observed in biopsy material. At certain sites, notably the oral cavity, it may be detected clinically in about two-thirds of cases. The nerve most commonly affected is the mandibular division of V; less frequently the tumours may invade the maxillary division of V, VI, VII, XII and branches of the cervical plexus. Involvement of nerves is sometimes multiple and sequential. Once tumour has penetrated the perineural spaces, carcinoma cells can extend centrally into the cranial cavity or peripherally - often into bone. Distances of 6-8 cm. or more may be traversed. Tumours growing within perineural spaces characteristically do not spread inwards and destroy the nerve trunks but, contrary to earlier views, it is now clear that involved nerves frequently develop degenerative changes in their myelin sheaths and axons and segmental infarction is occasionally observed. Such changes are not specific and are probably due to ischaemia following compression of the segmentally-arranged blood supply by columns of tumour cells.

Perineural spread by squamous carcinoma is an adverse prognostic feature mainly because it is associated with a high incidence of co-existing spread by lymphatics and blood vessels, and it has important bearings on clinical management (Carter and Pittam, 1980).

Direct invasion of bone

Compared to haematogenous skeletal metastases, direct spread of tumour into adjacent bone is generally uncommon. It is, however, a not infrequent finding in squamous carcinomas of the head and neck (Carter et al., 1980). In surgical material it is most often seen in association with tumours of the oral cavity and paranasal sinuses involving the jaws. The main routes of access are by direct spread from a contiguous primary carcinoma or nodal mass, and indirectly along perineural spaces - an important route of penetration of oral carcinomas into the mandible. Spread by way of periosteal lymphatics is rare.

The directional thrust of contiguous bone invasion is OUTWARDS → INWARDS - the reverse of skeletal metastases developing in the marrow spaces - and the process involves three phases:

1. The periosteum is breached.
2. Carcinoma cells interact with osteoclasts which then erode bone in front of the advancing tumour edge.
3. The tumour cells themselves infiltrate bone.

Most bone destruction is mediated by osteoclasts, and the capacity for tumour cells to invade bone unaided may be comparatively limited. Some osteoblastic activity is regularly seen and variable amounts of new bone are laid down, particularly in association with slowly growing carcinomas which penetrate only slowly into the bone substance. Local infection is not a pre-requisite for direct bone invasion.

A similar sequence of events is seen in the commoner clinical context of squamous carcinomas of the larynx infiltrating the laryngeal framework. It has long been known that ossified parts of the laryngeal cartilage are more susceptible to tumour invasion than intact cartilage - an apparent paradox which can now be readily explained (Carter and Tanner, 1979). The patches of metaplastic laryngeal bone faithfully reproduce normal bone, with trabeculae and marrow spaces. Osteoclasts are present which erode metaplastic bone in front of the advancing tumour in the same manner as in true bone.

The mechanisms underlying bone destruction are complex, but there is growing evidence that these squamous carcinomas release products which activate local osteoclasts. (1) High levels of prostaglandin-like materials have recently been extracted from a series of squamous carcinomas of the head and neck (Bennett et al., 1980). Prostaglandins of the E series predominated and the materials all appeared to be produced locally, no activity being demonstrable in jugular venous plasma - the main venous effluent from most tumours in the head and neck. (2) Culture media from eight lines of squamous carcinoma cells, established by Drs. D.M. and G.C. Easty, have shown variable degrees of osteolytic activity measured _in vitro_ by release of ^{45}Ca from isotopically-labelled calvaria from newborn mice. The osteolysis is variably reduced by indomethacin, an inhibitor of prostaglandin synthetase, strengthening the view that both prostaglandin and non-prostaglandin osteolysins are likely to be involved (Easty, Easty, Tsao and Carter: in preparation).

METASTASIS TO REGIONAL LYMPH NODES

The anatomical distribution of regional lymph node metastases from squamous carcinomas of the head and neck is closely dependent on the site of the primary tumour. Most surgical dissections of the neck in the United Kingdom are performed in previously irradiated patients, and the patterns and growth of nodal metastases are distinctive in such cases (Tanner et al., 1980; Carter and Pittam, 1980). Meticulous dissection of surgical specimens gives a high total yield of lymph nodes but the numbers of involved lymph nodes are characteristically small - about 1-3 per dissection. Most of the lymph nodes are completely replaced by carcinoma and about 90% of such nodes show transcapsular spread of tumour, varying from microscopic infiltration of the nodal capsule to gross invasion of local structures. It may occur in partly involved lymph nodes, making any simple mechanical explanation difficult to sustain. Transcapsular spread on this scale is not found with other carcinomas; and it is an adverse prognostic feature when extensive and when occurring in nodal groups lying close to the surgeon's resection lines. Keratin granulomas are commonly found in irradiated necks, co-existing with metastatic carcinoma or occasionally alone, unaccompanied by any demonstrable intact tumour. These lesions are uncommon in non-irradiated tissues, and their importance lies in the fact that they may form palpable masses which simulate nodal metastases. The morphological features in uninvolved regional lymph nodes in the irradiated neck are of no prognostic significance.

12

REFERENCES

    Details of the work summarized here, and a full bibliography, may
be found in the following publications:

Bennett, A., Carter, R.L., Stamford, I.F. and Tanner, N.S.B., 1980.
    Prostaglandin-like material extracted from squamous carcinomas of
    the head and neck. Brit. J. Cancer, 41: 204.
Carter, R.L., Tanner, N.S.B., Clifford, P. and Shaw, H.J., 1979.
    Perineural spread in squamous cell carcinomas of the head and
    neck. Clin. Otolaryngol., 4: 271.
Carter, R.L. and Tanner, N.S.B., 1979. Local invasion by laryngeal
    carcinoma - the importance of focal (metaplastic) ossification
    within laryngeal cartilage. Clin. Otolaryngol., 4: 283.
Carter, R.L., Tanner, N.S.B., Clifford, P. and Shaw, H.J., 1980.
    Direct bone invasion in squamous carcinomas of the head and neck:
    pathological and clinical implications. Clin. Otolaryngol., 5:
    107.
Carter, R.L. and Pittam, M.R., 1980. Squamous carcinomas of the
    head and neck: some patterns of spread. J. Roy. Soc. Med., 73.
Tanner, N.S.B., Carter, R.L., Dalley, V.M., Clifford, P. and Shaw, H.J
    1980. The irradiated radical neck dissection in squamous carcinoma
    a clinico-pathological study. Clin. Otolaryngol., 5.

THE RELATIONSHIP BETWEEN MALIGNANT MELANOMA MORPHOLOGY, METASTASES AND PATIENT SURVIVAL

B. Boeryd, J. Eldh and L.-E. Peterson

INTRODUCTION

Human cutaneous malignant melanoma is in many respects an interesting tumour, not the least owing to its metastazising behaviour. Much attention has been paid to its dissemination to regional lymph nodes and to the management of clinically uninvolved nodes. However, it should be noted that melanomas often disseminate to distant organs without affecting regional lymph nodes.

In a clinical morphological and multivariate analysis of prognostic factors in cutaneous malignant melanomas in stage I the location of the tumours and their thickness were found to be of most prognostic value. In addition, the levels of infiltration, presence of ulceration and mitotic activity influenced the prognosis (Eldh et al., 1978). In this communication the relationship between location of the tumours, their thickness, presence of ulceration and vascular invasion will be correlated to the incidence of metastases as well as to the time of their appearance and for death.

MATERIAL AND METHODS

The material comprises 277 patients treated for malignant melanoma during the years 1959-1973 at the Department of Plastic Surgery, Sahlgrenska Sjukhuset, Göteborg, Sweden. The treatment consisted of widely localized excision and skin graft. The regional lymph nodes were left intact in all cases. Postoperatively all patients were followed at the Department of Plastic Surgery at intervals of 3 months for the first 3 years and then every 6 months for up to 10 years (Eldh et al., 1978). When patients noted changes in lymph nodes or other symptoms between the follow up intervals, they were instructed to contact the hospital immediately. Regional lymph node metastases were excised as soon as they were diagnosed clinically if the examination did not show dissemination to distant organs, which occurred in 4 cases.

RESULTS

At the end of the year 1978 all patients had been observed for at least 5 years. During the observation period 68 patients died, 8 of certified intercurrent diseases and 60 of malignant melanomas. Nine of these died more than 5 years after excision of the primary tumour. Thus the corrected 5 year survival was 81.0 %. Lymph node metastases developed in 48 patients and 30 of these died later of dissemination to distant organs, while 18 were alive at the end of 1978 after at least 73 months observation. The 5 year survival rate after excision of lymph node metastases was 35.9 %. All 30 patients with metastases primarily in distant organs died.

Melanomas on the trunk metastazised more frequently primarily to distant organs than to lymph nodes, in contrast to melanomas in the other locations. The total incidence of metastases increased from melanomas on the arm, hand and leg, head and neck, trunk and foot, in that order (Table 1). Lymph node metastases from melanomas on the trunk appeared later and these patients survived longer as compared to patients with other locations. The thickness of the tumour did not seem to influence either the time for appearance of the lymph node metastases or the time for death of these patients (Table 2). In the 18 patients who, after treatment of the lymph node metastases, were still alive at the end of 1978 these metastases appeared later than in those who died (Table 3).

The primarily distant metastases were diagnosed later than the primary lymph node metastases and there were no obvious differences between patients with melanomas on the various locations, except for melanomas on the foot from which metastases appeared earlier. Further, the average time for death was rather similar for all patients irrespective of the locations of the tumours. However, metastases from melanoma > 3 mm in thickness were diagnosed much earlier and killed the patients earlier than did the thinner melanomas (Table 4).

Metastases to lymph nodes or distant organs from melanomas with diagnosed vascular invasion did not appear earlier than metastases from melanomas without obvious vascular invasion. Of the 269 patients 90 had ulcerated tumours (33 %). Almost half of these patients (41) died.

Within 12 months after excision of the primary tumour, lymph node metastases appeared in 25 of 48 patients and of these 21 died later with distant metastases. Of the 23 patients with lymph node metastases diagnosed later than 12 months after excision of the primary tumour 14 survived the observation period. During the first 3 years when the patients were followed up every third month, 40 of 48 patients had developed lymph node metastases.

DISCUSSION

The morphological parameter most significantly related to the prognosis is the thickness of the tumour (Eldh et al., 1978; Balch et al., 1978). In this material the incidence of metastases primarily to lymph nodes as well as to distant organs was much higher from thicker melanomas than from the thinner ones. This was not the case for metastases to lymph nodes from melanomas on the foot and for metastases to distant organs from melanomas on head and neck.

The material is limited and the times for excision of lymph nodes metastases, for diagnosis of distant metastases and for death show wide ranges. However, the data do allow some interpretations. The average time for death was similar for patients with or without regional lymph node metastases. This may indicate that

Table 1

Incidence of metastases primarily in lymph nodes (L) or distant organs (D) in 269 patients with malignant melanoma in different locations and with different thickness. Within brackets incidence of metastases in per cent.

Thickness of melanoma (mm)	Arm, hand, leg			Head and neck			Trunk			Foot		
	Total	L	D	Total	L	D	Total	L	D	Total	L	D
≤ 3.00	84	9 (11)	1 (1)	43	5 (12)	4 (9)	80	7 (9)	12 (15)	10	6 (60)	
> 3.00	15	6 (40)	3 (20)	11	6 (55)	1 (9)	12	4 (33)	5 (42)	14	5 (36)	4 (29)
All thickness	99	15 (15)	4 (4)	54	11 (20)	5 (9)	92	11 (12)	17 (18)	24	11 (46)	4 (17)

in the patients with lymph node metastases tumour cells also had disseminated to distant organs from the primary tumour, through the lymph nodes (Hewitt & Blake, 1975) or directly by venous vessels. Tumour cells could also have disseminated from lymph node metastases. In patients who died after treatment of lymph node metastases, the thickness of the tumours seemed not to influence the time of appearance of the lymph node metastases or death of these patients in contrast to the patients who died of primarily distant metastases. This fact suggests different mechanisms for dissemination of tumour cells and/or development of metastases in patients with or without regional lymph node metastases. Half of the patients who died did not develop regional lymph node metastases, and it can be questioned whether tumour cells from tumours in these patients passed through lymph nodes, whether they were arrested there but succumbed or if the tumour cells disseminated only via the blood. Similarly it can be asked if tumour cells disseminated only to regional lymph nodes in those patients, who after excision of late appearing regional lymph node metastases, survived the observation period.

Table 2

Number of patients dead after excision of lymph node metastases,
average time for their excision and for death.

Location of melanoma	Number of patients	Average time for excision of metastases[1] (Range)	Average time for death[1] (Range)
Arm, hand, leg	6	10 (1-26)	31 (9-54)
Head and neck	8 (2)[2]	10 (1-27)	32 (5-72)
Trunk	8 (2)[2]	22 (6-60)	42 (9-104)
Foot	8	13 (7-33)	29 (15-44)
All locations	30 (4)[2]	14 $\frac{\leq 3.00 \quad >3.00^{3)}}{16 \qquad 13}$	34 $\frac{\leq 3.00 \quad >3.00^{3)}}{35 \qquad 33}$

1) Months after excision of the primary tumour
2) Number of patients dead after >5 years
3) Thickness of melanoma (mm)

Table 3

Number of patients alive after excision of lymph node metastases,
average time for their excision and for observation.

Location of melanoma	Number of patients Thickness of melanoma		Average time for excision of metastases[1] (Range)	Average observation time[1] (Range)
	≤ 3.00	>3.00		
Arm, hand, leg	7	2	30 (5-89)	114 (74-197)
Head and neck	2	1	23 (7-46)	98 (73-120)
Trunk	3		39 (18-62)	125 (80-156)
Foot	3		35 (6-66	125 (108-152)

1) Months after excision of the primary tumour

Table 4

Number of patients dead of primarily distant metastases and
average time for their diagnosis and for death.

Location of melanoma	Number of patients	Average time for diagnosis of distant metastases[1] (Range)	Average time for death[1] (Range)
Arm, hand, leg	4	32 (11-46)	33 (12-47)
Head and neck	5 (1)[2]	32 (6-82)	37 (18-84)
Trunk	17 (4)[2]	29 (1-73)	36 (3-77)
Foot	4	21 (3-34)	39 (22-57)
All locations	30 (5)[2]	$29 \dfrac{<3.00 \quad >3.00^{3)}}{37 \qquad 19}$	$36 \dfrac{<3.00 \quad >3.00^{3)}}{43 \qquad 27}$

1) Months after excision of the primary tumour
2) Number of patients dead after > 5 years
3) Thickness of melanoma (mm)

   In the discussion of the value of prophylactic lymph node dissection it has to
be realized that, in a certain number of patients who died of malignant melanoma,
lymph node metastases never developed. Further, in the majority of patients with
lymph node metastases our data indicate that tumour cells disseminated not only
to lymph nodes but also to distant organs. In evaluating the results of different types of treatment it seems important to have a sufficiently long observation period.
   The data illustrate the difference in metastazising behaviour between
malignant human tumours such as malignant melanoma and experimental tumours.
To be able to mimic the dissemination of human tumours, improved experimental
models are needed.

REFERENCES

Balch, C.M., Murad, T.M., Soong, S., Ingalls, A.L., Halpern, N.B. and Maddox,
    W.A., 1978. A multifactorial analysis of melanoma: I. Prognostic histo-
    pathological features comparing Clark's and Breslow's staging methods.
    Ann. Surg. 188: 732-742.
Eldh, J., Boeryd, B. and Peterson, L.-E., 1978. Prognostic factors in cutaneous
    malignant melanoma in stage I. A clinical, morphological and multivariate
    analysis. Scand. J. Plast. Reconstr. Surg., 12: 243-255.
Hewitt, H.B. and Blake, E., 1975. Quantitative studies of translymphnodal
    passage of tumour cells naturally disseminated from a non-immunogenic murine
    squamous carcinoma. Br. J. Cancer 31: 25-35.

ANIMAL TUMOUR MODELS: THE INTRUSION OF ARTEFACTS

H.B. Hewitt

Such are the technical and ethical limitations imposed on the clinical
observer that our knowledge of the mechanisms of metastasis and our development and assessment of methods of restraining disseminated disease are very
dependent on the use of experimental animal tumour systems. They are 'models'
in the sense that they are intended to represent the clinical situation. The
similar pathogenesis of cancer in different mammalian species gives the
experimental cancer researcher great scope in confidently extrapolating his
findings to clinical practice. But his confidence in interspecies analogy is
merited only when there is scrupulous avoidance of the many laboratory
contingencies which can and do compromise the validity of an animal model.
By 'artefact' we here refer to features or conditions which are peculiar to
the model and do not prevail in the clinical situation. Artefacts may be
intrinsic to the model or can result from its technical handling. The
commonest and most influential artefacts are avoidable, and should be avoided.
Others are unavoidable using the small rodent models to which most researchers
are confined by their need to use isotransplants; they mostly relate to the
large differences of body size and tumour growth rate which distinguish man
and laboratory rodents. These scale differences have to be prudently
accommodated in attaching clinical relevance to the results of animal experiments. For example, occult metastases in the mouse will usually merit the
description 'micrometastases' whereas occult clinical metatases commonly
given this description are usually quite sizeable tumours which have not yet
attained detection by non-invasive imaging techniques.

To meet the need for quantitation and repeatability the experimenter
requires an animal tumour to be transplantable. And if there is to be any
reliance on the isogenicity of the transplants all but a very few researchers
will be confined to the use of mouse or rat tumours; logistic considerations
favour the prevailing large preference for mouse tumours. A dominant consideration in the selection of a system is the immunological status of the
host/tumour relationship. This is so because the advent of metastases is
analogous to the application of a 'second set' skin graft: immunity generated
by growth of the primary tumour will be exerted against the early metastases
from it. We shall here set aside the somewhat controversial issue as to the
immunogenicity of clinical tumours by confining attention to sources of
artefactual immunogenicity in the model - those which are peculiarly associated with certain laboratory methods of tumour induction or with breaches of

the conditions required for truly isogenic transplantation. Depending on the strength of any artefactual immunogenicity in a system, metastases may be totally suppressed or they may undergo spontaneous regression; with relatively weak immunogenicity, there may be potentiation of the effect of cytotoxic agents against metastases or conference of artefactual susrepti-bility to immunotherapy.

Since about 2/3 cancer patients develop disseminated disease, we might expect a rather large commitment of experimental cancer research to study of the mechanism and control of metastasis; but such studies are, in fact, poorly represented in the contemporary cancer literature. We analysed the contents of 4 leading cancer journals published during 1978 (Brit.J.Cancer, Cancer Res., Europ.J.Cancer, and Cancer) and found that the proportion of space allotted to this topic was, overall, only 1.8%. One discouragement may be the realisation that clinical metastasis is usually well established by the time patients first present with symptoms of the primary tumour, and that laboratory knowledge of the mechanisms of dissemination and seeding can therefore have no clinical application. This reservation is valid: over 50% of cases of cancer of the breast, prostate, head and neck, and lung have evidence of metastases at the time of diagnosis; from reasonable assumptions, it can be calculated that the pulmonary metastases from osteogenic sarcoma are usually seeded before the primary tumour has attained to 1 mm^3 in size.

A more compelling discouragement to experimental study of metastasis is the fact that a large proportion of the most readily available transplantable animal cancers do not exhibit natural metastasis on account of their immuno-genicity. We ascertained the origin and status of 46 animal tumour systems employed in the metastasis studies reported in the 1978 sample of the litera-ture referred to above. The Table records the distribution of these systems among categories having significance for their prospective validity as models of spontaneous clinical cancer. We can preface a discussion of the Table by observing that clinical cancer is not induced by local application of high concentrations of powerful chemical carcinogens, that no form of clinical cancer has yet been proved to be caused by an oncogenic virus, and that allo-graft status can be accorded only to trophoblastic cancer or to the very rare cases of foetal acquisition of maternal cancer.

The allografted tumours in the Table were all examples of the 70 year-old Ehrlich tumour or the 52 year-old Walker tumour. Numerous comparative studies reported during the last 30 years have established that practically all chemically induced tumours are immunogenic, whereas spontaneous tumours are rarely so. All the UV-induced tumours in the sample were transplantable

TABLE   Status of 46 Animal Tumour Models (1978)

Category		No.	%
Allograft		4	9
Chem.- or UV-induced		17	37
Virus-induced		4	9
'Old' spontaneous	(B16 Mel.)	6)	26
	(Lewis L.T.)	6)	
	(Other	2	4
'Recent' spontaneous		7	15

only to immunosuppressed mice. Tumours originally induced in adult animals
by oncogenic viruses are invariably immunogenic (Klein and Klein,1977). The
contemporary usage of 'old' tumours, albeit of spontaneous origin in inbred
animals, is associated with a very high risk of transplantation across histocompatibility barriers between divergent substrains. Twenty-six per cent of
the models in the sample were either the 28 year-old Lewis lung tumour or the
B16 melanoma. Neither tumour now boasts any feature which justifies its
preferential use over more recently isolated spontaneous tumours; their
current popularity as models now denotes a cult gaining adherents only by the
ever widening availability of these two tumours. The fact that our sample
contains only a small proportion of tumours having reasonable prospects of
freedom from artefactual immunogenicity betrays the persistent neglect of long
established principles which should govern the adoption of animal tumours to
serve as models of spontaneous autochthonous cancer.

In 56% of the experiments contributing to our sample, 'artificial
metastasis' was the technique used, whereby countable lung nodules are
produced by the i.v.injection of dispersed tumour cell suspensions.
Ostensibly used to allow study of influences on seeding independently of
natural dissemination, the device is most often resorted to because the immunogenic tumour used fails to exhibit natural metastasis. It must be emphasised
that this procedure represents not the secondary phenomenon of metastasis but
primary transplantation of tumour to the lung by the intravascular route. It
would be incautious to conclude that what influences the seeding of an
injected bolus of cells, subject to packing and productive of severe pulsed
hydraemia, has necessary relevance to the seeding of naturally disseminated
cells leaking into the circulation at relatively low density over a period of
months or years.

A further device commonly employed to elude the prohibitive limitations
of a non-metastasising immunogenic system is to immunosuppress tumour graft

recipients by their preliminary exposure to sublethal whole-body irradiation (WBI). The convenient assumption that immunosuppression is the only significant effect of WBI on metastasising potential cannot be sustained: several authors (e.g. Withers and Milas,1973) have demonstrated temporary enhancement of metastasis by local pre-irradiation of the target organ; and we (Hewitt and Blake,1977) have demonstrated very marked enhancement of metastasis to the regional node by preliminary exposure of mice to WBI. This effect was systemic because it could not be induced by local pre-irradiation of the tumour bed and/or the regional node. It was not, however, a manifestation of immunosuppression: the tumour was not immunogenic; the effect could not be cancelled by restoration of the mice with normal isogenic lymphocytes; and it persisted for at least 6 months after WBI – till long after immunocompetence would have returned. Clearly, the conduct of metastasis studies using immunogenic tumours in WBI mice invites a complex of interacting artefacts of very doubtful relevance to the behaviour of a non-immunogenic tumour in an un-irradiated patient.

It is concluded that current selection of animal models of human cancer for metastasis studies, as revealed in the Table, betrays widespread indifference to the intrusion of immunological artefacts. Ubiquitous veteran tumours appear to be favoured in the mistaken belief that their use permits comparability of results from different laboratories. This is denied, however, by the histocompatibility divergence between substrains of named animal strains separately propagated often over several decades. 'Isogenic' has come to signify a nominal rather than a real condition. A reform of current practice is indicated. It would be difficult to fault an assertion that the ideal model tumour is one which is non-immunogenic and was of spontaneous origin in the inbred substrain of animals providing transplant recipients. Comparable information from equally valid models maintained in different laboratories would have more clinical relevance than that from a common invalid model.

Among artefacts inseparable from the use of tumours in small rodents are those which arise from the approximately 2500-fold difference of body weight between man and mouse. A modest 1 cm diameter mouse tumour is equivalent, as a tumour load, to a 1.3 kg clinical tumour. Beyond this size, tumours in the mouse commonly induce systemic depredation (anaemia, cachexia,etc) which can influence the growth of metastases and their response to therapy. Whilst the mouse researcher must accept an unrealistic tumour load if he is not to become a microoncologist, humane and technical requirements dictate reasonable restraint in the maximum tumour size allowed. Reports have appeared of primary mouse tumours being allowed to attain tumour loads equivalent to a

20 kg tumour in man!

Finally, reference is made to increasing public concern to reduce the amount of distress to which experimental animals are subjected. The common procedure in metastasis studies of transplanting the primary tumour to the foot and ablating it by amputation is an unaesthetic and disabling procedure before and after operation. An experimental design which serves the requirement of the experimenter equally well but which is more acceptable consists in growing the primary implant intradermally in the flank and removing it by an elliptical excision of the tumour-bearing skin.

REFERENCES

Hewitt,H.B. and Blake,E.R., 1977. Facilitation of nodal metastasis from a non-immunogenic murine carcinoma by previous whole-body irradiation of tumour recipients. Br.J.Cancer,36,23-34.
Klein,G. and Klein,E., 1977. Rejectability of virus-induced tumors and non-rejectability of spontaneous tumors - a lesson in contrasts. Transpl. Proc.,9,1095-1104.
Withers,H.R. and Milas,L., 1973. Influence of pre-irradiation of lung on development of artificial pulmonary metastases of fibrosarcoma in mice. Cancer Res.,33,1931-1936.

MODELS OF PROSTATE, BREAST, LUNG, AND INTESTINAL CARCINOMAS WHICH METASTASIZE IN RATS

M. Pollard

The optimal model tumor system should manifest the following characteristics: the tumor should simulate the human counterpart disease. It should be organ-related, autochthonous, and malignant. The tumor cells should multiply non-synchronously, have multiple karyotypes, and metastasize spontaneously from extravascular sites. Control animals should not develop other tumors spontaneously in the course of experimental procedures. Model systems have been developed and used in this laboratory in mice with reticulum cell sarcoma (SJL/J strain), lymphatic leukemia (AKR strain), mammary adenocarcinoma (C3H strain), and lupus-like disease in Haas strain mice (Pollard & Sharon, 1970, Pollard, et al, 1976b). Model systems do not usually comply with all of the above characteristics. In the present report, model adenocarcinomas (CAs) of prostate, lung, breast, and intestine are described in germfree (GF) and in conventional rats (Table I).

Model Systems: Nine aged GF Lobund Wistar (LW) rats developed metastasizing prostate CAs "spontaneously" (Pollard, 1973, 1975a). In addition, this tumor has been observed in 2 conventional LW rats (Pollard, 1979a). Three transplantable cell lines, derived from the GF rats (designated PA-I, II, III), have been cloned and propagated in vitro. They reproduce the original tumor type after inoculation into only LW rats (Pollard & Luckert, 1975b). The transplanted tumors metastasize spontaneously from many implant sites through predetermined routes to specific target organs (Pollard & Luckert, 1979b). Multiple metastatic foci of tumor cells can be demonstrated in the lungs of rats within 3 weeks after subcutaneous inoculation of tumor cells.

*Supported in part by funds from the US Public Health Service Grants RR-00294 and CA 17559, and the Ambrose and Gladys Bowyer Foundation.

The lung CA was derived from a tumor which developed "spontaneously" in one GF LW rat. It has been demonstrated that the transplanted tumor cells spread ipsilaterally from the inoculated hind footpad of LW rats via lymph channels through sequences of lymph nodes to the lungs in which they produce large CAs. The cells are being propagated in monolayer cultures (Pollard, 1979a

A similar pattern of tumor spread is manifested in rats by 3 lines of breast CAs which were derived from Lobund Sprague-Dawley (S-D) rats in which breast CAs were induced by 1 oral dose (20 mg in sesame oil) of 7, 12 dimethylbenz(a)-anthracene (DMBA) (Pollard, 1972). While the rates of metastatic spread are slower than those manifested by the prostate CAs, they produce extensive lesions in the ipsilateral lymph nodes and in the lungs. Thus far, no "spontaneous" breast CA has been observed in GF rats (Pollard, 1972).

Autochthonous intestinal CAs can be induced in 100% of S-D rats by 5 weekly doses of 1, 2 dimethylhydrazine (DMH), administered by gavage (30mg/Kg B. W. / week). At 20 weeks after the first dose of DMH, all rats have CAs in the colon and less frequently in the small intestine and rectum (Pollard & Luckert, 1979c). The CAs are of several sizes and morphological types; and in about 5% of tumor-bearing rats, tumor cells had spread to adjacent lymph nodes and less frequently to the lungs. No "spontaneous" intestinal CA has been observed in S-D, nor in L-W, rats.

Patterns of Metastasis: In order to demonstrate if tumor cells are in the blood, individual rats with an extensive metastatic prostate, breast, or lung tumor were anesthetized and exsanguinated from the heart. Blood from each exsanguinated donor rat was then inoculated intravenously (1. 5 ml) into young rats which, 8 weeks later, were killed and examined for lung tumors. Within the sensitivity of this assay procedure it was demonstrated that all of the prostate, the breast and the lung CAs spread ipsilaterally via lymphatic channels and lymph nodes to the lungs. In addition, PA-II cells spread via circulating blood to multiple visceral organs (lungs, liver, spleen) and to the bone marrow. Numerous PA-II cells can be observed microscopically in stained blood smears, and tumors can be transplanted by transfusion of as little as 0.025 ml of blood to new rats (Pollard, 1979b).

The lung and breast CAs metastasize uniformly from inoculated footpads via lymphatic channels to the lungs. Occasionally, contralateral lymph nodes (lumbar, renal) were enlarged with tumor cells. By contrast, tumor cells implanted S.C. in the dorsal area of the body developed rapidly into large tumors, which rarely spread from that area to the lungs.

Modulation experiments: The experimental protocol for modifying the pattern of metastasis was performed, as follows: tumor cells were inoculated quantitatively into a hind footpad; and, at intervals thereafter, groups of the rats were treated with one of the modulating test agents. Treated and control tumor-bearing rats were killed and examined after 30 days (PA-I, II, III), after 80 days (breast CA and lung CA), and after 140 days (intestinal CA). The effects of treatments were based on comparative weights of right and left footpads (tumor weight), individual lymph nodes, and by numbers of tumor foci in the lungs. With PA-II, the assay was based on the same criteria plus weights of liver, spleen, and on white blood cell counts. The assay with intestinal CA was determined by comparative numbers of tumors in the intestinal tract of each DMH-treated rat.

Rats with the tumor model systems have been subjected to modulation trials involving cyclophosphamide (CPA), killed Corynebacterium parvum, heparin, ICRF-159, Na barbiturate, aspirin and indomethacin (IND); and by a combination of total body lethal x-irradiation plus allogeneic bone marrow transfusions (Pollard, 1979a). The latter procedure did not alter the patterns of metastasis of the solid tumors, nor of the sizes of the primary tumors.

It was demonstrated that the rate and extent of PA I, II, & III metastasis was retarded, but not cured, by treatments with CPA (Pollard & Luckert, 1976b), by killed C. parvum and by aspirin and IND, and that the spread of tumor cells was accelerated by administrations of Na barbiturate (0.1%) in the drinking water (Pollard, et al, 1977a, b). Similarly, metastasis of breast tumor cells from the foot-pad to the lungs was accelerated by Na barbiturate.

A promotional effect of orally-administered Na barbiturate was demonstrated in rats which had been treated with DMH (Pollard & Luckert, 1979d): the barbiturate-treated rats had tumors which were increased in numbers and sizes compared to the tumors in untreated control DMH-treated rats. However, there was no evidence that barbiturate enhanced the metastatic spread of DMH-induced intestinal tumors. Rats with DMH-induced intestinal tumors were treated with orally-administered IND which resulted in 50% reduction of tumor-bearing rats and a significant reduction of tumor numbers and sizes in the rest of the IND-treated rats (Pollard, 1979b).

REFERENCES

Pollard, Morris, 1972. Spontaneous and induced neoplasms in germfree rats. In: Environment and Cancer, The Williams and Wilkins Co., Baltimore, 394-406
Pollard, Morris, 1973. Spontaneous prostate adenocarcinomas in aged germfree Wistar rats. J. Nat. Cancer Inst., 51:1235-1241.
Pollard, Morris, 1975a. Prostate adenocarcinomas in Wistar rats. Medical Bulletin (Rush-Presbyterian-St. Luke's), 14(1):17-22.
Pollard, Morris, 1979a. Unpublished information.
Pollard, Morris, Burleson, G.R. and Luckert, P.H., 1977a. Factors that modify the rate and extent of spontaneous metastases of prostate tumors in rats. In: Cancer Invasion and Metastasis: Biologic Mechanisms and Therapy (Ed: S.B. Day et al), Raven Press, N.Y., pp 357-366.
Pollard, Morris, Chang, C.F., and Burleson, G.R., 1977b. Investigations on prostate adenocarcinomas in rats. Cancer Treatment Reports, 61(2):153-156.
Pollard, Morris and Luckert, P.H., 1975b. Transplantable metastasizing prosta adenocarcinomas in rats. J. Nat. Cancer Inst., 54(3):643-649.
Pollard, Morris and Luckert, P.H., 1976a. Chemotherapy of metastatic prostate adenocarcinomas in germfree rats. Cancer Treatment Reports, 60:619-621.
Pollard, Morris and Luckert, P.H., 1979b. Patterns of spontaneous metastasis manifested by three rat prostate adenocarcinomas. Jr. Surg. Oncology, 12:371-37
Pollard, Morris and Luckert, P.H., 1979c. Indomethacin treatment of rats with dimethylhydrazine-induced intestinal tumors. Cancer Treatment Reports, In press.

Pollard, Morris and Luckert, P.H., 1979d. Promotional effect of sodium
   barbiturate on intestinal tumors induced in rats by dimethylhydrazine. Jr.
   Nat. Cancer Inst., 63:1089-1092.
Pollard, Morris and Sharon, N., 1970. Chemotherapy of spontaneous leukemia
   in germfree AKR mice. Jr. Nat. Cancer Inst. 45:677-680.
Pollard, Morris, Truitt, R.L., and Ashman, R.B., 1976b. Mouse Leukemia
   and solid tumors treated with bone marrow grafting. Transplant. Proc.
   8:565-567.

TABLE I. Model Adenocarcinoma Systems in Lobund Rats

A. Transplanted Tumors

Origin	Etiology	Organ	In vitro Culture	Metastasis from Footpad Through	Target Organ
GF Wistar* (PA-I)	Spontaneous	Prostate	Monolayer	Lymphatics	Lungs
GF Wistar* (PA-II)	Spontaneous	Prostate	Monolayer	Lymphatics Blood	Lungs, liver, bone marrow
GF Wistar* (PA-III)	Spontaneous	Prostate	Monolayer	Lymphatics	Lungs
GF Wistar*	Spontaneous	Lung	Monolayer	Lymphatics	Lungs
GF Sprague-* Dawley	7,12 DMBA	Breast	Monolayer	Lymphatics	Lungs

B. Autochthonous Tumors

Origin	Etiology	Organ	In vitro Culture	Metastasis from Footpad Through	Target Organ
GF and conv. Sprague- Dawley	1,2 DMH	Intestine	ND	Lymphatics	Lymph nodes

* Originally derived from GF rats and transplanted in Conv. rats.

A NEW IN-VITRO MODEL TO STUDY TUMOUR CELL INVASION

R. Tchao, A.B. Schleich, M. Frick, and A. Mayer

INTRODUCTION

There is an urgent need to develop suitable models to study tumour cell in-
vasion in tumour metastasis, however, there are only few available models
(Leighton and Kline, 1954; Easty and Easty, 1963, 1974; Schleich et al., 1974;
De Ridder et al., 1977; Kramer and Nicolson, 1979).

The first steps in tumour cell invasion are the interaction of the tumour
cells with the normal epithelium and the underlying basement membrane, followed
by the penetration of the basement membrane (for review see Fidler et al.,
1978; Mareel, 1979). In this paper we describe a new in-vitro model of a normal
human epithelium - the amnion epithelium, growing on a basement membrane. We
have studied the interaction of amnion epithelial cells with several human
epithelial cell lines derived from human tumours and a fibroblastic cell line
derived from normal human decidua.

METHODS AND MATERIALS

Detailed description of the culture method and the cell lines will be published else where. Briefly, amnion was obtained after the delivery of foetus
by caesarean section, and was carefully separated from the chorion. Pieces of
this membrane were floated onto stainless steel grids coated with agar.

In this report we will describe two tumour cell lines: HeLa I, obtained
from Dr. G. Gey in 1954 and HT29, a colon adenocarcinoma cell line, kindly
supplied by Dr. L.M. Franks. The decidua cell line was developed by Schleich
et al. Two drops of culture medium containing tumour cells in aggregates, prepared by Moscona's method, were put on the amnion membrane. A slight depression in the grid allowed the aggregates to remain in place. The culture were
incubated in a CO_2 incubator at $35^{\circ}C$ and were fed every two days.

After 3-7 days the cultures together with the grids were fixed in Bouin for
18 hours. The amnion membrane was processed and sectioned at 5 μ vertically
through the membrane, and stained with H&E.

RESULTS

The amnion is an uniform epithelium of one cell layer. Using a dissecting
microscope we selected those pieces without any tears or acellular patches for
culture. Mitotic figure was rare.

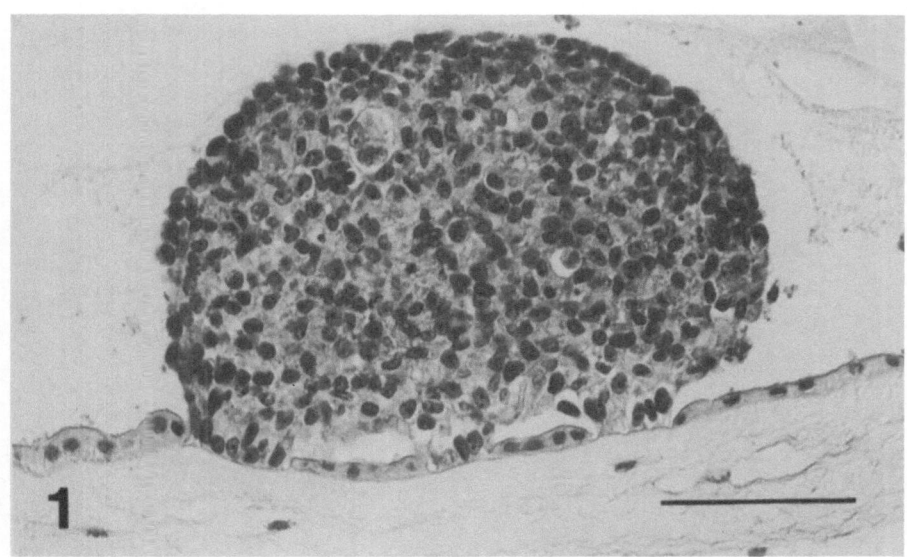

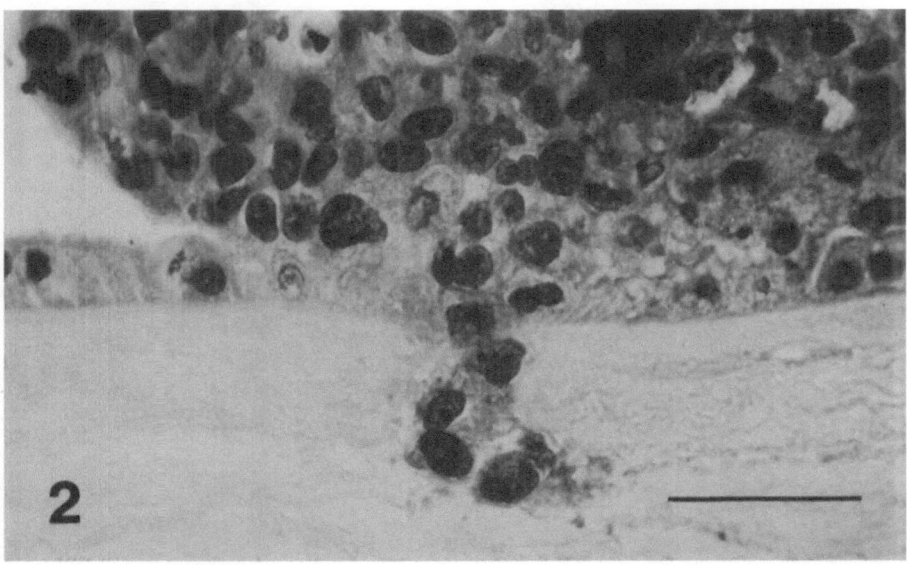

Legend: Cultures of HeLa cells as aggregates on human amnion epithelium.
Fig. 1 shows a 7 day culture, HeLa cells have attached at several
points to the basement membrane. Bar = 100 µm. Fig. 2 shows a 7 day
culture, HeLa cells have broken through the basement membrane and
have infiltrated into the collagenous tissue. Bar = 50 µm.

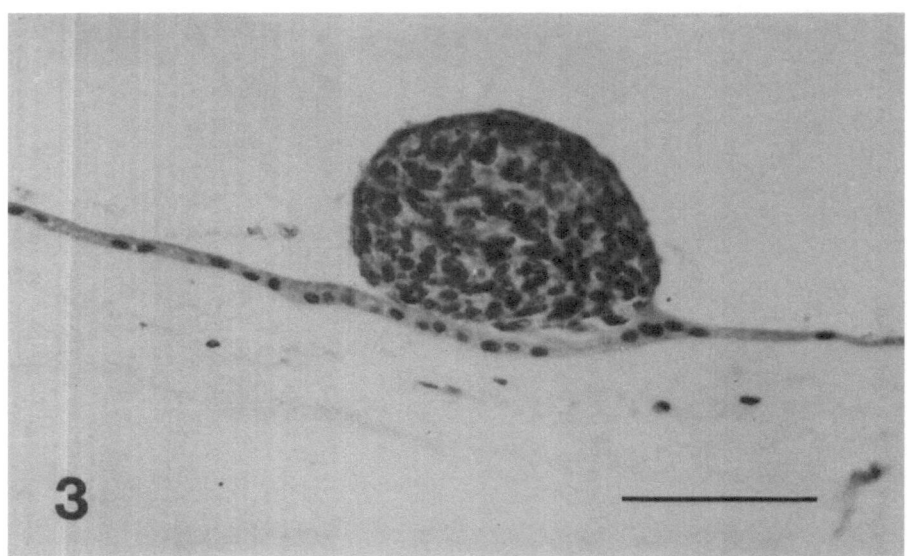

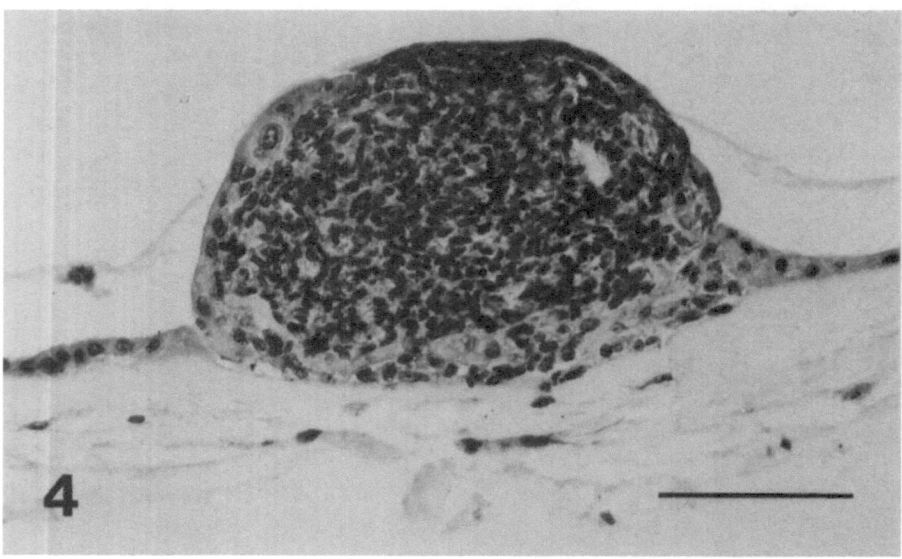

Legend: Cultures of decidua cells as aggregates on human amnion epithelium. Fig. 3 shows a 3 day culture, there is no invasion of the amnion epithelium by the decidua cells. Fig. 4 shows a 7 day culture, the amnion epithelial cells have migrated over the top of the decidua aggregate. Bar = 100 μm.

The amnion appeared very healthy in culture up to 7 days. When aggregates of HeLa I cells were added to the amnion, in the first 2-3 days the tumour cells stayed as aggregates on top of the amnion epithelium. In occasional places, HeLa cells put out processes in between the amnion epithelial cells and pushed the amnion cells away from each other. After 5-7 days the HeLa cells still remained in aggregates but the lower cells in contact with the amnion have inserted cell processes between the amnion cells at several points and have established good contact with the underlying basement membrane, as shown in figure 1. The amnion epithelial cells were quite healthy where no tumour cells overlaid. Immediately beneath the aggregate of HeLa cells, some amnion epithelial cells were dead or dying.

In some cultures HeLa cells apparently broke through the basement membrane and grew into the underlying collagenous tissue as shown in figure 2.

HT29 aggregates did not remain intact, the tumour cells dispersed and invaded the amnion epithelium individually, by inserting processes between the amnion cells and lifting off these cells.

The decidua aggregates remained intact on the amnion. The cells did not invade the amnion epithelium as shown in figure 3. However, after 5-7 days culture, the decidua aggregates became an integral part of the amnion membrane and the amnion epithelial cells migrated over the decidua cells as shown in figure 4. Some cells from the decidua aggregate also grew into the collagenous layer. This migration of the amnion epithelial cells over the aggregate explant were never observed with tumor aggregates.

DISCUSSION

When a tumour has penetrated its underlying basement membrane, it is generally regarded by pathologists as malignant and has the potential to metastasize. It has been shown in-vitro that tumour cells may be less adhesive to each other, more motile, and may secrete proteolytic enzymes or collagenases (for review see Fidler et al., 1978; Liotta et al., 1980). However, the major problem has been the establishment of a suitable model to test these hypotheses. This amnion model, by virtue of it consisting of a living monolayer of epithelial cells with intact basement membrane and collagenous connective tissue, may help us to study many of the factors involved in tumour cell invasion.

The response of the amnion epithelial cells to normal fibroblasts showed that this epithelium was active, capable of the typical epithelial movements seen in organ cultures. Schor (1979) has observed that epithelial cells do not migrate into a collagen gel whereas fibroblasts do. In this study, we have repeatedly observed HeLa I cells to break through the basement membrane and infiltrate the collagen layer, which is unlike the reconstituted collagen gel.

Ultrastructural studies are now in progress.

In this preliminary study we have only cultured the amnion up to 7 days it is possible that longer time is necessary for most cells to penetrate into the collagen layer. It may also be necessary to improve the culture of amnion cells by using EGF and FGF. In some preparations we have used PAS stain to visualize the basement membrane, it will be interesting to study whether new membrane material is being synthesized and whether its penetration by tumour cells follows at first by the dissolution of the basement membrane. An important question that may also be answered by this model is whether all the cells in a tumour cell line are capable of invasion or only a fraction have this capability.

REFERENCES

De Ridder, L., Marel, M. and Vakaet, L., 1977. Invasion of malignant cells into cultured embryonic substrates. Arch.Geschw.Forsch. 47: 7-27.
Easty, G.C. and Easty, D.M., 1963. An organ culture system for the examination of tumour invasion. Nature, 199: 1104-1105.
Easty, D.M., and Easty, G.C., 1974. Measurement of the ability of cells to infiltrate normal tissue in-vitro. Brit.J.Cancer, 29: 36-49.
Fidler, I.J., Gersten, D.M. and Hart, I.R., 1978. The biology of cancer invasion and metastasis. Adv.Cancer Res., 28: 149-250.
Kramer, R.H. and Nicolson, G.L., 1979. Interaction of tumor cells with vascular endothelial cell monolayer: A model for metastatic invasion. Proc.Natl.Acad. Sci. USA, 76: 5704-5708.
Leighton, J. and Kline, I., 1954. Studies on human cancer using sponge matrix tissue culture. Texas Rep.Biol.Med., 12: 847-864, 865-873.
Liotta, L.A., Tryggvason, K., Garbisa, S., Hart, I., Foltz, C.M. and Shafie, S., 1980. Metastatic potential correlates with enzymatic degradation of basement membrane collagen. Nature, 284: 67-68.
Mareel, M., 1979. Is invasion in vitro characteristic of malignant cells? Cell Biol.Int.Rep., 3: 627-640.
Schleich, A.B., Frick, M. and Mayer, A., 1974. The confrontation of normal tissue and malignant cells in vitro, human decidua graviditatis and HeLa cells. A model for studies on tumor invasion. Z.Krebsforsch., 82: 247-255.
Schor, S.L., 1979. Cell migration through three-dimension gels of native collagen fibers. J.Cell Biol., 83: 471a.

Acknowledgement: R.T. thanks the Deutsche Krebsforschungszentrum for a research fellowship.

INVASIVENESS AND THE 'METASTATIC POTENTIAL' OF TUMOUR CELLS

C. Meyvisch, P. Van Hoorde and M. Mareel

INTRODUCTION

Local invasion from the primary tumour is the first, although not a sufficient step in the formation of metastases. We have developed an experimental
model in which spheroidal aggregates of malignant cells were used to study
invasion in vitro (Mareel et al., 1979) and in vivo (Meyvisch and Mareel, 1979).
Using this aggregate model it was found that invasion and growth were separate
activities of malignant cells (Storme and Mareel, 1980).

Pretreatment of the aggregates before implantation with drugs which inter-
fered with directional migration (microtubule inhibitors) inhibited tumorigenicity more than drugs which allowed directional migration, although the effect
of both on growth was similar (Meyvisch et al., 1980). Further work with drug
treated aggregates (Meyvisch et al., in preparation) supported our hypothesis
that the invasive capacity of transplanted malignant cells is important for the
development of a local tumour. A model was set up to assess if this invasive
capacity is also related with the metastatic potential of these cells.

MATERIALS

Mice

Female C3H/He mice from an inbred colony maintained at the animalarium of
the Katholic University of Louvain were used when 8-15 weeks old. They were
kept on a standard pellet diet and drinking water ad libitum.

Tumour cells

MO_4 cells were grown from a C3H mouse cell line (MO) after transformation in
vitro by Kirsten murine sarcoma virus (Billiau et al., 1973). The MO_4 cells
do not produce infectious virus, they are highly invasive when confronted with
embryonic chick tissues in vitro and they produce invasive tumours after subcutaneous or intramuscular inoculation in the syngeneic host (inbred C3H mice)
(Mareel et al., 1975). They form progressively growing lung nodules after
intravenous injection (De Brabander et al., 1974).

METHODS

Tissue culture procedures

The MO_4 cells were cultured in Eagle's minimum essential medium (MEM, Flow
Laboratories, Ltd, Irvine, Scotland) plus 10% fetal bovine serum and 0.05%

glutamine. They were routinely passaged by short trypsinization.

Spheroidal aggregates of MO_4 cells were harvested from gyrotory shaker cultures after 48 hrs as described by Mareel et al. (1979). Aggregates with a diameter of 0.3 mm containing approximately 30.000 cells were selected under a stereomicroscope and washed three times with fresh culture medium to discard loose cells.

Implantation

A single MO_4 aggregate was implanted subcutaneously in the tail of **syngeneic** mice at 4.5 cm from the tip with the aid of a MICROPETTER (SMI Scientific Manufacturing Industries, Emeryville, Cal.) as described in Meyvisch et al. (1980).

Tumour volume

Two caliper measurements at right angles were taken and the volume of the ellipsoid tumours was calculated with the formula derived by Attia and Weiss (1966) : volume = 0.4 (ab^2) where a and b represent the larger and smaller diameters, respectively.

Histology

Aggregates of MO_4 cells were fixed in glutaraldehyde 2.5% in veronal acetate buffer, with postfixation in osmium tetroxide (1% in the same buffer), embedded in Araldit, sectioned into 1 μm thick sections and stained with hematoxylin and eosin.

Tail tumours were fixed in Bouin's solution. Lungs were prelevated in toto and fixed in buffered formalin solution. Tissues were embedded in paraplast and serially sectioned. The sections (8 μm thick) were stained with hematoxylin-phloxin-safranin.

OBSERVATIONS
Primary tumour

After subcutaneous implantation of an MO_4 aggregate in the tail nearly all mice developed a palpable tumour ($\pm$ 1 mm diameter) from the second week on. The tumour take in three separate groups of mice was : 20/20 - 9/9 - 8/9.

The increase in volume of these tumours was followed during 10 weeks (Fig. 1). Large variations in the growth rate of individual tumours were obvious.

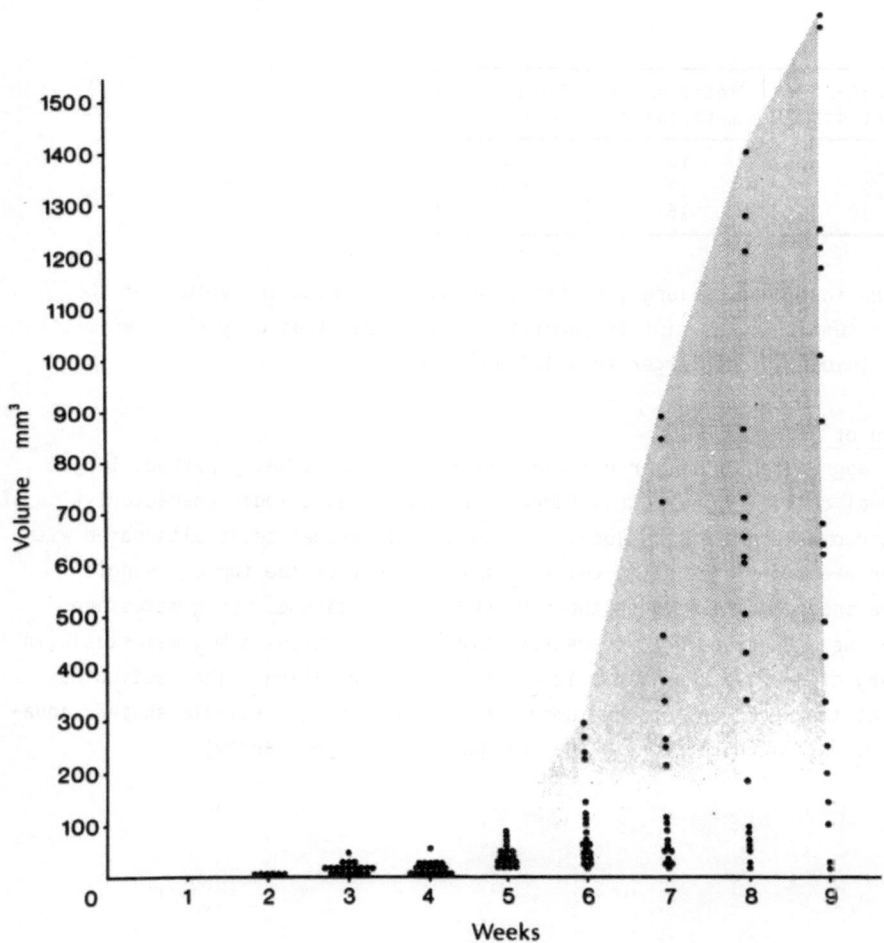

Fig. 1. Growth of the primary tumour in the tail. Ordinate : volume in mm^3; abscissa : time in weeks. Each point represents an individual measurement.

Incidence of lung metastases

Mice bearing a primary tumour in the tail remained in good general health for the first 10 weeks, even with a tumour volume up to 1500 mm^3. When thereafter a few of the animals showed signs of health deterioration the whole group was sacrificed. The incidence of lung metastases is shown in Table 1.

TABLE 1

No of animals with metastases	Total no of metastases	Range per animal
5/9	14	1-4
6/9	12	1-3
10/18	15	1-3

When the incidence of lung metastases was compared with the volume of the primary tumour at the time of sacrifice it appeared that only those animals with a tumour volume larger than 400 mm^3 showed metastases.

Pattern of invasion

MO_4 aggregates in shaker culture were built up by tightly packed, large polygonal cells. Primary tail tumours showed the histologic characteristics of fibrosarcomas; bundles of closely packed spindle shaped cells alternated with smaller areas of large plump cells. At the border of the tumours single spindle shaped cells invaded the surrounding host tissue. Lung metastases showed the same histologic characteristics. Fig. 2 shows a MO_4 metastasis in the lung of a mouse sacrificed 12 weeks after inoculation. The section was taken at the periphery of the tumour nodule where single spindle shaped, invasive MO_4 cells can be seen in the pulmonary parenchyma (arrow).

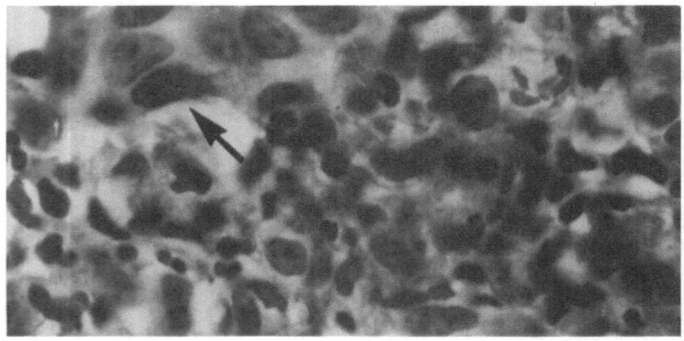

Fig. 2. Light micrograph from a lung metastasis .

CONCLUSIONS AND DISCUSSION

After subcutaneous implantation in the tail of an aggregate of the highly invasive MO_4 cells, a progressively growing tumour developed near the implantation site from which lung metastases were formed. The volume of the primary tumour appeared to determine the incidence of lung metastases. Histologically no difference was seen in the pattern of invasion of MO_4 cells from an aggregate immediately after implantation (Meyvisch et al., 1979), as compared to invasion from the primary tumour in the tail or from the lung metastases.

We have prefered to use aggregates of MO_4 cells instead of cell suspensions because no single MO_4 cells, which could give a false impression of invasion, are present (Meyvisch et al., 1979). As the implantation site in the tail is exactly known we have a model that allows us to follow invasion of MO_4 cells from the earliest steps in loco up to the formation of lung metastases. The localization of the primary tumour in the tail offers the advantage of easy, not too traumatic amputation at a definite distance from the original implantation site.

Using this aggregate model we are now implanting MO_4 cells that have been pretreated with anti-invasive drugs in order to assess the importance of the invasive capacity of malignant cells in the process of metastasis formation.

REFERENCES

Attia, M.A. and Weiss, D.W., 1966. Immunology of Spontaneous Mammary Carcinomas in Mice. V. Acquired Tumor Resistance and Enhancement in Strain. A Mice Infected with Mammary Tumor Virus. Cancer Res., 26: 1787-1800.
Billiau, A., Sobis, H., Eyssen, H. and Van Den Berghe, H., 1973. Non-infectious intracisternal A-type particles in a sarcoma-positive leukemia-negative mouse cell line transformed by murine sarcoma virus (MSV). Arch. Ges. Virusforsch., 43: 345-351.
De Brabander, M., Aerts, F. and Borgers, M., 1974. The Influence of a Glucocorticoid on the Lodgement and Development in the Lungs of Intravenously Injected Tumour Cells. Europ. J. Cancer, 10: 751-755.
Mareel, M., De Ridder, L., De Brabander, M. and Vakaet, L., 1975. Characterization of Spontaneous, Chemical and Viral Transformants of a C3H/3T3-type Mouse Cell Line by Transplantation Into Young Chick Blastoderms. J. Natl. Cancer Inst., 54: 923-929.
Mareel, M., Kint, J. and Meyvisch, C., 1979. Methods of Study of the Invasion of Malignant C3H-Mouse Fibroblasts Into Embryonic Chick Heart in Vitro. Virchows Arch. B Cell Path., 30: 95-111.
Meyvisch, C. and Mareel, M., 1979. Invasion of Malignant C3H Mouse Fibroblasts from Aggregates Transplanted Into the Auricles of Syngenic Mice. Virchows Arch. B Cell Path., 30: 113-122.
Meyvisch, C. and Van Cauwenberge, R., 1980. Invasiveness of Malignant Mouse Fibroblasts in Vivo. In: M. De Brabander et al. (Editors), Cell Movement and Neoplasia. Pergamon Press, Oxford and New York, pp. 179-185.
Storme, G. and Mareel, M., 1980. Effect of Anticancer Agents on Directional Migration of Malignant C3H Mouse Fibroblastic Cells in Vitro. Cancer Res., 40: 943-948.

ACKNOWLEDGMENTS

This study was supported by a Grant from the Algemene Spaar- en Lijfrentekas, Brussels, Belgium.

A POSSIBILITY OF PREDICTING THE METASTATIC POTENTIAL OF TUMOURS BY IMPLANTATION INTO CHICK EMBRYO BLASTODERMS

G.V. Sherbet and M.S. Lakshmi

1. INTRODUCTION

The ability of a tumour to invade and metastasize may be considered as an intrinsic biological property of its component cells. Although the expression of malignant behaviour may be influenced by the host, it may be helpful in the clinical management of patients if it were possible to determine the potential of a primary tumour to dissem: nate and form metastases. Recently Carter (1978) has argued that the available methods for assessing metastatic potential are inadequate. It would appear that the morphological criteria of site, size and histology of the primary tumour which are relied upon heavily may not be fully indicative of its metastatic potential. It is of utmost importance, therefore, that new methods of assay are developed which can determine the metastatic potential. Our investigations of the interactions between chick embryonic tissue and tumour cells have resulted in the development of an assay system by which it appears possible to distinguish between normal and neoplastic cells, and also to determine the degree of malignancy of tumours (Sherbet and Lakshmi, 1968, 1969, 1974a,b, 1978; Sherbet et al., 1969). Tumour cells implanted between the cell layers of the chick blastoderm elicit three major cellular responses, of which the most characteristic are the histogenetic responses from the embryonic ectoderm and/or the endoderm which appear to occur with increased intensity with increase in the malignancy of the implanted cells.

In the present paper, we describe the correlation observed betwee the metastatic ability of the implanted tumours and the intensity of the histogenetic responses which they induce.

2. MATERIALS

2.1. Morris hepatomas

Six Morris minimum deviation hepatomas with varying metastatic abilities were used (Sherbet et al., 1969, 1970).

2.2. Metastasizing (ML) and non-metastasizing (NML) lymphosarcomas

Two homotransplantable lymphosarcomas (Carter and Gershon, 1966) were used. They were maintained by serial transplantation in 2 - 4 month old inbred Syrian cream hamsters (Guy et al., 1977). Tests were carried out both on the undissociated tumours and on viable tumour cells isolated from the tumours by collagenase disaggregation (Guy et al., 1977) followed by sedimentation of the cells on a mixture of Ficoll-Hypaque (Mavligit et al., 1973).

2.3. Human breast tumour series

A short series of human breast tumours were investigated, which comprised fibroepithelial hyperplasias and carcinomas. The specimens investigated were supplied by Professor I.D.A. Johnston, Dr. P.A. Riley and Mr. R.G. Wilson.

3. METHODS

3.1. Embryo culture and tumour implantation

16 - 18 hr old chick embryo blastoderms were explanted in vitro as described by New (1955). The tumour tissues being investigated were implanted between the ectodermal and endodermal layers of the blastoderms as described by Waddington (1932). After implantation the embryos were incubated for a further period of 18 hr, when they were fixed, sectioned serially, stained and examined histologically. Each tumour being tested was implanted into about 15 embryos (two 0.3 mm^3 grafts per embryo), making a total of about 30 grafts of each tumour.

3.2. Assessment of histogenetic responses

The frequency of occurrence and the intensity of the histogenetic responses were assessed and scored according to the following scheme (Sherbet and Lakshmi, 1974a).

	% Positive of total no. of implants	Score
Frequency of induction of response	100 - 75	3
	74 - 50	2
	49 - 25	1
	<25	
Intensity of response	Moderate	1
	High	2

4. RESULTS AND DISCUSSION

4.1. Morris hepatomas

Normal liver tissue produced a histogenetic response score of 3.
The hepatomas 9633 and 9618B which possessed no ability to metastasize
were found to be comparable with normal liver as regards the histogenetic responses induced. Two other hepatomas, No. 7794A and 7787,
which were able to produce a few metastases, induced histogenetic
responses of grade 4. Also hepatoma No. 7793, which could produce
many large metastases, induced histogenetic responses of grade 4.
Tumour No. 5123C, which also was highly metastatic, produced grade
5 histogenetic responses. Although the metastatic ability of the
tumours was assessed in an arbitrary fashion (Hruban et al., 1971),
an increase in the ability to metastasize seems to correspond clearly
with increased ability of these tumours to induce histogenetic responses (Fig. 1).

4.2. Hamster lymphosarcomas

The non-metastasizing form of the lymphosarcoma produced a grade
3 (tissue pieces) or grade 4 (viable cells isolated from the tumour)
histogenetic response. In sharp contrast with this, the metastasizing
form induced histogenetic responses of grade 7 (tissue pieces) or
grade 9 (viable cells). This marked difference is consistent with
the differences in their metastatic ability which have recently been
demonstrated unequivocally by Sherbet et al. (1980).

4.3. Human mammary tumours

The fibroepithelial hyperplasias investigated produced histogenetic
responses ranging from grade 0 - 3 (Fig. 2). On the other hand, the
histologically proven carcinomas induced histogenetic responses ranging
between grades 3 - 10. At the lower end of the scale (histogenetic
score 3 - 6) the patients were found to be disease-free for 4 - 7 years
following mastectomy. In contrast, three patients whose tumours had
induced responses of grades 8 and 10 had died of disseminated disease
about three years after mastectomy had been performed (Fig. 2). One
patient with grade 7 tumour has had a recurrent carcinoma. Although
these observations may be deemed as preliminary, it would appear that
in these carcinomas the metastatic abilities of the primary cancers
may be reflected in their histogenetic response scores.

From these data relating to three diverse tumour models, one may
reasonably conclude that the ability to induce histogenetic responses
in the chick embryo blastoderm may be an indicator of the metastatic
potential of tumours and that these tests may be helpful in the
clinical management of patients.

42

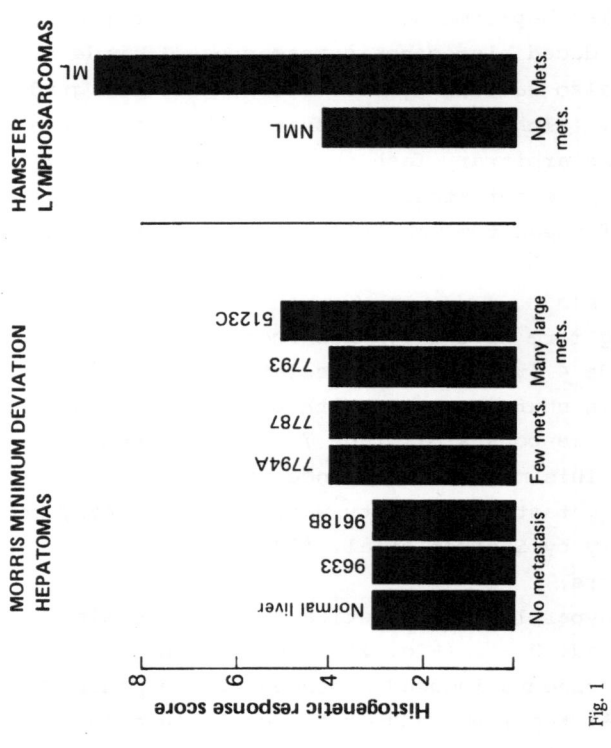

Fig. 1

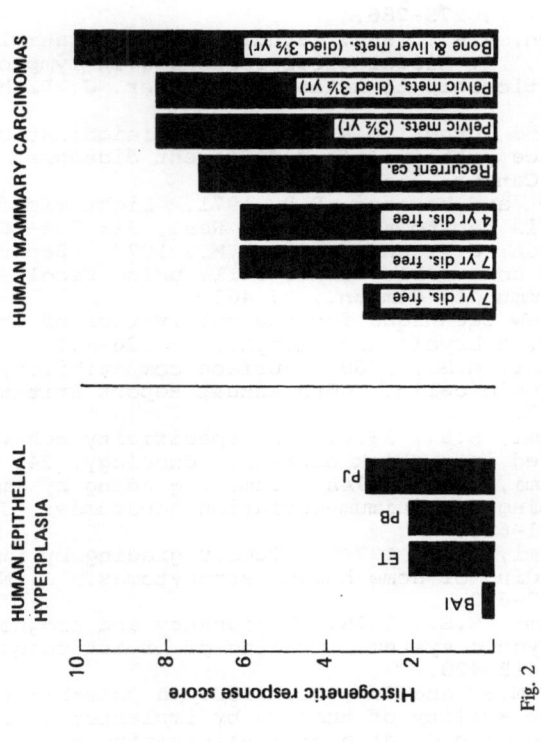

Fig. 2

44

5. ACKNOWLEDGMENTS

The authors wish to thank the North of England Cancer Research Campaign and the Manpower Services Commission for generous financial support.

REFERENCES

Carter, R.L., 1978. Metastatic potential of malignant tumour. Invest. Cell Pathol., 1: 275-286.

Carter, R.L. and Gershon, R.K., 1966. Studies on homotransplantable lymphomas in hamster. I. Histological responses in lymphoid tissues and the relationship to metastasis. Amer. J. Path., 49: 637-655.

Guy, D., Latner, A.L. and Turner, G.A., 1977. Radioiodination studie of tumour cell surface proteins after different disaggregation procedures. Br. J. Cancer, 36: 166-172.

Hruban, Z., Morris, H.P. and Meranze, D.R. 1971. Light microscopic observations of Morris hepatomas. Cancer Res., 31: 752-762.

Mavligit, G.M., Gutterman, J.V. and Hersh, E.M., 1973. Separation of viable cells from non-viable tumour cells using Ficoll-Hypaque density solution. Immunol. Commun., 2: 463.

New, D.A.T., 1955. A new technique for the cultivation of chick embryos in vitro. J. Embryol. exp. Morph., 3: 326-331.

Sherbet, G.V. and Lakshmi, M.S., 1968. Surface compatibility between neoplastic and embryonic cells. 46th Annual Report British Empire Cancer Campaign, p.57.

Sherbet, G.V. and Lakshmi, M.S., 1970. The specificity behaviour of tumour cells implanted into chick embryos. Oncology, 24: 58-67.

Sherbet, G.V. and Lakshmi, M.S., 1974a. Tumour grading by implantati in embryos. I. Grading of minimum-deviation hepatomas. J. Natl. Cancer Inst., 52: 681-686.

Sherbet, G.V. and Lakshmi, M.S., 1974b. Tumour grading by implantati in embryos. II. Grading of some human astrocytomas. J. Natl. Cancer Inst., 52: 687-692.

Sherbet, G.V. and Lakshmi, M.S., 1978. Malignancy and prognosis evaluated by an embryonic system. Grading of breast tumours. Eur. J. Cancer, 14: 415-420.

Sherbet, G.V., Lakshmi, M.S. and Guy, D., 1980. A possibility of predicting metastatic ability of tumours by implantation into chick embryos. Epigenetic grading of metastasizing and non-metastasizing forms of a hamster lymphosarcoma. Eur. J. Cancer (in press).

Sherbet, G.V., Lakshmi, M.S. and Morris, H.P., 1969. Behaviour of minimum-deviation hepatomas implanted into chick embryo blasto-derms. 47th Annual Report British Empire Cancer Campaign, p.109.

Sherbet, G.V., Lakshmi, M.S. and Morris, H.P., 1970. Behaviour of minimum-deviation hepatomas implanted into chick embryo blasto-derms. J. Natl. Cancer Inst., 45: 419-428.

Waddington, C.H., 1932. Experiments on the development of chick and duck embryos in vitro. Proc. Roy. Soc. London, 221: 179-230.

AN EXPERIMENTAL STUDY ON THE BARRIER FUNCTION
OF LYMPH NODES TO TUMOR CELLS

K. Kohno, T. Yamaguchi and T. Takahashi

Intralymphatic inoculation of rat ascites hepatoma AH130 has been carried out to elucidate the function of regional lymph nodes as a barrier for tumor spread. Tumor cells reaching regional lymph nodes decreased in number 48 to 72 hr. after inoculation. Ten per cent of tumor cells injected into lymphatic vessels appeared in the thoracic duct within 3 hr. after injection. Bioassay tests revealed that transnodal tumor cells were viable in the thoracic duct.

MATERIALS AND METHODS

Animal and tumor. Male donryu rats, weighing 200-240g, were used. The tumor was the Ascites Hepatoma (AH 130), which contained both free cells and clumps of cells. Rats, on the fifth day after intraperitoneal injection of 1×10^6 tumor cells, were injected intraperitoneally with 0.5 μci/g of ^{3}H-thymidine 5 times every 5 hr. Labelled tumor cells were washed twice and suspended in Hanks solution.

Injection procedure. Intralymphatic inoculation of tumor cells was made into the left testicle. A small amount of 10% Evans Blue and 0.2-0.3ml of physiologic saline was injected blindly into the left testicle. Lymphatic puncture was made under the dissecting microscope using a 27 gauge needle with a 15 μl Hamilton microsyringe. The injected volume was exactly 0.05ml in each instance. Shortly after inoculation, the spermatic cord was ligated and the testicle was removed.

Collection of lymph from the thoracic duct. A silicon rubber tube, 1.0mm in diameter, was inserted into the thoracic duct just below the diaphragm to collect thoracic lymph continuously. The rat was then placed in a cage in a semi-restrained position and maintained on a standard diet with 0.5% saline solution. The lymph was collected into an iced bottle.

RESULTS. Detection of labelled tumor cells into the lymph nodes and thoracic duct lymph

Labelled tumor cells were inoculated into the left testicular lymphatics, then from the left lumbar node and renal nodes and the thoracic duct lymph was taken at intervals of 1, 3, 6, 12, 24, 48, 72, 96, 120, 168 and 240 hr after inoculation. Radioactivity of the specimens was counted by a liquid scintillation counter.

Serial detection of radioactivity in the lymph node between 1 and 240 hr is shown in Fig.1. One hr after inoculation, maximum radioactivity, with a mean level of 6840 CPM, was recorded. Forty-eight hr after inoculation, the radioactivity of lymph node had dropped abruptly to a mean level of 682 CPM, about one tenth of the maximum CPM. This finding indicates that tumor cells lodging in the regional lymph node decreased markedly in number between 24 and 48 hr

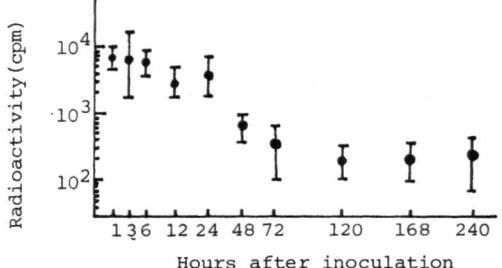

Fig. 1. Sequential radioactivity of tumor cells in the regional lymph nodes after intralymphatic inoculation of 1 x 10^5 tumor cells.

Serial detection of radioactivity in the thoracic duct lymph after inoculation of 1 x 10^5 and 1 x 10^6 labeled tumor cells is shown in Fig.2 and Fig.3, respectively. Peak radioactivity occurred between 1 and 3 hr, then decreased erratically.

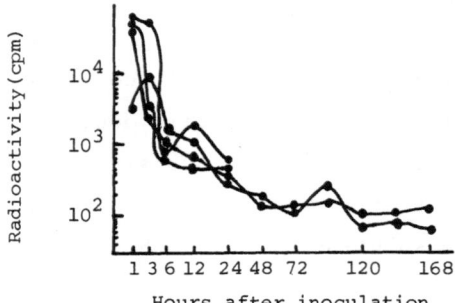

Fig. 2. Sequential radioactivity of tumor cells in the thoracic duct after intralymphatic inoculation of 1 x 10^5 tumor cells.

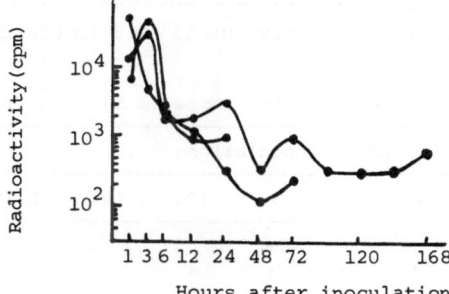

Fig. 3. Sequential radioactivity of tumor cells in the thoracic duct
after intralymphatic inoculation of 1 x 10^6 tumor cells.

In the first 3 hr after inoculation, the number of tumor cells
appearing in the thoracic duct lymph was approximately 10% of the
total injected, as shown in Fig.4.

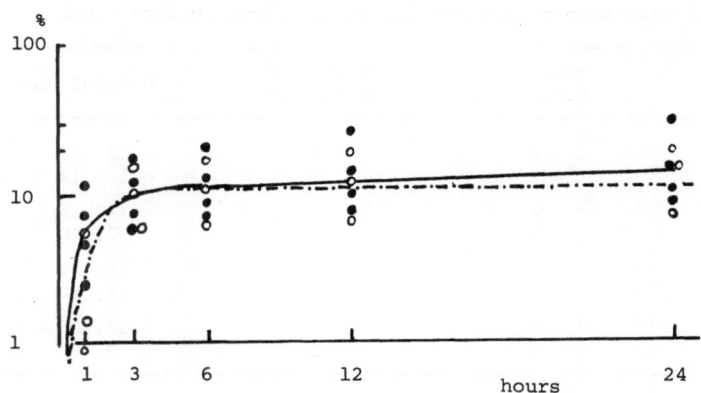

Fig. 4. Transnodal passage of tumor cells in the thoracic duct after
intralymphatic inoculation of tumor cells.
● —— ● : 1 x 10^5 tumor cells
o -·- o : 1 x 10^6 tumor cells

Detection of tumor cells by autoradiography

After injection of 1 x 10^6 labelled tumor cells into the testicular lymphatics, thoracic duct lymph was collected at intervals of 1,
3, 6, 12, 24, 48, 72, 96, 120 and 148 hr. Autoradiograms were prepared by dipping the slides in emulsion (Sakura MR-N$_2$). One hr after

injection, tumor cells had already appeared in the thoracic duct
lymph and thereafter were detected continuously until 168 hr(Table 1)

TABLE 1. Autoradiographic detection of tumor cells in the thoracic duct lymph

Rat No.	Hours after inoculation										
	1	3	6	12	24	48	72	96	120	144	168
No. 1	+	+	+	+	+	+	+	+			
No. 2	+	+	+	+	+	+	+	+	+	+	+
No. 3	+	+	+	+	+	+	+	+	+	+	

Biologic detection of tumor cells in the thoracic duct lymph

Samples of thoracic duct lymph collected at 3 and 24 hr after
the injection of 1×10^6 tumor cells were inoculated into the peritoneal cavity of rats to test for the presence of viable tumor cells.
All recipients revealed positive tumor growth and died in 7 to 16
days (Table 2).

TABLE 2. Biological detection of tumor cells in the thoracic duct lymph

Donor rat		Number of recipients	Number of dead rats	Survival days
No. 1	3 hr	2	2	15, 16
	24 hr	2	2	12, 14
No. 2	3 hr	2	2	12, 15
	24 hr	2	2	7, 10
No. 3	3 hr	2	2	15, 16
	24 hr	2	2	14, 16
No. 4	3 hr	2	2	13, 15
	24 hr	2	2	9, 10

DISCUSSION

Zeidman and Buss(1954) and Kurokawa(1970) who injected various
tumor cells into the lymphatics of rabbits and rats suggested that
lymph nodes act to a considerable extent as a mechanical barrier.
On the contrary, Fisher and Fisher(1966) demonstrated that lymph
nodes are not an effective barrier to the dissemination of tumor cells

In the present experiments to see whether lymph nodes can be a
completely effective filter preventing passage of tumor cells, quantitative examination was carried out using direct inoculation of labelled
tumor cells into afferent lymphatics.

Radioactivity of the lymph node reached a maximum one hr after inoculation of labelled tumor cells and thereafter decreased markedly, falling to a level of about one-tenth maximum value within 48 hr. This indicates that the regional lymph node acts as a mechanical barrier and catches the entering tumor cells temporarily after which lodging tumor cells decrease markedly in number between 24 and 48 hr. Labelled tumor cells were observed in the thoracic duct lymph shortly after intralymphaic inoculation. Within 3 hr, approximately 10% of the injected tumor cells had appeared in the thoracic duct lymph; thereafter radioactivity gradually decreased during the period of the experiment. Moreover, autoradiographic and biologic detection confirmed the viability of tumor cells in thoracic duct lymph. Of course, this result using only one strain of tumor cannot immediately lead to a general conclusion. However, it may be reasonable to presume that regional lymph nodes do not always act as a complete barrier to the spread of tumor cells.

REFERENCES

Fisher, B.& Fisher, E.R., 1966. Transmigration of lymph nodes by tumor cells. Science, 152: 1397-1398.
Kurokawa, Y., 1970. Experiments on lymph node metastasis by intralymphatic inoculation of rat ascites tumor cells, with special reference to lodgement, passage, and growth of tumor cells in lymph nodes. Gann, 61: 461-471.
Zeidman, I. & Buss, J.M., 1954. Experimental studies on the spread of cancer in the lymphatic system. (I) Effectiveness of lymph nodes as a barrier to the passage of embolic tumor cells. Cancer Res., 14: 403-405.

METASTASES FROM DMBA-INDUCED CARCINOMAS IN HAMSTER CHEEK POUCH

G.T. Craig

INTRODUCTION

Chemically-induced carcinomas in Syrian hamster cheek pouch mucosa were first described by Salley (1954), who found that topical applications of 0.5 per cent 9, 10-dimethyl-1, 2-benzanthracene (DMBA) in either acetone or benzene for a period of 16 weeks with 9 weeks additional observation resulted in the development of squamous cell carcinomas; regional lymph node metastases occurred in 18 out of the 19 surviving animals. Although the hamster cheek pouch has subsequently been subjected to a variety of experimental regimes covering most aspects of carcino-genesis (Homburger, 1969, 1972 and Shklar, 1972), apart from one isolated example (Rwomushana et al., 1970) it would appear that metastases have never been reported consistently again. The few indisputable regional lymph node metastases known to the author have arisen more than 20 weeks after the initial painting with carcino-gen. By contrast, the overwhelming majority of published reports of DMBA carcino-genesis in the cheek pouch are based on experiments lasting between 12 and 18 weeks. Since the paucity of metastases from this model has prevented its wider acceptance, it was decided to investigate the possibility that the incidence of metastases might be dependent upon survival time.

MATERIALS AND METHODS

The experimental group comprised 30 male Syrian hamsters (Mesocricetus auratus), 4-6 weeks old, who had their right cheek pouches painted thrice weekly for 10 weeks with a 0.5 per cent. solution of 7, 12-dimethylbenz (α) anthracene in liquid paraffin B.P. Ten age- and sex-matched hamsters painted with liquid paraffin BP alone provided the control group. The carcinogen was applied with six strokes of a number four sable brush to the medial wall of the right pouch just behind the anterior vein. At weekly intervals each animal was weighed, the cheek pouches were examined visually and regional lymph nodes were palpated. Between week 10 and week 30, exophytic tumours greater than 0.5 cm diameter were surgically excised from the carcinogen-treated cheek pouches. Animals were killed when in obvious discomfort or following progressive weight loss to below 60g. Surviving control animals were killed coincident with the last experimental animal. At death a record was made of the number, approximate sizes, distribution and morphological character of the carcinogen induced tumours; the ipsilateral and contralateral superficial cervical lymph nodes were removed, specimens were taken from both cheek pouches and an autopsy was performed. Conventional methods were employed to prepare tissues for histological examination.

RESULTS

Two experimental and one control animal died before the experiment commenced. In addition, the early attempts at tumour-removal were associated with significant mortality and 5 out of the 28 carcinogen-treated animals failed to survive their first operation. At the end of the experiment 11(48%) of the 23 experimental animals showed histologically confirmed, metastatic deposits of squamous cell carcinoma confined to the ipsilateral superficial cervical lymph node. The extent of the metastases varied from discrete, sometimes multiple, foci occupying the peripheral sinus and outer cortex of the node to almost total effacement of the nodal architecture with extensive necrosis. On histological criteria, 10 of the metastases represented moderately differentiated keratinizing squamous cell carcinomas and 1 comprised a poorly differentiated squamous cell carcinoma. The contralateral lymph nodes appeared essentially normal and the autopsy showed no evidence of spread beyond the ipsilateral lymph nodes. In the remaining 12(52%) experimental animals the ipsilateral lymph nodes contained no metastatic deposits and the contralateral nodes resembled their counterparts in the animals with metastases.

Of the surviving 23 experimental animals, 19 were subjected to a total of 45 individual operations for the removal of 85 exophytic tumours. The necessity for, and frequency of, tumour-removal operations (Fig.1.) varied as did the number of tumours excised at any one operation.

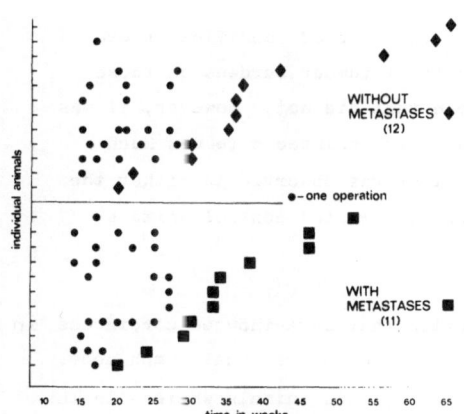

Fig.1. No. of operations and age at death for animals with and without metastases

A comparison of those animals with and without metastases in respect of tumour removal operations and numbers of tumours removed (Table 1) suggested that there were no striking differences between the groups.

TABLE 1

The influence of tumour-removal operations on metastatic yield.

	With Metastases (11 animals)	Without Metastases (12 animals)
Number of animals operated upon	11	8
Total number of operations	23	22
Total number of tumours removed	37	48

Furthermore, there appeared to be no significant correlation either within each group or between the two groups, concerning the time elapse from the last tumour-removal operation to the time of death (Fig.1). It was also evident that the range of ages at death was similar for both groups.

The excised tumours varied widely in histological appearance from nodules in which the surface epithelium showed differing degrees of dysplasia to frankly malignant nodules where the connective tissue core was invaded by squamous cell carcinoma. The exophytic lesions first appeared after about 6 weeks of carcinogen painting and arose, in the majority of cases, remote from the painted site. By contrast, from about 15 weeks onwards lesions began to develop in the region of the painted site; these were predominantly endophytic in nature and presented macroscopically as ulcerated and invasive carcinomas. Because of their morphological character, the latter were not amenable to surgical excision and their relentless growth was largely responsible for the decision to sacrifice experimental animals.

On the basis of the subjective evaluation at the time of sacrifice, there appeared to be no difference in the respective total tumour burdens of those animals that proved to have metastases and those that did not. However, it was clear that the incidence of endophytic lesions at the painted site was much greater in the group with metastases. No pathology was observed in either the cheek pouches or the lymph nodes of liquid paraffin-treated control animals.

DISCUSSION

The results confirm Salley's (1954) observation that DMBA-induced carcinomas in the hamster cheek pouch are capable of metastasizing to the regional lymph node. However, Salley obtained metastases in 95 per cent of his animals whereas in the study reported here the incidence was 48 per cent. A possible explanation for the difference in metastatic yield, apart from the important one of animal strain (Homburger, 1972) is related to the vehicle for the carcinogen. Salley originally used acetone as a solvent for the DMBA but subsequently (Salley, 1957) employed heavy mineral oil and was unable to detect metastases at the end of a somewhat shorter experimental period. More recently Marefat and Shklar (1977) have shown that carcinoma of Syrian hamster tongue can be much more readily and rapidly induced with DMBA in acetone as opposed to DMBA in heavy mineral oil.

The findings in the present study also suggest that metastasis in this model is, at least in part, survival time dependent and that this factor alone could account for the paucity of metastases from previous investigations. Wallace(1956) has also maintained that a short survival time limits the possibilities for spontaneous metastases to develop.

Although it would have been desirable to avoid the tumour-removal operations and thereby eliminate a possible influence on the metastatic process, it was known from previous experience of the model that ulceration and necrosis of the exophytic lesions would be significant factors governing the decision to kill animals during the early stages of tumour development. If the number of tumour-removal operations per animal had constituted a significant metastasis promoting factor, one would have expected those animals with metastasis to show the greater experience but this was not the case. Similarly, if surgical interference with a tumour was associated with an increased incidence of metastasis, one would have expected to find that the average number of tumours removed per animal was greater in the metastasis group but this was not the case. In this context it is interesting to note that Shklar (1968) concluded that neither extensive manipulation nor surgical incision produced greater invasion or spread of DMBA-induced exophytic tumours in the cheek pouch.

DMBA carcinogenesis in hamster cheek pouch is an example of a multiple tumour model and as such, it might be anticipated that, for a given metastatic deposit it would be virtually impossible to identify the primary tumour responsible. However, the observation that endophytic, invasive carcinomas occured much more frequently in the metastasis group argued strongly in favour of their role as the metastasizing tumours. The longer latent period prior to development of the endophytic lesions coupled with the demonstration that metastasis itself is a relatively late phenomenon in this model, lend support to this interpretation.

It is generally accepted that experimental tumours seldom metastasize spontaneously and Kim (1971) suggested that metastatic potential was intimately linked with tumour immunogenicity, the lower the immunogenicity the higher the incidence of metastasis. Eccles and Alexander (1974) also demonstrated an inverse relationship between immunogenicity and metastatic capacity for a series of chemically induced rat sarcomata. In general, it appears that immunogenicity is strongest amongst chemically induced tumours that have a short latent period and require minimal doses of carcinogen for their production. On this basis, it might have been reasonable to attribute the paucity of metastases from DMBA-induced hamster cheek pouch tumours to their immunogenic status although direct evidence concerning the latter is not available. However, the clear demonstration of metastatic potential reported here would suggest that the level of immunogenicity varies from tumour to tumour within the pouch, a view consistent with that expressed by Kim (1971) for other multiple tumour models. Furthermore, it is tempting to speculate that tumour progression (Kerbel, 1979) may also be operating, since the tumours giving rise to metastases were considered to have longer latent periods and more frankly invasive morphological and histological appearances than the traditional exophytic cheek pouch tumours. In the present context it is relevant to note that tumour progression has been associated with an increased metastatic potential in both spontaneous as well as induced tumours (Rudenstam, 1968).

The unequivocal demonstration of metastases from DMBA-induced carcinomas in hamster cheek pouch mucosa justifies continued use of the model in studies related to the development and spread of human oral cancer.

REFERENCES

Eccles, S.A. and Alexander, P., 1974. Macrophage content of tumours in relation to metastatic spread and host immune reaction. Nature (Lond.), 250:667-669.

Homburger, F., 1969. Chemical carcinogenesis in the Syrian golden hamster - a review. Cancer, 23: 313-338.

Homburger, F., 1972. Chemical carcinogenesis in Syrian hamsters. In: F.Homburger (Editor), Progr.exp.Tumour Res.Karger, Basel, 16: 152-175.

Kerbel, R.S., 1979. Implications of immunological heterogeneity of tumours. Nature (Lond.), 280: 358-360.

Kim, U., 1971. Metastasizing mammary carcinomas in rats: Induction and study of their immunogenicity. Science, 167: 72-74.

Marefat, P. and Shklar, G., 1977. Experimental production of lingual leukoplakia and carcinoma. Oral Surg., 44: 578-586.

Rudenstam, C.-M., 1968. Experimental studies on trauma and metastasis formation. Acta chir.scand., Suppl. 391.

Rwomushana, J.W., Polliack, A. and Levij, I.S., 1970. Cervical lymph node metastasis of hamster cheek pouch carcinoma induced with DMBA.J.dent.Res., 49: 184.

Salley, J.J. 1954. Experimental carcinogenesis in the cheek pouch of the Syrian hamster. J.dent.Res., 33: 253-262.

Salley, J.J., 1957. Histologic changes in the hamster cheek pouch during early hydrocarbon carcinogenesis. J.dent.Res., 36: 48-55.

Shklar, G., 1972. Experimental oral pathology in the Syrian hamster. In: F.Homburger (Editor), Progr.exp.Tumor Res. Karger, Basel, 16: 518-538.

Shklar, G., 1968. The effect of manipulation and incision on experimental carcinoma of hamster buccal pouch. Cancer Res., 28: 2180-2182.

Wallace, A.C., 1956. The occurence of metastases in a group of related rat tumours. Brit.J.Cancer, 10: 724-732.

QUANTITATION AND CELLULAR GROWTH OF OCCULT METASTASES OF A RAT MAMMARY CARCINOMA

H. Speakman and B. Dixon

INTRODUCTION

The mammary carcinoma, LMC_1, arose spontaneously in a breeding female of John's strain Wistar rat. The kinetics and histology of the isogeneic transplanted tumour, now anaplastic have been described (Moore and Dixon, 1977a), and metastases develop when its growth is delayed by chemotherapy or irradiation (Moore and Dixon, 1977b, Dixon et al., 1979). Occult metastases are present in the superficial lymph nodes of 50% of rats when their transplanted tumour is excised at a mean diameter of 8-10 mm (Dixon and Speakman, 1979).

The cellular process of metastasis is difficult to quantitate in vivo. Dissemination of tumour cells may be assayed by the cannulation of efferent tumour lymphatics (Carr et al., 1979) or veins (Liotta et al., 1978), or by transplantation of lymph nodes (Hewitt and Blake, 1977). Transplantation of whole potentially tumourous nodes, and injection of monodisperse suspensions of LMC_1 cells have enabled us to estimate the numbers of occult tumour cells present in inguinal and axillary nodes from their initial spread from the primary tumour to the advent of measurable metastases. Thus we have quantitated microscopic spread and proliferation of LMC_1 cells indirectly by measuring macroscopic events.

MATERIALS AND METHODS

Three to six month old 100-150g virgin female isologous rats were used. Experimental primary tumours were prepared by the "sausage" method of Thomlinson (1960). Each "sausage" was implanted subcutaneously at the posterior right abdominal flank. Randomised groups of rats were killed 1 to 28 days after implantation. Their right axillary and inguinal lymph nodes were removed aseptically and implanted subcutaneously, 2 per rat, into fresh hosts. Each site was inspected for up to 100 days and tumours produced were measured daily across three perpendicular axes, from palpation to sacrifice of the host.

Other animals bearing experimental tumours were randomised into three groups. Those in groups 1 and 2 were killed at 12 and 24 days respectively after implantation of their tumours, when their right axillary and inguinal nodes were removed, transplanted and measured as above. Animals in group 3 had their primary tumour excised at 12 days (Dixon and Speakman, 1979). At 24 days post-implantation, i.e. 12 days after surgery, they were killed, their nodes transplanted and tumours produced measured as for groups 1 and 2.

Tumour tissue for the preparation of monodisperse suspensions of LMC_1 cells was obtained from the margins of primary tumours at post-mortem. The tissue was minced and agitated mechanically for 20 min at $37°C$ in 0.25% (W/V) trypsin in

Hank's Balanced Salt Solution (HBSS - Flow, Scotland). Fragments of tumour tissue were allowed to settle for 10 min and the supernatant was centrifuged at 180g for 5 min. The cell pellet obtained was then dispersed, using a Pasteur pipette, washe centrifuged and resuspended in fresh HBSS. A fresh solution of trypsin was added t the residual tumour tissue and the above procedures repeated, usually 4 times. Har vested cells were kept in HBSS on ice until the last incubation when all cell suspensions were pooled, counted and examined by microscopy to ensure that a monodisperse cell preparation had been obtained. Cell viability, usually 90-95%, was estimated by Trypan Blue exclusion. Inocula containing a mean number of 3.3×10^{-2} to 4.6×10^{6} LMC_1 cells in 0.2 ml of HBSS were prepared and injected subcutaneously at 4 abdominal sites per rat. Those sites which became positive for tumour, and th time taken for each growth to reach a mean diameter of 8-10 mm, were recorded - individual tumours being measured daily until sacrifice of the host.

RESULTS

Lymph nodes transplanted within 10 days of implantation of the primary never gave rise to LMC_1 in fresh hosts. Thereafter the percentage of lymph nodes positive for LMC_1 increased with time of removal after implantation of the primary in the original host (Table 1).

TABLE 1

Day of Assay	Number of nodes assayed	Percentage with tumour ($\pm$ s.d.)
1	20	0
3	24	0
6	26	0
10	20	50 $\pm$ 11
12	26	39 $\pm$ 9
15	20	60 $\pm$ 10
20	22	68 $\pm$ 9
24	28	71 $\pm$ 8
28	14	100

No significant differences in tumour production rates were obtained between axillary and inguinal lymph nodes. For injection with LMC_1 cells the TD_{50} was about 5 cells and inoculation with 35 or more produced a tumour in 90% or more site (Table 2) :-

No. of Cells	No. of Sites	% with Tumour
3.3×10^{-2}	80	0
3.3×10^{-1}	40	3 $\pm$ 2
3.4	28	42 $\pm$ 9
3.5×10	12	92 $\pm$ 8
4.0×10^{2}	16	88 $\pm$ 8
3.2×10^{3}	28	96 $\pm$ 4
2.0×10^{4}	20	100
3.2×10^{5}	20	100
4.6×10^{6}	8	100

Irrespective of the method of implantation, i.e. by the "sausage" technique, as dispersed cells or as cells within intact lymph nodes, all LMC_1 tumours had the same growth characteristics e.g. volume doubling times.

After injection with isolated cells, the mean time to reach 8-10 mm for tumours at positive sites was calculated and used to construct a standard curve (Fig. 1).

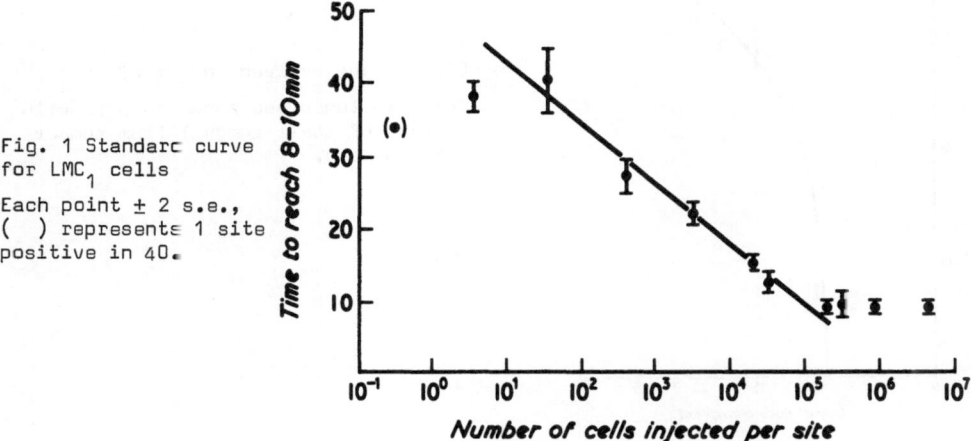

Fig. 1 Standard curve for LMC_1 cells

Each point ± 2 s.e., ( ) represents 1 site positive in 40.

For 50 to 5×10^5 cells per inoculum; there was a direct relationship between the logarithm of the number of cells injected and the time taken for tumours to reach 8-10 mm. Similarly, the time taken for positive nodes to produce 8-10 mm tumours was noted, but for these, the individual values were converted to equivalent tumour cell numbers using Figure 1. A mean value ± 2 s.e. was calculated for each group of tumourous nodes and either given in Table 3 for rats in groups 1,2 and 3

TABLE 3

	Group 1	Group 2	Group 3
No. of nodes assayed	12	12	12
Day to reach 8-10 mm	19.1 ± 4.5	9.5 ± 6.1	10.1 ± 7.7
Number of LMC_1 cells	7.9 ± 1.0 $(\times 10^3)$	1.3 ± 0.9 $(\times 10^5)$	7.9 ± 3.3 $(\times 10^4)$

or plotted as a function of the time of their removal and transplantation into fresh hosts (Fig. 2).

DISCUSSION

Alfieri and Hahn (1979) demonstrated a linear relationship between the number of fibrosarcoma cells injected and the time for tumours produced to reach a diameter of 1 cm. We have demonstrated a similar relationship for LMC_1 and this (Fig. 1), with lymph node transplantation, is a suitable method to quantitate metastasis and growth of clonogenic cells from primary tumours (Fig. 2).

58

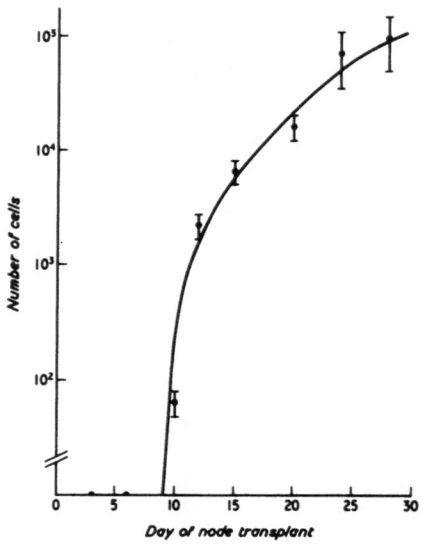

Fig. 2 The derived number of LMC$_1$ cells in tumourous nodes as a function of time of their removal from tumour bearing rats.

Dissemination of metastatic cells may be either continuous or episodic. If it is continuous, and the number of cells shed is related to the size of the primary tumour (Carr et al., 1979; Liotta et al., 1978) and therefore with time from implantation, the data (Figure 2) may merely reflect an increase in the number of LMC$_1$ cells transient and therefore present (Fisher and Fisher, 1967) in the nodes at the time of their removal. If dissemination is episodic, cells released soon after vascularisation of the primary may seed in the draining nodes and proliferat in situ. The increase in number of LMC$_1$ cells with time (Fig. 2) would then be explained by an increased number of tumour cell divisions before the nodes were removed for transplantation. Evidence against episodic dissemination is consid- erable (Hewitt and Blake, 1977; Carr et al., 1979; Liotta et al., 1978). However the number of LMC$_1$ cells in nodes at 24 days after tumour transplantation is appro imately the same whether tumours are excised at 12 days or are left in situ (Table 3). This suggests that it is the cells disseminated to nodes early in the development of a primary tumour which make the greatest contribution to the growth of a metastasis. In addition, the percentage of tumourous nodes increases with time (Table 1) and the most plausible explanation for this is that the continual shedding of cells, although not contributing significantly to the increase in number of LMC$_1$ cells in an involved node, does increase the probability of produci additional lymph node metastases.

If Fig. 2 represents an increase in cell number due to proliferation, these data suggest that the first tumour cell reaches a node about 9 days after implantation of the primary tumour. In previous experiments (Dixon and Speakman, 1979) lymph nodes were left _in situ_ for up to 100 days after excision (at 1-9 days) of the primary. Then distant metastases never occurred without an animal first developing a local recurrence. The present data (Fig. 2) further suggests that where seeding is successful, cell division ensues fairly rapidly and the population doubling time (PDT) of LMC$_1$ cells within the nodes increases from about 10 to 90 hr. From 11 to 12 days post-implantation, the PDT approximates to 18 hr, the mean cycle time for LMC$_1$ cells _in situ_ (Moore and Dixon, 1977a), suggesting that all are in cycle. Administration of an adequate dose of a cycle specific agent at this time should eliminate all occult metastases in axillary and inguinal nodes. Beyond 12 days the PDT of metastatic cells increases progressively to 4-5 times the cycle time (Fig. 2), suggesting a progressively diminishing growth fraction. This presumably will reduce the effectiveness of systemic therapy. The data reported here, are being used to design chemotherapy schedules to control metastasis and permit an improved treatment of the primary tumour.

REFERENCES

Alfieri, A.A. and Hahn, E.W., 1978. An in situ method for estimating cell survival in a solid tumour. Cancer Research, 38: 3006-3011.

Carr, J., Carr, I., Dreher, B. and Franks, C.R., 1979. Lymphatic metastasis of tumour: Persistent transport of cells. Experientia, 35: 825-826.

Dixon, B. and Speakman, H., 1979. Local recurrence and metastasis of excised breast carcinoma in the rat. J. Roy. Soc. Med., 72: 572-577.

Fisher, B. and Fisher, E.R., 1967. Barrier function of lymph nodes to tumour cells and erythrocytes. I Normal nodes. Cancer, 20: 1907-1913.

Hewitt, H.B. and Blake, E.R., 1977. Further studies of the relationship between lymphatic dissemination and lymphnodal metastasis in non-immunogenic murine tumours. Brit. J. Cancer, 35: 415-419.

Liotta, L.A., De Lisi, C., Vembu, D. and Boone, C.C., 1978. Micrometastasis: Model Systems. In: Pulmonary Metastasis. Weiss and Gilbert (Editors) G.K. Hall and Co. Boston, PP. 62-75.

Moore, J.V. and Dixon, B., 1977a. Serial transplantation, histology and cellular kinetics of a rat adenocarcinoma. Cell Tissue Kinet., 10: 583-590.

Moore, J.V. and Dixon, B., 1977b. Metastasis of a transplantable mammary tumour in rats treated with cyclophosphamide and/or irradiation. Brit. J. Cancer, 36: 221-226.

Thomlinson, R.H., 1960. An experimental method for comparing treatments of intact malignant tumours in animals and its applications to the use of oxygen in radiotherapy. Brit. J. Cancer, 14: 555-576.

COMPARISON OF NATURAL AND ARTIFICIAL LUNG METASTASES FROM A MURINE TUMOUR OF SPONTANEOUS ORIGIN

A.C. Begg and K.A. Smith

Abstract

The metastatic potential of the non-immunogenic CBA SA F tumour was investigated. Eradication of subcutaneous tumours of different sizes with 80Gy of X-rays resulted in lung metastases incidence increasing from 0 to 100% as the primary tumour size increased from 2 to 10mm. The number of metastases also increased and the average survival time decreased with increasing primary tumour size at treatment. The survival times suggested slower growth in lungs compared with subcutaneous sites. A bioassay for circulating tumour cells indicated there were less than 30 cells per ml venous blood in mice with tumours less than 12mm in diameter.

Experiments on 'artificial' metastases showed that lung colonies after intravenous injection of SA F cells had a higher colony forming efficiency and appeared later after smaller inocula. The difference in appearance times plus the observation of a wide range of colonies in the same lung for both natural and artificial metastases suggest a) a wide range of growth rates, or b) a multicell origin for some colonies, or c) a dormant period for some colonies. Correlations of these kinetic differences with treatment sensitivity are being investigated.

Introduction

Natural and "artificial" metastases, arising from subcutaneous tumours and intravenous injection of tumour cells respectively, were investigated in the belief that an increased understanding of the biology of metastases in these tumours will lead to improved treatments. The questions asked were whether artificial metastases mimicked spontaneous ones in characteristics such as their rate of growth, size distributions and times of appearance. If artificial metastases proved a good model for spontaneous ones, treatment studies using cells injected iv, an easier system to manipulate, could be carried out with increased confidence.

Materials and Methods

The CBA SA F, a tumour of spontaneous origin (Hewitt and Wilson, 1961) was used throughout. Recent studies have shown a failure to immunize mice against the tumour using lethally irradiated cells, demonstrating that it is non-immunogenic (Begg, A.C., unpublished data). Tumours for these experiments were grown from 10^5 to 10^6 cells in 0.05 mls inoculated subcutaneously on the lower back. Irradiation of tumours was performed using one of two Pantak

X-ray sets operating at 240 kV and 15 mA, with 0.24 mm Cu + 1 mm A1 filtration, giving a dose rate of approximately 350 rads/minute. Irradiation of cells, for addition to intravenous inocula of live cells, was achieved by giving 100 Gy of ^{60}Co gamma rays to the cell suspension at 330 rads/minute.

Locally cured mice were sacrificed either after becoming moribund due to their lung metastases, or after 3 months. Lungs were placed in Bouins solution for at least 24 hours before the number and sizes of the metastases were assessed. The same procedure was used for the artificial metastases.

To determine the number of tumour cells in blood, lymph nodes or lungs, tissues were transplanted subcutaneously to normal recipients from tumour bearing donors. The incidence of progressively growing tumours (takes) per inoculated site was scored. 0.4 mls blood was collected in a heparinized syringe from the right side of the heart or inferior vena cava and injected into 4 sites per recipient mouse; 0.1 mls per site. Lungs were rinsed in saline, minced in 0.4 mls saline and injected into 4 sites, 1 recipient per set of lungs. Subcutaneous flank lymph nodes were minced in a small volume of saline and injected into 2 sites per recipient.

The TD_{50} (number of cells required to produce 50% takes) was determined for tumour cells diluted in either saline or heparinized blood. Each dilution of the cell suspension was injected into 4 s.c. sites per mouse, 0.05 mls per site, and using 4 mice per dilution.

Results. Natural metastases. Subcutaneous primary tumours at 2,4,6,8 or 10 mm were eradicated by local irradiation with 80 Gy of X-rays. The resultant incidence of lung metastases was zero for 2 mm tumours increasing to 100% for 10 mm tumours (fig 1a). The survival times of mice with metastases decreased from approximately 70 to 20 days as the treatment size of the primary increased. This may partly reflect the greater number of metastases in mice treated at the larger sizes (fig 1b).

The transplantation bioassay data are shown in fig. 2. The incidence of takes, directly related to the average number of cells per inoculum, showed a pattern for lungs very similar to that for the metastases incidence shown in fig 1a. The non-zero incidence of takes from transplants of s.c. lymph nodes demonstrates the presence of tumour cells in transit through the node but not seeding there, since no lymph node metastases were observed. Blood transplantation produced no takes except at the largest primary tumour size. To test the sensitivity of the bioassay, a TD_{50} experiment was performed. Cells inoculated in heparinized blood or saline appeared to have similar "take" rates (fig 3a). The latent period data (fig 3b) show no significant difference between the saline and blood groups. From these data it would appear that 3 tumour cells or greater per inoculum could be detected in a transplantation

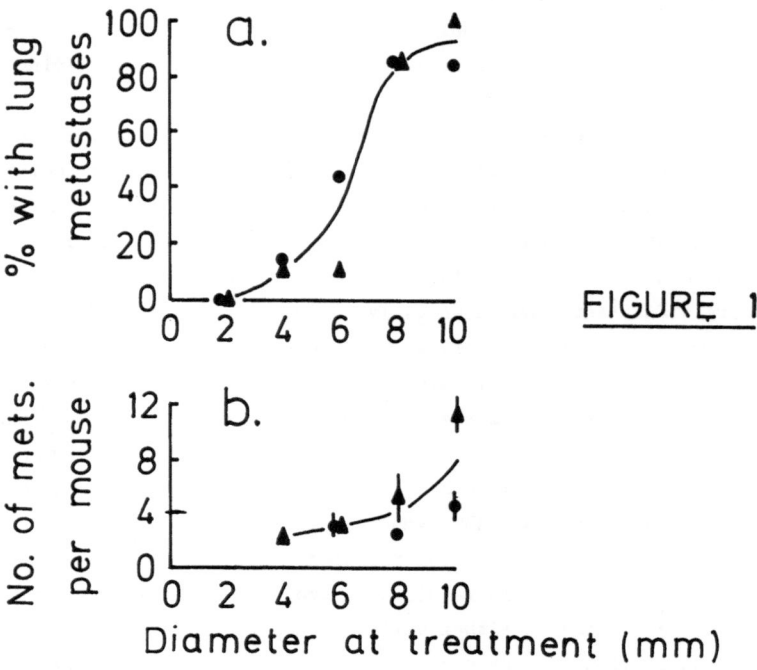

FIGURE 1

bioassay. Since the inoculum volume was 0.1 ml, the concentration of cells in the blood was probably less than 30 per ml in mice with tumours of less than 12 mm, and approximately 100/ml for mice with 12 mm tumours.

Artificial metastases. The efficiency of iv injected tumour cells in producing lung colonies is shown in fig 4. All live cell inocula contained 10^5 lethally irradiated cells. The time to reach a plateau of colony numbers was approximately 14 days longer for the 2.5×10^2 group compared with the 10^5 group (fig 4a). In addition, the final colony numbers achieved were not proportional to the number of cells injected (fig 4b), the colony forming efficiency (CFE) being approximately 10 times higher for the 2.5×10^2 group. The later appearance time from smaller inocula would not be expected if all colonies arose from a single cell regardless of the injected cell number.

The size distributions of both spontaneous and artificial metastases were wide. Different tumours in the same set of lungs often varied in diameter from less than 0.5 mm to 5 mm. The range of sizes was usually slightly greater, however, in the spontaneous metastases groups. This would be expected if there were a continual shedding of metastatic cells, in contrast to a single iv bolus

Discussion. The data on natural metastases suggest, firstly, that metastatic cells are not shed by the transplant procedure since mice cured of 2 mm tumours had zero metastases. Secondly, the long times between treatment and sacrifice

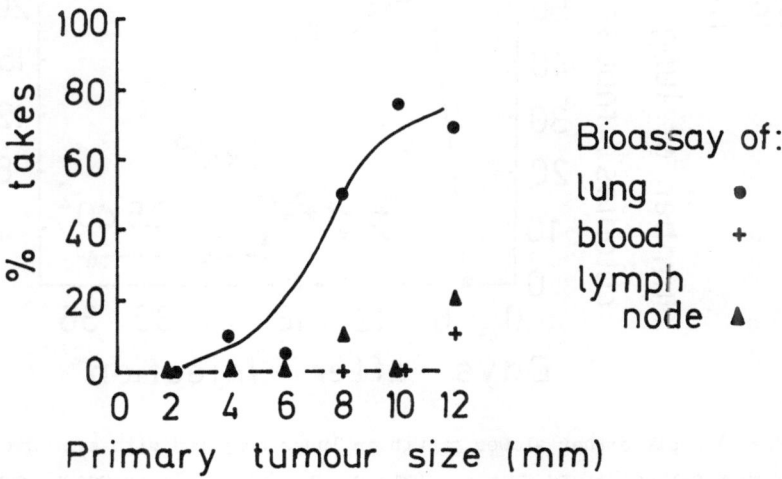

FIG. 2

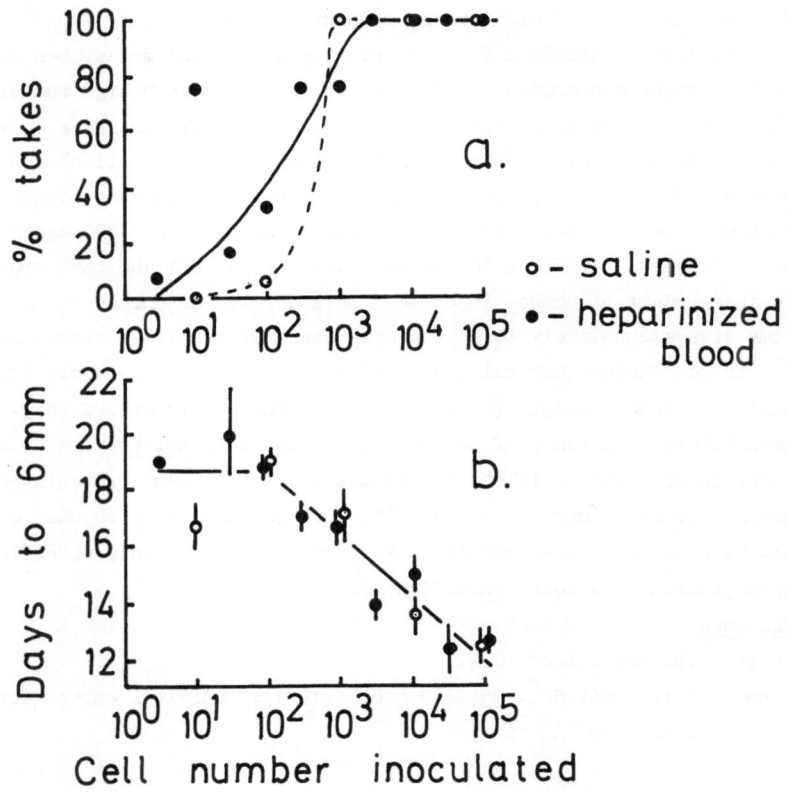

FIG. 3

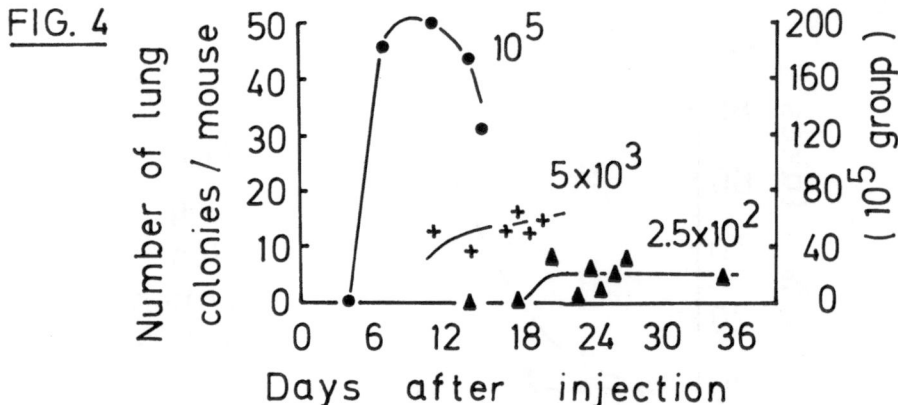

FIG. 4

(fig 1) imply either slower growth in lungs compared with s.c. sites, or a
dormant period before growth. Data of Dr. Sally Hill (personal communication)
on the same tumour show metastases occurring up to 110 days after locally
curative treatments. This suggests growth rates for some metastases up to 5
times slower than subcutaneous tumours (longest latent period approximately
20 days, fig 3b) if there were no dormant periods.

The most interesting finding from the artificial metastases experiments
was the longer appearance times after low compared with high numbers of injected
cells (fig 4). Possible causes include slower growth and/or a dormant period
after small inocula, or that colonies arise from multi-cell clumps after large
inocula. To account for the 14 day difference in appearance time, however,
colonies after 10^5 cells must start from clumps of over 1000 cells assuming
that colonies after 2.5×10^2 cells start from 1 cell and that growth rates
are independent of number injected. This appears an unrealistically large
clump size and unlikely to be the sole cause of the time discrepancy.

In conclusion, natural and artificial metastases from this tumour are
similar in some respects (e.g. size range) but not in others (e.g. the long
times before appearance of natural metastases have not been seen after iv
injection of cells). If natural metastases in the lung grow slower than s.c.
tumours, or have dormant periods, the question arises as to what effect this
will have on their chemosensitivity, particularly to cycle specific drugs.
These problems are being investigated.

Reference

Hewitt, H.B. and Wilson, C.W.

Anals N.Y. Acad. Sci. 95, 818 - 827 (1961). Survival curves for tumor
cells irradiated in vivo.

GROWTH INHIBITION OF SIMULATED METASTASES BY A LARGE PRIMARY TUMOR

S. Öhl, F. Schüning and C.G. Schmidt

INTRODUCTION

Cell cultures in diffusion chambers (DC) implanted into the abdominal cavity of host animals are a convenient method to study cell proliferation (Benestad 1970). Cell-to-cell interaction between cultured and host cells is prevented by the chamber walls, whereas the cultured cells may be freely exposed to humoral factors.

In this closed system the kinetics of experimental tumor cells (Cain et al 1974, Öhl et al 1980) have previously been studied. The object of the present experiments was to investigate wether the presence of a single solid Lewis lung carcinoma (LLC) may influence the proliferation of autologously grown LLC in DC on a somewhat unrelated Ehrlich ascites tumor (EAT) in DC.

Indeed reports of animal studies suggest that secondary tumors produce considerable effects on the growth of the primary inoculum (Dewys 1972). This paper reports on our current experiments on the influence of amputation of a large primary tumor on cell kinetics in DC after a prolonged coculturing period.

MATERIAL AND METHODS

LLC and EAT cells were passaged in a solid or ascitic form respectively. The transplantation procedure has been to inject trypsinized homogenates ($> 1 \times 10^6$ viable cells) unilaterally into the gastrocnemius muscle of the recipient mouse (LLC) or by obtaining the EAT from the peritoneal cavity 2 weeks after intraperitoneal inoculation of 1×10^6 to 1×10^9 cells.

Detailed accounts of most of the DC methods employed have been given elsewhere (Benestad 1970).

In brief: the chambers (DC) were made of lucite rings with a Millipore filter, pore size 0.22 μm on either side. Two chambers per animal were implanted into the peritoneal cavity of C57 Bl/6 mice under ether anaesthesia.

Varying numbers of LLC or EAT cells (1×10^5 - 1×10^6 cells) were implanted initially in all experiments. The chambers were removed and the cells harvested at different times after implantation (1 - 12 days). Clots were dissolved by shaking the chambers for 60 min. in a 0.5% Pronase and 5% Ficoll solution. After puncture of the DC and aspiration of the content, the total number of cells

I

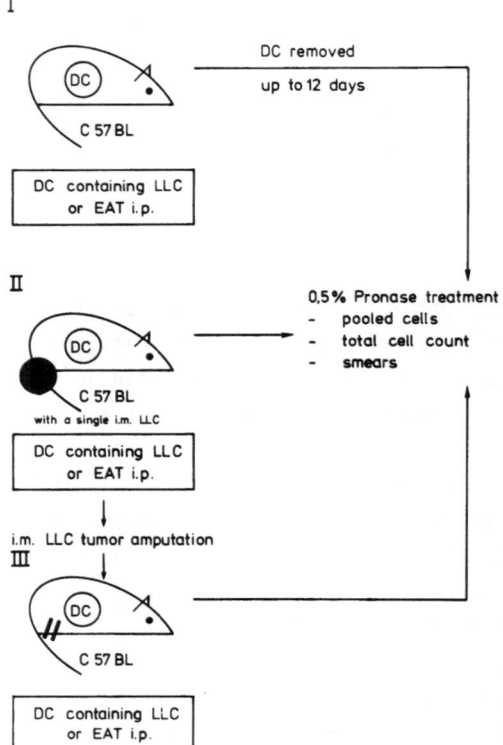

Figure 1
Experimental design

per DC was calculated and smears made to analyse cell morphology (see experimental
design, figure 1).
In one series of experiments C57 Bl/6 mice bearing single i.m. LLC (size > 7mm
to < 1.2 mm in diameter) were used as DC chamber host up to 5 days. The tumor
leg was then disjointed at the knee under phenobarbital anaesthesia and the skin
lesion closed with a silk thread. At periodic intervals, amputated mice were
killed and DC recovered as described above.

RESULTS
Figure 2 A-C shows the proliferation pattern of LLC or EAT cells in DC, in the pr
sence of a concomitant solid LLC (Figure 2 B) or after amputation of the solid
LLC tumor (Figure 2 C). The number of cells implanted in DC grew proportionally
when 0.1 x 10^6 to 1 x 10^6 cells were cultured in the absence of a solid primary

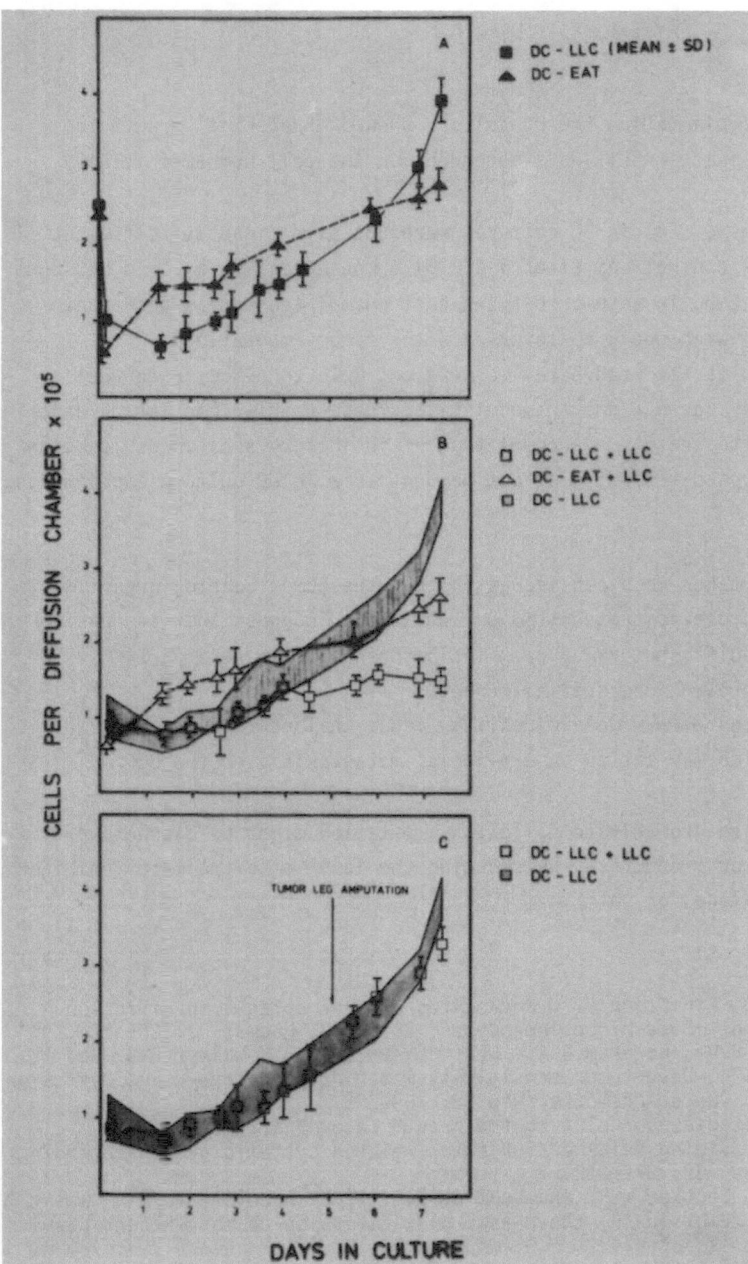

Figure 2 A-C. Growth of LLC or EAT cells in diffusion chambers. DC containing 10^5 cells were implanted into host mice with or without a single solid LLC tumor. Shaded area shows unmanipulated proliferation of LLC in DC. Each point represents the geometric mean of 6 DC cultures. The corresponding SDs are given as vertical bars.

tumor. Early after implantation the DC-culture showed exponential growth to reach a plateau phase after 5-11 days dependent on the cell number initially implanted.

Whereas growth curves of EAT in DC cultures were not significantly different whether cultured in a control animal or a C57 Bl/6 mouse bearing a solid LLC tumor, the incubation of LLC-DC in a tumor bearing host animal led to a significant growth deceleration, wich could be reversed after tumor amputation.

Based on the results reported here, we were not able to demonstrate what diffusible factor may cause a growth modulation. These double inoculation experiments seem to indicate that accumulation of inhibitory substances leads to a rather specific growth retarding effect demonstrable in DC culture experiments.

DISCUSSION

Although it must be taken into consideration that the tumor bearing organism represents a very complex situation, the present results may suggest that increasing concentration of specific humoral growth inhibitors be at least a partial explanation of the growth decelerating effect.

It might be speculated whether we are dealing with a chalone (Rytömaa and Kiviniemi 1968), which may act on an artificial metastasis i.e. the DC culture.

Finally, the increased growth rate following amputation might be caused by abolishing toxic tumor products or by reducing the level of a specific inhibitory agent, the tumor chalone, or both.

REFERENCES

Benestad, H.B., 1970. Formation of granulocytes and makrophages in diffusion chamber cultures of mouse blood leucocytes. Scand. J. Haemat. 7: 269-288.
Chain B.F., Calvely S.B., Boreham B.A., West C., Price N.A., Walker D.J. and Churchhouse M.J., 1974. Drug-tumor sensitivity matching procedure using diffusion chambers in vivo. Cancer Chemother Rep 58: 189-205.
Dewys, W.D., 1972. Studies correlating the growth rate of a tumor and its metastases and providing evidence for tumor related systemic growth retarding factors. Cancer Res. 32: 379-382.
Öhl, S., Seeber, S., Boecker W.R. and Schmidt C.G. 1980. A colony forming assay for experimental tumors using the plasma clot diffusion chamber. Recent Results Cancer Res. (in press).
Rytömaa, T. and Kiviniemi K., 1968. Control of granulocyte production. I. Calone and antichalone, two specific humoral regulators. Cell Tissue Kinet 1: 329-340.

Supported by Aktion "Kampf dem Krebs" (German Cancer Society)

QUANTITATIVE STUDIES ON METASTASIS USING YOSHIDA RAT ASCITES HEPATOMAS, WITH SPECIAL REFERENCE TO THE BIOLOGICAL CHARACTERISTICS IN METASTASIZABILITY AND DRUG SENSITIVITY

H. Sato, M. Suzuki and H. Satoh

A series of transplantable tumors of Yoshida ascites hepatomas have been used in various kinds of experimental studies in Japan, particularly on the mechanism of metastasis and chemotherapy in our laboratories.

In this paper the characteristics of this series of tumors are described, together with the historical origin, and the use of these tumors as either an experimental model for studying the mechanism of metastasis in cancer, or as a tool in experimental cancer chemotherapy.

ORIGINS

Yoshida ascites hepatomas of the rat are a series of transplantable ascites tumors, the first of which was established by ascitic conversion of azo dye-induced liver cancers in rats in Sendai (Yoshida et al., 1951). The tumor of this new cancer was found in an experiment which was carried out to reproduce the same type of tumor as the so-called Yoshida sarcoma because the origin of Yoshida sarcoma had been considered, at that time, as of reticuloendothelial cells of the liver. Following this unexpected discovery of a new type of ascites tumor, more than 50 strains of the ascites hepatoma were established by Yoshida's co-workers in the Sasaki Institute, Tokyo between 1952 and 1962. There are now about 80 strains of these tumors maintained in both of our laboratories. The method of maintaining these tumors is either by serial intraperitoneal transplantation or by frozen storage in liquid nitrogen.

The reason so many strains of the ascites hepatoma were established is because it was noted that each strain of these tumors possessed different characteristics in its malignant expression. Thus for example, morphological and biological characteristics of tumor cells are individually different even in each strain, which originated from different tumor nodules developed in the liver of a rat such as AH41A, AH41B and AH41C. A of AH41A means that this strain was established by transplanting tumor cells obtained from tumor ascites of a rat of No.41; B means that the initial transplantation was done with tumor cells obtained from a tumor nodule of the liver of the same animal, and C comes from another nodule of the animal.

Most of the ascites hepatomas are now considered as of hepatic cell origin. Furthermore even Yoshida sarcoma is now thought of as one of the ascites hepatomas.

ASCITIC CHARACTERISTICS

When tumor cells proliferate in the ascites, there are free cells, island cells and mixed type cells. The size of the islands varies. The smallest unit of island is a two cells complex which is called "pair". The percentage of free cell and island population is different in each strain, but the population is quite stable cytogenetically, although there were a few cases in which the ascitic population has changed from "island-forming" to "free cell" or vice versa, either suddenly or gradually.

TRANSPLANTABILITY

The rate of intraperitoneal transplantation is usually quite high and the LD50 value of intraperitoneal transplantation is around 10 days or less in many strains of these tumors. However, when it was transplanted either subcutaneously or intravenously, the rate varies in each strain.

SURVIVAL TIME

When transplanted intraperitoneally, survival days varied in each strain. In the usual transplantation for serial maintenance, about 0.02 to 0.05 ml of ascites containing about 2-5 million cells was drawn from the peritoneal cavity by using a glass pipette and inoculated into a new rat intraperitoneally. The shortest survival time after intraperitoneal transplantation is 6 days and the longest 22-25 days. In case of either subcutaneous or intravenous transplantation, survival times are characteristic of each strain.

METASTASIS AND TUMOR CELL APPEARANCE IN THE BLOOD

Appearance of tumor cells in the circulating blood occurs soon after transplantation in some strains, but late in others when transplanted intraperitoneally.

When transplanted intravenously, metastasis occurred only in the lungs in some strains, while it occurred in various sites spreading throughout the body in other strains, together with some other strains of intermediate type, in which metastasis was seen either in the lungs or some other sites.

Liberation of cells from the primary site of growth into the circulating blood seemed to be correlated with the transitional phase from logarithmic growth to plateau growth of cells, regardless of either rate or growth or site. Striking differences were noted in the frequency and number of tumor cells appearing in the blood among the strains examined. Furthermore the fatal decrease of tumor cells in the arterial blood was, interestingly, correlated with the rigidity of those cells measured.

MOTILITY AND DEFORMABILITY (RIGIDITY) OF TUMOR CELLS

These characteristics are different in the strains examined and relate to general spread of metastasis.

SENSITIVITY TO CHEMOTHERAPEUTIC DRUGS

Each strain of ascites hepatomas is characteristically different in drug sensitivity. It has been examined by the ip-ip system initially, then ip-iv, iv-ip, iv-iv, ip-po and iv-po systems have been used for testing the effects of drugs. This is known as the "Hepatoma spectrum" (Hiroshi SATOH); it can be used as an adequate model of human cancer.

SUMMARY

A series of rat ascites hepatomas studied are adequate models for the recognition of similarities and differences among various kinds of tumor cells in the light of the concept of "individuality in cancer" proposed by the late Professor Tomizo Yoshida about a quarter century ago. The final target in cancer research is human cancer. Considering the complicated problems in human cancer, comparative studies using these tumors could be a great help in understanding and solving those problems.

REFERENCES

Origin and ascitic characteristics

Isaka, H., Izumitani, M., Umehara, S., Sato, M. and Sato, H., 1967. Chromosomal features in ascites and metastatic lesions of cancer clones. Gann, 58: 167-175.
Odashima, S., 1964. Establishment of ascites hepatomas in the rat, 1951-1962. Ascites Tumors, Yoshida Sarcoma and Ascites Hepatoma(s), Yoshida T. and Sato H. (Eds), Nat. Cancer Inst. Monograph No. 16, pp.51-93.
Yoshida, T., Sato, H. and Aruji, T., 1951. Origin of the Yoshida sarcoma I. Experimental production of "Ascites Hepatoma" in the rat. Proc. Japan Acad. 27: 485-492.

Transplantability and survival

Sato,H., 1955. Intraperitoneal transplantation of the Yoshida sarcoma and the ascites hepatoma to various American strains of rats. J. Nat. Cancer Inst., 15(5): 1367-1378.
Sato, H., Essner, E. and Belkin, M., 1955. Experiments on an ascites hepatoma. II. Intraperitoneal transplantation of free tumor cells separated from island of the rat ascites hepatoma. Experim. Cell Res., 9(3): 381-392.
Satoh, H., 1964. Transplantability of Yoshida Sarcoma. NCI Monograph, 16: 7-49.

Sato, H., Satoh, H. and Kuroki, T., 1966. Quantitative analysis of malignancy. Evaluation of transplantability and survival. Gann Monograph, 1: 29-42.
Sato, H. and Fujii, K., 1967. Quantitative analysis of the acquired resistance in tumor bearing hosts. Tohoku J. exp. Med., 91: 397-407.

Metastasis and tumor cell appearance in the blood

Hori, K., Suzuki, M., Abe, I., Saito, S. and Sato, H., 1979. A model of lymph node metastasis by transplantation of tumor cells into rat ear. Gann, 70: 383-384.

Khato, J., Suzuki, M. and Sato, H., 1974. Quantitative study on thromboplastin in various strains of Yoshida ascites hepatoma cells of rat. Gann, 65: 289-294.

Khato, J., Nakadate, T., Suzuki, M. and Sato, H., 1975. Quantitative studies on lung metastases, with reference to the number and size of tumor nodures produced by intravenous inoculation of tumor cells. Sci. Rep. Res. Inst. Tohoku Univ. -C, 22(3-4): 69-76.

Khato, J., Sato, T., Sato, H., Abe, K., Endo, E., Ohta, E. and Fukuoka, Y., 1977. Hematological alterations in tumor-bearing rats, with reference to pathogenesis of chronic type of disseminated intravascular coagulation syndrome. Gann, 68: 797-804.

Kurokawa, Y., 1970. Experiments on lymph node metastasis by intralymphatic inoculation of rat ascites tumor cells, with special reference to lodgment, passage and growth of tumor cells in lymph nodes. Gann, 61: 461-471.

Narisawa, T., 1966. Tumor extension from the glomeruli to the tubuli in experimental kidney metastasis. Tohoku J. exp. Med., 88: 245-256.

Sato, H., 1959. Experimental studies on the mechanism of metastasis formation. Acta Path. Jap., 9: 685.

Sato, H., 1962. Cancer cells in the circulating blood with reference to cancer metastasis. Bull. Wld. Hlth. Org., 26: 675.

Sato, H., 1964. Cancer metastasis and ascites tumors. Nat. Cancer Inst. Monograph, 16: 241-261.

Sato, H. and Suzuki, M., 1973. Experimental studies on metastasis formation, with special reference to the mechanism of cancer cell lodgement in the microcirculation. Excepta Medica International Congress Series No. 269, ATHEROGENESIS-II, 168-176.

Takahashi, T., 1966. Experimental studies on lung tumor by implantation of tumor cells through the air passage. Gann, 57: 337-352.

Yamaura, H. and Sato, H., 1973. Experimental studies on angiogenesis in AH109A ascites tumor tissue transplanted to a transparent chamber in rats. Chemotherapy of Cancer Dissemination and Metastasis. Edited by S. Garattini and G. Franchi, Raven Press, New York, 149-175.

Yamaura, H. and Sato, H., 1974. Quantitative studies on the developing vascular system of rat hepatoma. J. Nat. Cancer Inst., 53: 1229-1240.

Motility and deformability

Essner, E., Sato, H. and Belkin, M., 1954. Experiments on an ascites hepatoma. I. Enzymatic digestion and alkaline degradation of the cementing substance and separation of cells in tumor islands. Experim. Cell Res., 7: 430-437.

Goto, M. and Sato, H., 1965. Studies on tissue culture of ascites tumors. III. Colony formation of Yoshida sarcoma cells in agar medium. Sci. Rep. Res. Inst. Tohoku Univ. -C, 12: 319-323.

Hosaka, S., Khato, J., Goto, M., Suzuki, M. and Sato, H., 1977. Quantitative study on the dispersiveness of cultured tumor cells, with reference to the invasiveness of cancer. Sci. Rep. of the Research Inst. Tohoku Univ. -C. 24(2-4): 61-67.

Hosaka, S., Suzuki, M., Goto, M. and Sato, H., 1978. Motility of rat ascites hepatoma cells, with reference to malignant characteristics in cancer metastasis. Gann, 69: 273-276.

Hosaka, S., Suzuki, M. and Sato, H., 1979. Leucocyte-like motility of cancer cells, with reference to the mechanism of extravasation in metastasis. Gann (JJCR), 70: 559-561.

Khato, J., Sato, H., Suzuki, M. and Sato, H., 1979. Filtrability and flow characteristics of leukemic and non-leukemic tumor cell suspension through polycar-
bonate filters in relation to hematogeneous spread of cancer. Tohoku J. exp.
Med., 128: 273-284.

Kuroki, T., Goto, M. and Sato, H., 1965. Studies on in vitro growth of Yoshida
sarcoma cells. I. Culture of a small number of cells with references to the
role of erythrocytes. Gann, 56: 35-47.

Nakadate, T., Suzuki, M. and Sato, H., 1979. Quantitative study on the liberation
of tumor cells into the circulating blood. Gann(JJCR), 70: 435-446.

Sato, H., Kuroki, T. and Goto, M., 1968. Tissue culture of rat ascites hepatomas
on fluid and agar media. Cancer Cells in Culture, Edited by Katsuta. University
of Tokyo Press, Tokyo, 35-47.

Sato, H., Goto, M. and Kuroki, T., 1966. Culture of rat ascites hepatoma cells in
agar medium and screening for anti-cancer substances. Gann Monograph, 2: 127-14C

Sato, H. and Suzuki, M., 1976. Deformability and viability of tumor cells by
transcapillary passage, with reference to organ affinity of metastasis in cancer
Fundamental Aspects of Metastasis, edited by Leonald Weiss, North-Holland
Publishing company, pp.311-317.

Sato, H., Goto, M. and Hosaka, S., 1977. Growth behavior of ascites tumor cells
in three-dimensional agar culture. Tohoku J. exp. Med., 122: 155-160.

Sato, H., Khato, J., Sato, T. and Suzuki, M., 1977. Deformability and filtrability
of tumor cells through "Nucleopore" filter, with reference to viability and
metastatic spread. GANN Monograph on Cancer Research, 20: 3-13.

Drug sensitivity

Abe, I., Sato, S., Watanabe, M. and Sato, H., 1978. Mechanism of natural resistance
of rat ascites hepatomas to 1-β-D-arabinofuranosylcytosine. Gann, 69: 557-564.

Abe, I., Sato, S., Watanabe, M. and Sato, H., 1978. Phosphorylation of 1-β-D-
arabinofuranosylcytosine by the cell-free extract of rat ascites hepatoma, in
relation to the mechanism of natural resistance. Gann, 69: 565-568.

Abe, I. and Sato, H., 1979. Dephosphorylation of nucleotides of 1-β-D-arabino-
furanosylcytosine in relation to the different drug sensitivity in tumor cells.
Tohoku J. exp. Med., 127: 281-288.

Isaka, H., 1964. Natural drug resistance of the ascites hepatoma in the rat. Nat.
Cancer Inst. Monograph, No. 16, pp.131-147.

Ishidate, M., Kobayashi, K., Sakurai, Y., Sato, H. and Yoshida, T., 1951. Experimental studies on chemotherapy of malignant growth employing Yoshida sarcoma
animals. (ii) The effect of N-oxide derivatives of nitrogen mustard. Proc.
Japan Acad., 27(8): 493-500.

Satoh, H., 1956. Studies on the ascites hepatoma. XI. Different responses by different strain of ascites hepatomas of rats to chemotherapeutic treatment. Gann,
47: 334-337.

Sato, H., 1959. Experimental studies on the effect of nitromin (Nitrogen mustard
N-oxide) upon tumor growth with special respect to inhibition of metastasis
formation. Acta U.I.C.C., XV, pp.253.

Sato, H., 1960. Experimental studies on the role of cancer chemotherapy for prevention of recurrence and metastasis formation in malignant tumors. Acta U.I.C.C.,
XVI, pp.763.

Sato, H., 1961. Studies on the role of cancer chemotherapy for prevention of lymph
node metastasis. Cancer Chemother. Rep., 13: 33-40.

Sato, H. and Suzuki, M., 1977. Metastasis and chemotherapy, with reference to
permeability of microcirculation system. Cancer Invasion and Metastasis: Biologi
Mechanisms and Therapy, edited by S.B.Day et al., Raven Press, New York,
pp. 145-149.

Terui, S., 1975. Experimental study on drug sensitivity of the rat ascites hepatoma
cells in embryonated eggs, Sci. Rep. Inst. Tohoku Univ. -C, 22(1-2): 10-17.

CANINE OSTEOSARCOMA AND CANINE MAMMARY CARCINOMA

L.N. Owen

The main criteria for spontaneous cancer models are:-

1. The histological type of tumour should resemble the human tumour.
2. The biological behaviour, particularly growth rate and metastasis, should be similar.
3. The size of the animal should permit the required clinical investigations.
4. The tumour incidence should be high enough to study a large number of cases.

The dog fulfills these requirements for some tumours, in particular for osteosarcoma and certain mammary carcinomas.

Comparison of major features of osteosarcoma (Owen 1969a)

	Man	Dog
Frequency	Infrequent	Not uncommon in 'giant' breeds. Uncommon in small dogs.
Age	Second decade	Middle aged and old.
Site	Metaphysis of long bones particularly distal femur and proximal tibia	Metaphysis of long bones particularly distal radius and ulna (weight bearing).
Radiography	Same both species	-
Histological appearance	Same both species	-
Metastasis	Lungs and bones	Lungs in particular
Survival	Amputation alone 5 - 20% at 5 years	Amputation alone, median survival 4 months

Studies made or planned

Prognosis	Serum alkaline phosphatase (Owen & Stevenson 1962)
	Clq serum levels - good potential (Segal-Eiras et al., 1980)
Tissue Culture	T.C.199 + 10% foetal calf serum
	Cell lines available (Owen, Doyle & Littlewood, 1980).
Transplantation	Nude mice - successful but no metastasis (Oughton & Owen, 1974)
	Foetal or immuno-suppressed dogs (A.L.S.) (Owen, 1969b)
	When cells injected i/v many tumours appear in skeleton
Surgery	Preservation of limb by prostheses theoretically possible but technically difficult
Radiotherapy	Megavoltage. Regression 4-12 months. No cures (Owen & Bostock, 1973; Owen, Bostock & Lavelle, 1977)
	Uptake of misonidazole in canine osteosarcoma 70% of plasma levels 1 - 3 hours after i/v injection (White et al., 1979)

International WHO trials in progress on value of radiosensitizers for primary tumour and prophylactic lung irradiation..

Chemotherapy

Results using limited number of drugs - cyclophosphamide, doxorubicin, methotrexate - folinic acid were variable, median survival after amputation 10 months (Henness et al., 1977).

Immunotherapy

Delay in onset of lung metastasis after i/v B.C.G. (Owen, Bostock & Lavelle, 1977). Macrophages activated by B.C.G. showed greater cytotoxicity to osteosarcoma cells in vitro than non-activated macrophages (Gorman, 1977).

CANINE MAMMARY CARCINOMA

The mammary gland of the experimental Beagle dog rapidly develops hyperplastic and neoplastic nodules following administration of large doses of progestational compounds.

It has consequently been found an unsatisfactory animal model for carcinogenicity testing of such hormones (Owen & Briggs, 1977).

The spontaneously arising carcinomas of the mammary gland however, particularly the invasive tubular, invasive solid and anaplastic carcinomas greatly resemble the invasive carcinomas in the human breast in many respects, particularly metastasis, and are excellent models for many studies including therapy.

COMPARISON OF MAJOR FEATURES OF BREAST TUMOURS IN WOMEN AND BITCHES (OWEN, 1979)

	WOMEN	BITCH
Frequency	Frequent	Age adjusted is 3 times as common as women
Age (carcinomas)	Middle aged and old	Old
Incidence in male	1% of number in women	2% of number in bitches
Relative incidence - malignant tumours	+ - 60%	30 - 40%
Cell of origin - malignant tumours	Secr. epithelial (myoepithelial uncommon and mesenchymal rare)	Secr. epithelial, myoepithelial or both. Mesenchymal less common.
Most frequent benign tumour	Fibroadenoma	Mixed tumour
Effect of irradiation on incidence	Increased	Developed earlier
Prognostic factors (carcinomas)		
Clinical stage	++	++
Size	++	++
Lymph node metastasis	++	-+-
Mitotic frequency	++	?
Tubule formation	++	?
Sinus histiocytosis	+	
Metastasis		
Regional nodes	+	+
Distant nodes	+	+
Lungs	+	+
Pleura	+	++
Liver	+	-+-
Bones	+	
Oestrogen receptors	Some tumours	Some tumours
Hormonal therapy e.g. oöphorectomy or hormone administration	Regression in 15-40% of tumours in actively menstruating women	Regression not proven. Early oöphorectomy has sparing influence on breast cancer.
Effect of menopause on therapy	Important	No menopause

Studies made or planned

Prognosis (Carcinomas)

POSTMASTECTOMY SURVIVAL TIME OF BITCHES WITH HISTOLOGICALLY CONFIRMED
MAMMARY CARCINOMAS*

Tumour Type	ONE YEAR SURVIVAL (%)		MEDIAN SURVIVAL TIME (WEEKS)	
	Invasive	Well-defined	Invasive	Well-defined
Papillary	50	86	65	128
Tubular	44	74	38	110
Solid	26	73	26	82
Anaplastic	24	-	11	-

* Tumours were apparently completely excised and there was no clinical
evidence of metastasis at the time of surgery, based on biopsy material
from 220 mammary carcinomas (Bostock, 1975).

Tissue Culture

Trypsinisation at 20°C.

T.C. 199 + 20% foetal calf serum.

Cell lines available (Owen, Doyle & Littlewood, 1980)

Transplantation

Nude mice. Successful but no metastasis.

A.L.S. Immuno-suppressed dogs (Owen et al., 1977).

Radiotherapy

Little information is available.

Chemotherapy

Following mastectomy.

A combination of cyclophosphamide and 5-fluoracil is being evaluated
(Theilen & Madewell, 1979).

Immunotherapy

The effect of intravenous B.C.G. on the median survival time and death
rate of bitches following excision of an invasive mammary carcinoma (Bostock
& Gorman, 1978).

Group	No. of dogs	Median survival (weeks)
Control surgery only	11	24
Surgery and placebo	10	24
Surgery and B.C.G.(i/v)	13	100

Following these encouraging results an International WHO trial is planned using B.C.G. and intravenous C. parvum. If these trial results are similarly successful the effect of immuno-stimulating agents less toxic to man will be evaluated.

REFERENCES

Bostock, D.E. and Owen, L.N. 1970. Transplantation and tissue culture studies of Canine Osteosarcoma. Europ. J. Cancer, 6: 499-503.

Bostock, D.E. 1975. The prognosis following the surgical excision of canine mammary neoplasms. Europ. J. Cancer, 11: 389-395.

Bostock, D.E. and Gorman, N.T. 1978. Intravenous B.C.G. therapy of mammary carcinomas in bitches after surgical excision of the primary tumour. Europ. J. Cancer, 14: 879-883.

Gorman, N.T. 1977. Aspects of intravenous B.C.G. therapy of tumours in the dog. Ph.D. Thesis, University of Cambridge.

Henness, A.M., Theilen, C.H., Park, R.D. and Buhles, W.C. 1977. Combination therapy for canine osteosarcoma. J. Am. Vet. Med. Ass. 170: 1076-1081.

Oughton, S.M.J. and Owen, L.N. 1974. Transplantation of dog neoplasms into the mouse mutant Nude. Res. vet. Sci. 17: 414-416.

Owen, L.N. and Stevenson, D.E. 1961. Observations on canine osteosarcoma. Res. vet. Sci. 2: 117-129.

Owen, L.N. 1969a. Bone Tumours in Man and Animals. Butterworths, London, 200 pp.

Owen, L.N. 1969b. Transplantation of canine osteosarcoma. Europ. J. Cancer 5: 615-620.

Owen, L.N. and Bostock, D.E. 1973. Prophylactic X-irradiation of the lung in canine tumours with particular reference to osteosarcoma. Europ. J. Cancer 9: 747-752.

Owen, L.N. and Briggs, M.H. 1976. Contraceptive steroid toxicology in the Beagle dog and its relevance to human carcinogenicity. Current Med. Res. and Op. 4: 309-329.

Owen, L.N., Morgan, D.R., Bostock, D.E. and Flemans, R.J. 1977. Tissue culture and transplantation studies on canine mammary carcinomas. Europ. J. Cancer, 13: 1445-1449.

Owen, L.N., Bostock, D.E. and Lavelle, R.B. 1977. Study on therapy of osteosarcoma in dogs using B.C.G. vaccine. J. Amer. Radiol., 18: 27-29.

Owen, L.N. 1979. A comparative study of Canine and Human Breast Cancer. Invest. Cell. Pathol.,2: 257-275.

Owen, L.N., Doyle, A. and Littlewood, T.D. 1980. Long term cultures and cell lines of neoplasms in domesticated animals. J. Comp. Path. (in the press).

Segal-Eiras et al. 1980. To be published.

Theilen, G.H. and Madewell, B.R. 1979. In Veterinary Cancer Medicine. Lea and Febiger, Philadelphia, p.200.

White, R.A.S., Workman, P., Owen, L.N. and Bleehen, N.M. 1979. The penetration of Misonidazole into spontaneous canine tumours. Br. J. Cancer, 40: 284-294.

SELECTION OF A HUMAN MALIGNANT MELANOMA X HAMSTER HYBRID CELL LINE BY METASTASIS

J.F. Watkins

Hybridisation of human tumour cells with cells of another species can be regarded as a form of 'heterogenisation' (1) or 'xenogenisation'(2). Experiments with hybrids of mouse tumours (3) suggest that such hybrids of human tumours may be worth trying as immunotherapeutic agents in human cancer.

The main technical problem in producing a suitable hybrid line arises from the fact that human chromosomes are preferentially lost from interspecific hybrids. Hybrid cell lines can be selected for the retention of certain human enzymes (e.g. thymidine kinase), but no selection methods exist for selecting hybrid cell lines which retain human tumour antigens.

If tumour antigens are present in human tumour cells they may or may not be essential for in vivo survival, or growth, or metastasis of tumour cells. If they are essential then selection for in vivo growth or metastasis of hybrid cells would increase the probability that any hybrids obtained would be expressing tumour antigens, although there may be no collateral method of demonstrating their presence.

Attempts to select hybrids from fusion mixtures by growth in inbred or athymic mice of hybrid tumours from fusion mixtures of mouse embryo cells and human tumour cells have been unsuccessful. An attempt was therefore made to use metastasis to select a hybrid line by injection into hamsters of a fusion mixture of a hamster cell line (BHK-21) (of low oncogenicity and low metastatic potential) with a human melanoma line (Mel 364) (of high metastatic potential).

BHK-21 CELLS:

DERIVATION: From the original isolate (4) from baby hamster kidney cells. The line used has had many passages in vitro, and is now oncogenic.

ONCOGENICITY: A few small pulmonary metastases (1-3mm diameter) were found in one of five hamsters killed 70 days after subcutaneous injection of 10^6 cells.

KARYOTYPE: See Fig. 1A.

PLASMINOGEN ACTIVATOR: See Fig. 4.

MEL 364 CELLS:

DERIVATION: (by Dr. R. Whitehead, Dept. of Surgery, Welsh National School of Medicine) from metastases in inguinal lymph glands of a male patient eighteen months after the appearance of primary malignant melanoma on the ankle.

ONCOGENICITY: Five weeks after subcutaneous injection of 10^6 cells into two athymic mice nodules about 3 mm in diameter were present at the injection site. Histologically they resembled the original tumour, and occasional cells stained positively for melanin. No tumours developed within 3 months of subcutaneous injection of 10^6 cells subcutaneously into 3 hamsters.

KARYOTYPE: See Fig. 1B and Fig. 2.
PLASMINOGEN ACTIVATOR: See Fig. 4.
ELECTRON MICROSCOPY: Melanosomes were present in many cells.

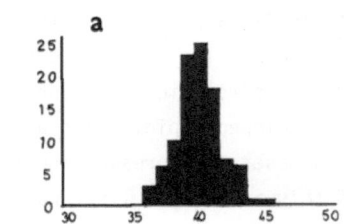

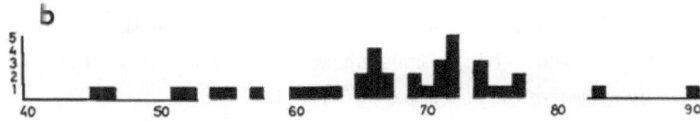

Fig. 1: Chromosome distribution of (a) BHK and (b) Mel 364. (Ordinate: no. of metaphases; abscissa: no. of chromosomes).

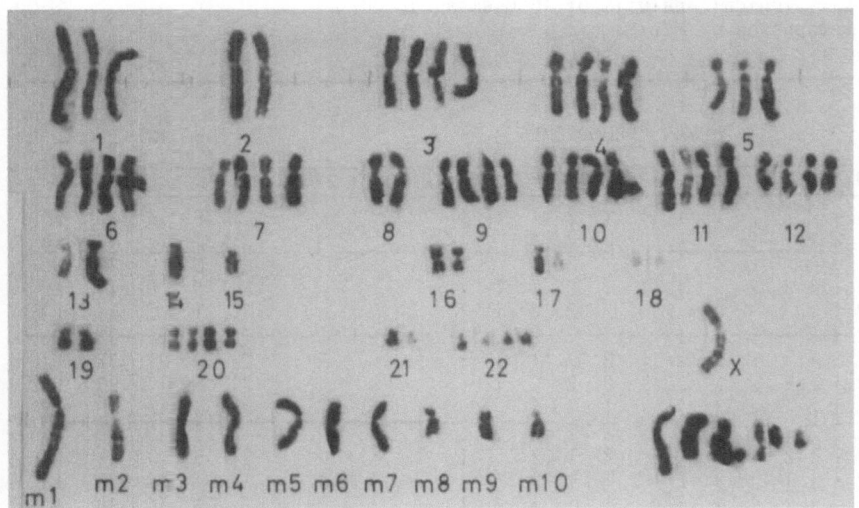

Fig. 2: Representative karyotype of Mel 364.

MTL/2:

DERIVATION: A confluent monolayer of 10^6 BHK-21 and 10^6 Mel 364 cells was fused with polyethylene glycol (5). The fusion culture was grown in vitro in 10% foetal calf serum and Minimal Essential Eagle's Medium for a further 10 days, when the culture flasks contained about 10^8 cells. The whole culture was injected subcutaneously into a hamster. A tumour developed rapidly, attaining a size of about 6 cm in diameter in 41 days. The hamster was then killed and large pulmonary metastases were seen. The subcutaneous tumour was subcultured in vitro, and after 2 days 10^6 cells were injected subcutaneously into a second hamster. Once again a tumour developed rapidly, and after 55 days the hamster died. Extensive pulmonary metastases were present and these were subcultured in vitro. A single colony of this in vitro culture was removed and grown up to form the line MTL/2.

ONCOGENICITY: Local tumours were first detected about 7 days after subcutaneous injection of 10^6 - 10^7 MTL/2 cells into 11 hamsters. The animals died or were killed within 25-45 days of inoculation, and large pulmonary metastases were present in all eleven. MTL/2 thus showed a very considerable increased tendency to pulmonary metastasis compared with BHK-21.

KARYOTYPE: See Fig. 3 and Table 1.

PLASMINOGEN ACTIVATOR: See Fig. 4.

ELECTRON MICROSCOPY: Occasional single melanosomes were present.

TABLE 1: Karyological analysis of 16 Giemsa-banded metaphases of MTL/2.

HUMAN CHROMOSOMES																									TOTAL HUMAN	UNIDENTIFIED	TOTAL HAMSTER	TOTAL CHROMOSOMES
1	2	3	4	5	6	7	8	9	10	11	12	13	14	15	16	17	18	19	20	21	22	X	Y	A				
1		2			1	1	2	2	2	2	1	1	1	2	1	1	1							2	39	15	40	94
1		2	2	1	2	2	2	2	2	2	2	2	2	1		1								1	31	2	43	76
	2		2				2				2			1										2	20	9	27	56
2		1	2	1	2	1	1	2	2	1	1	1	2	1	1		2							2	36	9	44	89
2	2	2	2	1	2	2	1		2	2	1	1												1	31	7	43	81
2	2	1	1		2	1	2	1	1	1	1	1	2	2	1	1	1	1						2	42	16	32	90
2		2	1	1	2	2	2	2	2	1	2	1	1	1	1			1						2	37	7	37	81
2	2	2	2	1	1	1	2	2	2	2	1	2	2	2	1		1				2			2	45	11	39	95
2		2	1		1	1	2	2	2	1	1	1	2				1							2	36	14	38	88
2	1		2	1	3	2	2	1	2	2	1	1	1	3				1						1	35	9	38	82
	2	2	3	2	1	1	2	1	2	2	2	1	2		1						2			2	35	7	44	86
2	1	3	2	2	1	1	1	1	1	2	1	1	2		1		1	2			2			2	37	10	40	87
2		1	1	1	2	1	1	1	2	1	1	1	1	2	1	2	1	1			1			3	41	16	32	89
1		2	1		2	1	2	1	1	1		1			1									2	25	8	39	70
	2	1				1	1	1	1	1						1								2	28	15	37	80
1		1		1	1	1	1	1	1				1											1	31	18	33	82

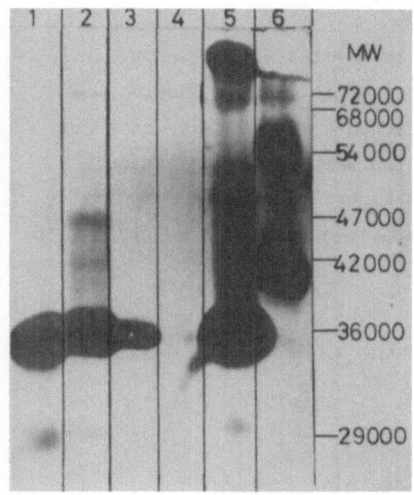

Fig. 3:
      Plasminogen activator profiles of BHK-21
(Channel 1), MTL/2 (Channel 2) and MEL 364
(Channel 6). Plasminogen activator preparations (standardised against urokinase) were
made from serum-free medium overlying cells
and subjected to electrophoresis on SDS-
acrylamide. The gel (treated to remove SDS)
was laid on a casein-agarose gel containing
plasminogen and incubated for 10 hrs. at
37°C. Clear bands in the casein-agarose
indicate the presence of plasminogen activator.
MTL/2 produced at least 5 bands not produced
by BHK-21. MEL 364 produced bands in roughly
similar positions to these 5. (Channels 3,
4 and 5 were produced by other cell lines
which are not relevant to this paper).

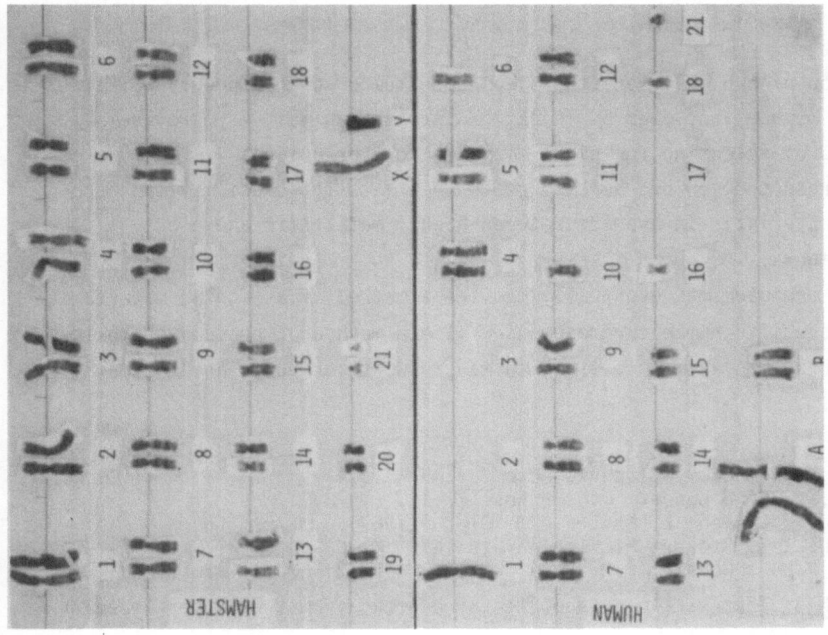

Fig.4: Karyotype of MTL/2. The large marker chromosome labelled
A was present in all metaphases examined. Its Giemsa-banding
pattern resembles that of marker M1 in MEL 364.

84

In collaboration with Prof. L. Hughes (Dept. of Surgery, Welsh National School of Medicine) MTL/2 cells were injected into two patients with advanced malignant melanoma with multiple metastases.

2.5 x 10^7 cells were injected intradermally at 4 sites in both upper arms and both thighs. The injections were repeated one month later. Nodules developed at the sites of inoculation. These reached a maximum size at about 5 days (Fig. 5) and had regressed completely by two weeks after injection.

No obvious clinical benefit in the existing tumours has resulted in the 4 months since injections began. No further metastatic deposits have appeared in either patient in that period.

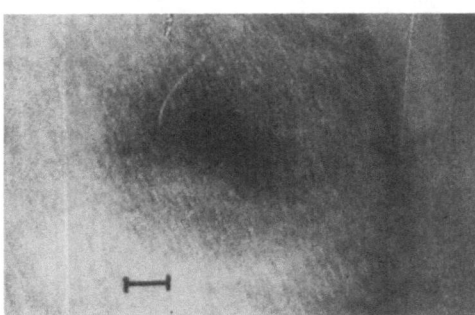

Fig. 5:
Nodule on forearm of patient 5 days after i.d. injection of MTL/2 (Bar = 1 cm).

CONCLUSIONS

(1) Fusion of a highly metastasising human tumour with a poorly metastasising animal tumour, followed by injection into the animal, may provide a general method of selecting for highly metastatic hybrid lines.

(2) The result described here suggests that metastatic ability may be a dominant characteristic in hybrids between highly metastatic and poorly metastatic tumours.

(3) This approach may eventually provide a method of assigning metastatic ability to a specific human chromosome and also a method of producing hybrids of human tumours with animal cells which may be worth using in attempts at immunotherapy.

REFERENCES

1. Lindenman, J. Biochem. Biophys. Acta 355:49. (1974).
2. Kobayashi, H. GANN Monogr. Cancer Res. 21:21. (1978).
3. Watkins, J.F. & Chen, L. Nature 223:1018. (1969).
4. Macpherson, I. & Stoker, M. Virology 16:147. (1962).
5. Davidson, R.L. & Gerald, P.S. Somat. Cell Genet. 2:165. (1976).

ACKNOWLEDGEMENTS: This work was supported by a grant from the Cancer Research Campaign.

MORPHOLOGICAL ASPECTS OF THE INTERACTION OF BLOOD COAGULATION AND TUMOUR DISSEMINATION

K.P. Dingemans

Numerous pathological and clinical investigations suggest an association between blood coagulation and tumour dissemination and frequently even lead to the assumption that blood coagulation is an intrinsic part of the metastatic process. Although there is a growing body of opinion which would dispute this point, many mechanisms have been proposed to explainthe influence of blood coagulation on tumour dissemination. Some of these lend themselves to morphological examination and will be briefly discussed. Two points should be emphasized: first, the methodology used in the present experiments (for references, see Roos and Dingemans, 1979) consisted of intravascular injection of tumour cell suspensions rather than spontaneous metastasis; hence the validity of the observations under natural conditions remains to be established. Second, only a limited number of tumour types was studied (M 8013, TA3/Ha, and TA3/St mammary carcinomas, B16/F1 and B16/F10 melanomas, and MB 6A lymphosarcoma), and even these showed great variations in their behaviour.

A general picture of thrombus formation around embolic tumour cells is given in Figs. 1-4, taken from an experiment in which B16/F10 melanoma cells were injected into tail veins of syngeneic mice, resulting in almost instantaneous trapping in the lungs. Most tumour cells with adherent thrombi are situated in capillaries directly branching from larger vessels (Fig. 1). Closely associated with the tumour cells are platelet pseudopods and masses of fibrin that often shows, even within 5 minutes after the injection, the characteristic 20 nm periodicity (Figs. 2,3). Further on the tumour cell surface, degranulated platelets predominate, whereas newly arrived, fully granulated platelets are especially found along the free edges of the thrombus (Fig. 2). In places, the tumour cell surface may be intimately intertwining with platelets (Fig. 4).

Perhaps the most obvious explanation of a stimulating effect of blood coagulation on metastasis formation is the theory that fibrin coating the tumour cells acts as a glue, facilitating the adhesion of tumour cells to endothelium (Weiss, 1977). Our observations do not support such a mechanism since no fibrin was ever found in the narrow space separating the surfaces of tumour and endothelial cells; indeed, these spaces invariably looked empty (Fig. 5). Also the theory that the initial contact between tumour emboli and endothelium is mediated via platelets (Gastpar, 1970) is not supported by our observations: when tumour emboli adhered to the walls of larger vessels, platelets predominantly accumulated at the side of the vascular lumen rather than inserting themselves between the tumour cells and the endothelium (Fig. 6). The same figure shows, in addition, that also blocking of vessels by thrombi — which has

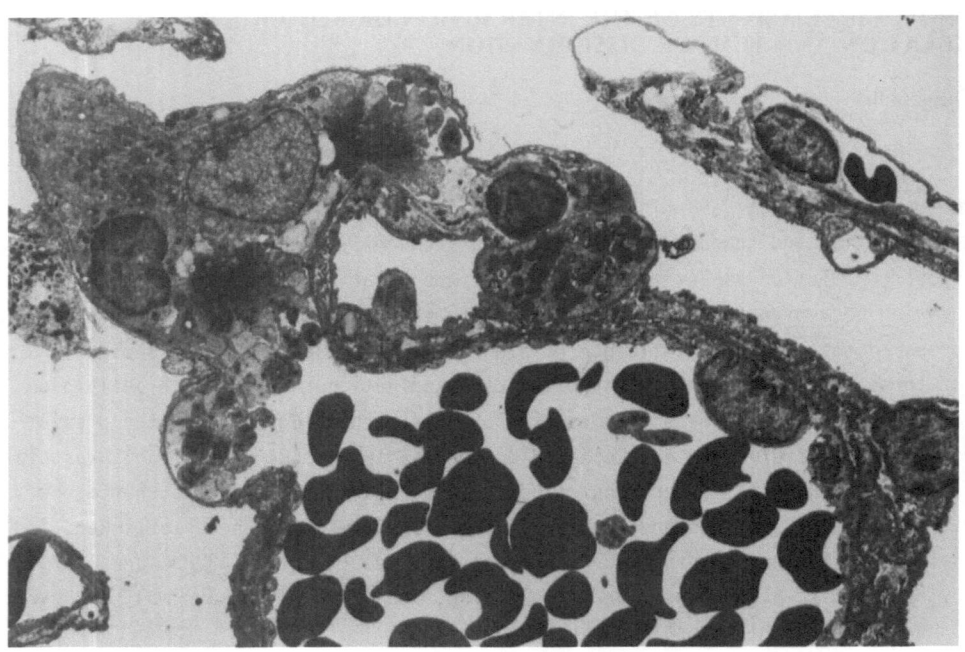

Fig. 1. Lung capillary (upper left), branching from larger lung vessel, 5 min after injection of B16/F10 melanoma cells into a tail vein. Embolus blocking capillary
consists of tumour cell (large, pale nucleus), leucocyte, and thrombus. X 2450.

been proposed as another metastasis-promoting mechanism (Johnson et al., 1973) — is
by no means necessary for tumour emboli to be trapped in vessels. Finally, Fig. 6
shows that tumour emboli are only partially covered by thrombi, which strongly suggests that thrombi do not play an important role in protecting the tumour cells from
friction forces of the streaming blood (Lione and Bosman, 1978).

It is conceivable that platelets and fibrin protect tumour cells from host defenc
mechanisms. As for a possible action of leucocytes against tumour cells (Pickaver et
al., 1972), it can be seen in Fig. 6 that leucocytes adhere to the thrombi rather
than to the tumour cells. This might give the tumour cells a prolonged opportunity t
to escape from the vessel and to initiate the formation of a metastasis. Wood (1958)
suggested another effect of leucocytes: in his experiments leucocytes quickly migrat
ed under the thrombi and penetrated the endothelium whereas tumour cells followed
only later, probably utilizing the same opening. Among the hundreds of tumour emboli
in the lung and the liver constituting the present material, such an activity of leu
cocytes was never observed.

Many authors have drawn attention to the fact that platelets release inflammatory
substances such as histamine and serotonin which are known to increase the vascular
permeability (Gasic et al., 1976). In our material, morphological signs of endo-

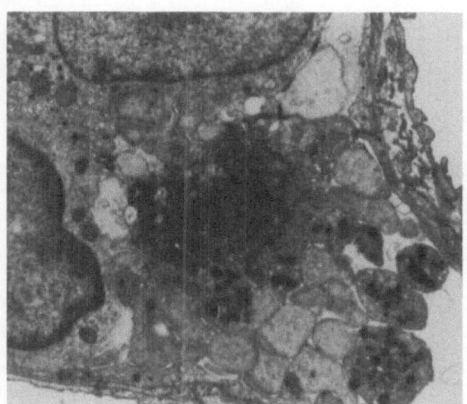

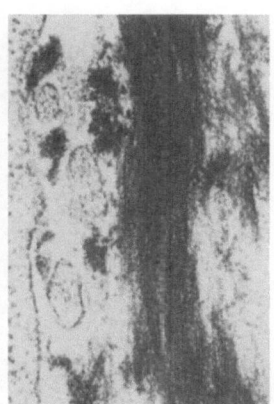

Fig. 2   Fig. 3

Fig. 2. Part of embolus illustrated in preceding figure. Dark central area consists of platelet pseudopods and fibrin. To the lower right, degranulated platelets
and newly arrived, granulated platelets can be seen. X 7100.
Fig. 3. Fibrin strand in tumour embolus, showing 20 nm periodicity. X 55.500.

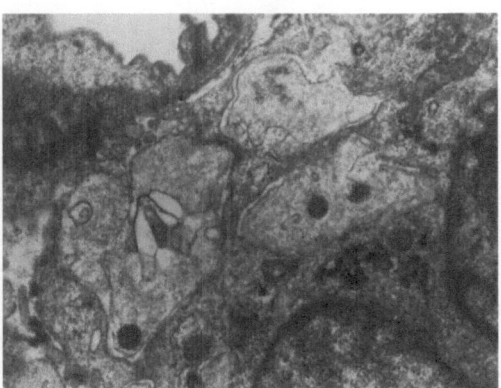

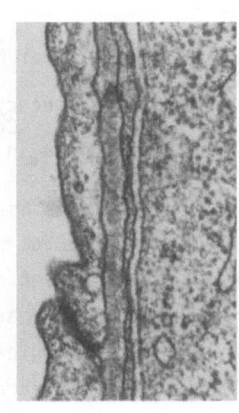

Fig. 4   Fig. 5

Fig. 4. Part of tumour embolus illustrated in Fig. 1, showing intertwining of tumour cell surface with partially degranulated platelets. Small electron-dense dots in
tumour cell cytoplasm represent intracisternal A-type virus particles. X 16.500.
Fig. 5. Detail of B16 melanoma cell trapped in lung capillary, showing apparently
empty space separating tumour cell from endothelial surface. X 51.000.

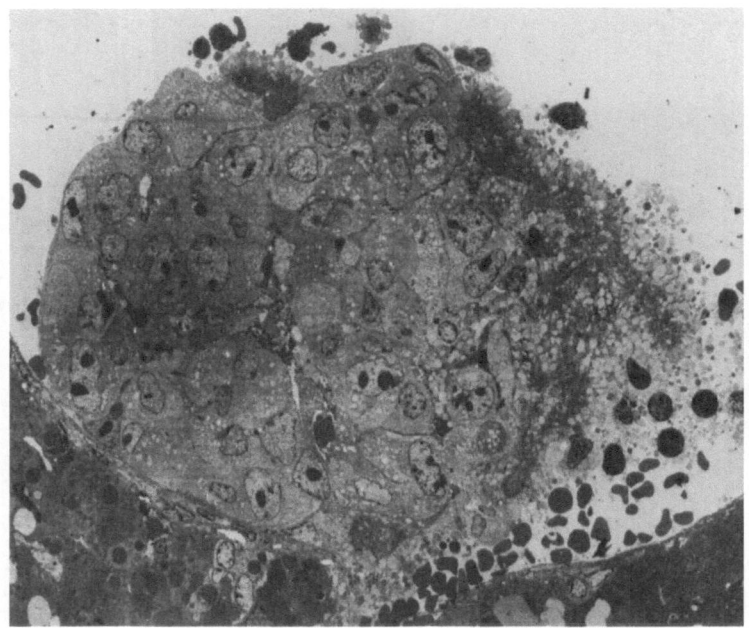

Fig. 6

Fig. 6. Embolus of M 8013 mammary carcinoma cells adhering to wall of portal ves
2.5 h after injection of tumour cells into portal system. Note thrombi covering par
of embolus, and leucocytes adhering to the thrombi rather than to the free surfaces
of the tumour cells. Contact with endothelium is mainly directly by tumour cells;
only small thrombus in lower centre is situated near vascular wall. X 900.

thelial alterations associated with the presence of thrombi have never been detecte

The last mechanism to be discussed relates to the hypoxia that can be brought
about by the blocking of blood vessels by tumour emboli. Even when the totally non-
thrombogenic TA3 mammary carcinoma cells were trapped in the liver, a fast accumulation of lipid droplets in the cytoplasm of hepatocytes indicated a state of hypox
in extensive tissue areas (Fig. 7). Indeed, sinusoids with a defective sinusoidal linii
could be readily detected in such areas (Fig. 8). It seems obvious that such hypoxii
induced tissue damage will be further promoted by thrombus formation.

In conclusion, morphological observations seem to support only a few of the mechanisms that can be conceived to explain a stimulating influence of blood coagulatioi
on tumour dissemination. However, it should be realized that pure morphology can on
partially answer the functional questions in this field.

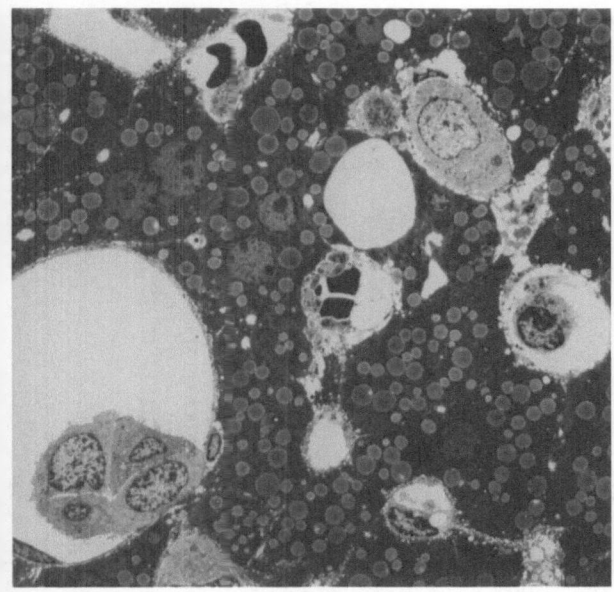 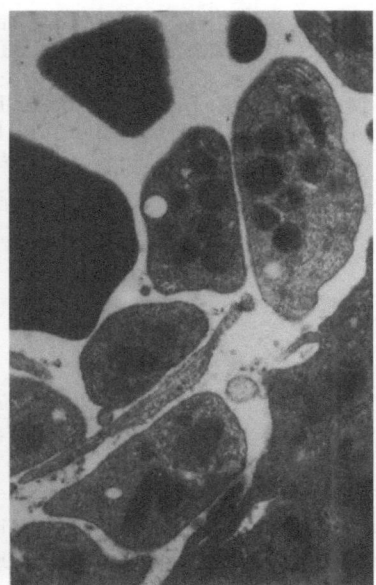

Fig 7   Fig. 8

Fig. 7. Area of liver tissue containing trapped TA3 cells, 1 h after their injection into portal system. Accumulation of lipid droplets indicates hypoxic state of extensive tissue areas. X 1100.
Fig. 8. Part of central sinusoid in preceding figure, showing platelets escaping
from sinusoidal lumen along remnant of endothelium. X 15.000.

REFERENCES

Gasic, G.J., Koch, P.A.G., Hsu, B., Gasic, T.B., and Niewiaroaski, S., 1976. Thrombo-
    genic activity of mouse and human tumors: effects on platelets, coagulation, and
    fibrinolysis, and possible significance for metastases. Z. Krebsforsch., 86:263-277.
Gastpar, H., 1970. Stickiness of platelet and tumor cells influenced by drugs. Throm-
    bos. Diathes. Haemorrh., Suppl. 42: 291-303.
Johnson, T., Gasic, T., and Gasic, G., 1973. Platelet aggregation by fibroblasts and
    its enhancing effect on metastasis in mice. In: S. Garrattini and G. Franchi (Edi-
    tors), Chemotherapy of Cancer Dissemination and Metastasis. Raven Press, New York,
    pp. 107-117.
Lione, A. and Bosman, H.B., 1978. The inhibitory effect of heparin and warfarin
    treatments on th intravascular survival of B16 melanoma cells in syngeneic C57
    mice. Cell Biol. Int. Rep., 2: 81-86.
Pickaver, A.H., Ratcliffe, N.A., Williams, A.E., and Smith, H., 1972. Cytotoxic ef-
    fects of peritoneal neutophils on a syngeneic rat tumour. Nature New Biol., 235:
    186-187.
Roos, E. and Dirgemans, K.P., 1979. Mechanisms of metastasis. Biochim. Biophys. Acta,
    560: 135-166.
Weiss, L., 1977. A pathbiologic overview of metastasis. Semin. Oncol., 4: 5-17.
Wood, S., 1958. Pathogenesis of metastasis formation observed in vivo in the rabbit
    ear chamber. Arch. Path., 66: 550-568.

CANCER CELL PROCOAGULANT ACTIVITY, WARFARIN AND EXPERIMENTAL METASTASES

M. Colucci, F. Delaini, G. de Bellis Vitti, D. Locati,
A. Poggi, N. Semeraro and M.B. Donati

It has long been suspected that the coagulation mechanism may be involved in the pathogenesis of primary and especially metastatic cancer growth. This concept was initially based on the histological evidence showing a close association between cancer cells and fibrin in experimental or human malignancies and is further suggested by the inhibitory effect of anticoagulant treatment on tumor metastases in some experimental models (reviewed by Donati and Poggi, 1980). Several investigations have indeed indicated that induction of hypocoagulability in animals prior to the intravenous injection of viable tumor cells reduced the number and incidence of lung nodule formation (Hilgard and Thornes, 1976).However, different results were obtained when the same drugs were used in "spontaneous" metastasis models which better mimicked the clinical conditions of dissemination from a primary tumor site (Poggi et al., 1980; Hilgard,1980).

Table 1 summarizes the experience we have collected on treatment of mice bearing the Lewis Lung Carcinoma (3LL) with drugs influencing at various levels the host's hemostatic system. It can be observed that all the drugs studied (an anticoagulant, a defibrinating enzyme and two platelet aggregation inhibitors) share some inhibitory effect on the "artificial" metastasis model, whereas only warfarin treatment is also effective in markedly reducing "spontaneous" metastasis formation (Poggi et al.,1980). These observations, in agreement with those reported by Hilgard (1980) would argue against the concept of warfarin's antimetastatic effect being mediated only by plasma anticoagulation. It has been recently shown that 3LL cells possess a peculiar procoagulant activity, which has been partially characterized (Curatolo et al., 1979; Colucci et al., 1980). These cells, either harvested directly from tumor masses or obtained from primary cultures, shortened the recalcification time of normal, factor VIII-and factor VII-deficient, not factor X-deficient plasma, and generated thrombin when mixed with a source of prothrombin and factor X, factor V, phospholipid and calcium chloride. These data indicated that 3LL cells possessed an activity directly activating coagulation factor X, without requiring the mediation of factors of either the extrinsic or the intrinsic pathway (Curatolo et al., 1979).

TABLE 1

Effect of prolonged treatment with various drugs on artificial and spontaneous metastasis growth of 3LL (induced and evaluated as described by Poggi et al.,1977). For each drug considered, the results are expressed as the percentage of the values measured in the respective control group. Twenty animals per group were studied.

Experimental Group	LUNG COLONIES		SPONTANEOUS METASTASIS	
	Number	Weight	Number	Weight
	PERCENT OF RESPECTIVE CONTROLS			
Warfarin[a]	10.9	3.4	34.2	18.2
Batroxobin[b]	59.4	n.d.	159.4	122.2
Acetylsalycilic acid[c]	50.7	64.2	100.0	94.0
Ditazole[d]	51.2	69.4	104.2	148.0

[a]0.2-5 mg/kg b.w. in drinking water (day -2 to sacrifice)
[b]17.5 NIH u/kg b.w. twice per day i.p. (day 0 to sacrifice)
[c]100 mg/kg b.w. twice per day i.p. (day 0 to sacrifice)
[d]200 mg/kg b.w. twice per day i.p. (day 0 to sacrifice).

More direct evidence for the existence of such an activator, was obtained from experiments showing that 3LL cells, when mixed with Factor X and calcium chloride, generated an activity capable to split a synthetic substrate, Bz-Ile-Glu-Gly-Arg-pNa (S-2222, Kabi Diagnostica, Stockholm), which is specific for activated factor X.

It is conceivable that such a procoagulant activity of 3LL cells could contribute to the fibrin deposition observed, at the primary tumor site (Poggi et al., 1977), and possibly modify the metastatic capacity of 3LL cells. We therefore investigated whether warfarin treatment of 3LL bearing mice influenced the tumour cell's proccagulant (factor X activating) activity. 3LL cells (1×10^5 per mouse) were injected i.m.into the hind paw pad of C57Bl/6J male mice at day 0. Warfarin (Coumadin[R], Erdo laboratories, Garden City, N.Y., USA) was given in drinking water from day 7 according to a schedule capable of maintaining prothrombin complex activity (measured by the Thrombotest, Immuno S.p.A., Pisa, Italy) at less than 5% of control values (Poggi et al., 1978). Treatment was continued till the animals were killed, on day 22, when the primary tumour weight was similar in control and warfarin-treated mice. In these conditions both the number and the weight of lung metastases was significantly reduced in treated animals (Table 2). At sacrifice of the animals, primary tumour cells were obtained **from necrosis-free** fragments, washed extensively (4x) with phosphate buffered saline, suspended in the same buffer at the desired concentration and immediately tested. Procoagulant activity was assayed by a one-stage recalcification time of human factor VII-deficient plasma containing less than 1% factor VII:

TABLE 2

Effect of chronic warfarin treatment on Thrombotest levels and on primary and metastatic 3LL growth. Means $\pm$ S.E. of values obtained from 20 animals per group.

Experimental Group	Thrombotest (%)	Primary tumor (g)	Lung metastases Number	Weight (mg)
Control	90 - 110	9.8 $\pm$ 0.6	19.3 $\pm$ 3	260 $\pm$ 49
Warfarin (day 7-22)	< 5	9.5 $\pm$ 0.2	9 $\pm$ 3*	45 $\pm$ 12*

$p < 0.01$ at Student's t test.

----

the clotting time of a mixture of cell suspension, plasma substrate and 0.025 M $CaCl_2$ was determined in plastic tubes at $37^{\circ}C$; this experimental system was espe-cially deviced for assaying direct factor X activating activity (Curatolo et al., 1979). Table 3 shows that cells from warfarin-treated mice had significantly lower factor X activating activity (longer recalcification times) than those from untreated mice. When vitamin K_1 (Konakion, Roche, Milano, Italy) was added (4 mg/kg b.w.) to the drinking water of warfarin-treated mice, for three days before killing, a complete normalization of both prothrombin complex activity and 3LL cell procoagulant activity was observed (Table 3).

TABLE 3

Effect of chronic warfarin treatment on blood prothrombin complex activity (Thrombotest) and on 3LL cell $(15 \times 10^6/\text{ml})$ procoagulant activity (measured as recal-cification time); means $\pm$ S.E. of data obtained from 15 animals per group.

Experimental Group	Thrombotest (sec)	Recalcification time (sec)
Control	23.9 $\pm$ 1.1	46.6 $\pm$ 1.6*
Warfarin	> 180	81.7 $\pm$ 2.4
Warfarin + Vitamin K_1	23.8 $\pm$ 1.1	48.5 $\pm$ 1.1*

* $p < 0.001$ compared to the warfarin group (Student's t test for independent values).

In none of the conditions considered did _in vitro_ addition of warfarin (at various concentration up to 1 mg/ml) to the test system, influence the recalcifi-cation times.

This study shows therefore that the specific procoagulant activity of 3LL cells is significantly reduced in mice treated with a warfarin schedule capable to inhibit metastasis formation. This effect cannot be ascribed to a direct _in vivo_ cytotoxic activity of warfarin on 3LL cells, considering that the primary tumor weight was the same in treated and control mice at the time of cell harvest.

Most probably, warfarin may induce some selective alteration of the cells' metabolism that impairs their ability to synthesize the procoagulant activity. The observed correction by vitamin K of this warfarin effect strongly suggests that the synthesis of the specific procoagulant activity of 3LL cells is a vitamin K-dependent phenomenon.

It has been shown that vitamin K deficiency is as effective as warfarin treatment in inhibiting 3LL metastasis formation, thus suggesting a crucial role for this vitamin in the modulation of cancer cell capacity to disseminate (Hilgard, 1977). Studies are in progress to evaluate whether vitamin K deficiency also influences 3LL cells procoagulant activity. The present observation of a "cellular" anticoagulant effect of warfarin on cancer cells could shed fresh light **on** our understanding of the antimetastatic activity of the drug and of the involvement of fibrin in dissemination processes.

Acknowledgements

This work was performed within the frame of the Cell-fibrin Interaction Subgroup of the Tumor Invasion Group of EORTC. The partial support of Italian National Research Council (Contract 80.01621.96) is gratefully acknowledged. The Authors with to thank Prof. P.M. Mannucci, Milan University, Medical School, for kindly supplying plasma from a factor VII-deficient patient. Warfarin was a gift from Endo Laboratories, Garden City, N.Y. USA. Judith Baggott, Gigliola Brambilla, Vanna Pistotti helped prepare this manuscript.

References

Colucci, M., Curatolo, L., Donati, M.B. and Semeraro, N., 1980, Cancer cell procoagulant activity: Evaluation by an amidolytic assay. Thromb. Res., in press.

Curatolo, L., Colucci, M., Cambini, A.L., Poggi, A., Morasca, L., Donati, M.B. and Semeraro, N., 1979, Evidence that cells from experimental tumours can activate coagulation factor X, Br. J. Cancer, 40: 228-233.

Donati, M.B. and Poggi, A., 1980, Malignancy and haemostasis, Br. J. Haematol., 44: 173-182.

Hilgard, P., 1977, Experimental vitamin K deficiency and spontaneous metastases, Br. J. Cancer, 35: 891-892.

Hilgard, P., 1980, The use of oral anticoagulants in tumour therapy. In:
    M.B. Donati, J.F. Davidson and S. Garattini (Editors), Malignancy and the
    Hemostatic System. Raven Press, New York, in press.

Hilgard, P. and Thornes, R.D., 1976, Anticoagulants in the treatment of cancer,
    Eur. J. Cancer, 12: 755-762.

Poggi, A., Donati, M.B. and Garattini, S., 1980, Fibrin and experimental cancer
    cell dissemination: Problems in the evaluation of experimental models.
    In: M.B. Donati, J.F. Davidson and S. Garattini (Editors), Malignancy and
    the Hemostatic System. Raven Press, New York, in press.

Poggi, A., Mussoni, L., Kornblihtt, L., Ballabio, E., de Gaetano, G. and
    Donati, M.B., 1978, Warfarin enantiomers, anticoagulation and experimental
    tumour metastasis, Lancet, 1: 163-164.

Poggi, A., Polentarutti, N., Donati, M.B., de Gaetano, G. and Garattini, S.,
    1977, Blood coagulation changes in mice bearing Lewis lung carcinoma, a
    metastasizing tumor, Cancer Res., 37: 272-277.

MOLECULAR MECHANISM OF FIBRINOLYSIS AND ITS POTENTIAL ROLE IN METASTASIS

S.A. Cederholm-Williams

INTRODUCTION:

Increased blood clotting and increased fibrinolytic activity are known to be associated with malignant tumors and certain tumors, particularly those of the prostate, are capable of inducing total clinical defibrination by over stimulation of the fibrinolytic mechanism. Interaction of malignant cells with the haemostatic system is receiving increased attention (1) and with a new understanding of the molecular mechanisms of fibrinolysis and coagulation,phenomena such as cancer cell growth, tumor shedding, invasion and lodgement in target tissues may soon be better explained.

Plasminogen activation is one of the mechanisms for the production of localized extracellular proteolytic activity involved in cell mobility, inflammation, macrophage function and tissue remodelling. In culture, malignant cells synthesize and release large quantities of plasminogen activator following transformation and for some cells the presence of plasminogen is necessary before the morphological changes characteristic of transformation are expressed (2). Protease inhibitors of serum and synthetic antifibrinolytic agents reduce cell motility and delay the expression of certain malignant characteristics (3). The exact role of fibrin in the spread or containment of tumor cells is a subject of current debate.

Fibronectin, a major cell surface protein of fibroblasts and other cells, is responsible for cell adhesion to collagen, basement membrane and artificial surfaces. This protein is lost from the cell surface following transformation and its levels have been related to the capacity of cells to induce invasive tumors. Fibronectin carries fibrin(ogen) binding sites and is a substrate for plasmin (4).

Though the role of fibrinolysis in malignant transformation and metastasis is uncertain and the significance of the interaction of fibronectin with fibrin and plasmin unknown, progress has been made in the elucidation of the molecular mechanism of fibrinolysis. This work has clear relevance to the investigation of the metastasising cell.

Molecular Mechanism of Fibrinolysis:

Following the proteolytic action of thrombin or other thrombin like enzymes, fibrinogen spontaneously polymerises forming the insoluble macromolecular structure of fibrin. This structure is subsequently covalently crosslinked by thrombin activated plasma transglutaminase, and becomes the primary substrate of the fibronolytic enzyme plasmin.

The fibrinolytic proenzyme plasminogen is normally present in plasma and is
converted to the powerful protease by cleavage of an arginine-valine bond
followed by the release of an N-terminal peptide. Active plasmin is a two chain
enzyme of molecular weight 84,000 in which the active centre is located on the
smaller light chain and regulatory site(s) on the larger heavy chain. Though
plasmin has a wide proteolytic specificity the activity is normally confined
to fibrin by the action of the regulatory site(s) (5). One of these sites has
binding activity which allows the formation of stable plasminogen-fibrin
complexes.

The plasminogen activator responsible for vascular fibrinolysis is released
from the vascular endothelium following injury or other stimulation. This enzyme
also has a high affinity for fibrin and rapidly becomes fibrin bound. Fibrin
bound activator converts fibrin bound plasminogen to fibrin bound plasmin. The
high proteolytic activity of plasmin is confined to fibrin by the co-ordinated
actions of the fibrin binding site of the plasmin heavy chain and circulating
α-2-antiplasmin.

Plasma contains two protease inhibitors which possess significant antiplasmin activity. Of these, the primary plasmin inhibitor is α-2-antiplasmin
(6) and is responsible for 90% of the total plasma antiplasmin activity. The
remaining antiplasmin is exerted by α-2-macroglobulin. α-2-antiplasmin is
a single chain glycoprotein of molecular weight 70,000 which inhibits plasmin
in a very rapid two step reaction:

$$P + AP \xrightleftharpoons{k_1} P\text{-}AP \xrightarrow{k_2} P\text{-}AP^*$$

The first step involves the formation of a reversibly associated bimolecular
complex followed by an intramolecular rearrangement resulting in the formation of
a covalent bond between plasmin and antiplasmin. The first step of the reaction is
exceedingly fast (k_1 = 2-4 x $10^7 M^{-1} Sec^{-1}$) and is amongst one of the fastest
known protein-protein interactions (7). This inhibition step is so fast that
under normal circumstances plasmin does not have any appreciable existence as
a free enzyme in plasma. The speed of this reaction is determined by the
regulatory site (5) of the plasmin heavy chain (8). Removal or blockage of these
regulatory residues reduces the speed at which plasmin is inactivated.

These same residues of the heavy chain are closely involved in binding
plasmin(ogen) to fibrin and interact with the antifibrinolytic lysine analogues
e-aminocaproic acid and t-aminomethyl cyclohexanoic acid. These synthetic
inhibitors bind to the fibrin binding site of plasmin(ogen) causing the
competitive dissociation of fibrin-plasmin(ogen) complexes at very low inhibitor

Figure 1: MODEL FOR THE MECHANISM OF FIBRINOLYSIS:

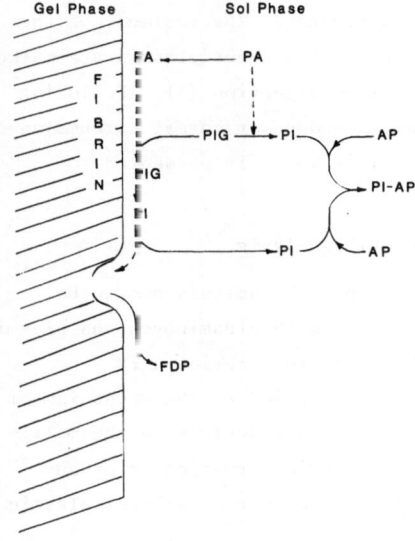

Fibrin bound plasminogen activator
(PA) and plasminogen (PlG) generate
active plasmin (Pl) on the
surface of fibrin in an environment protected from the inhibitory
action of antiplasmin (AP).
Following fibrin degradation
(FDP) plasmin is released and
immediately inhibited (Pl-AP).

Figure 2: MODEL FOR PLASMINOGEN ACTIVATION ON THE MALIGNANT CELL SURFACE:

Plasminogen from the external
medium binds to a specific cell
surface component (represented
by the oblong blocks) where
plasminogen activator (PA)
from the malignant cell
induces plasmin (Pl) generation
on the cell surface. Because
of the involvement of the
lysine sensitive regulatory
sites of the Pl heavy chain
this plasmin is protected from
antiplasmin (AP) but is
dissociated from its receptor by
e-aminocaproic acid (e-ACA).

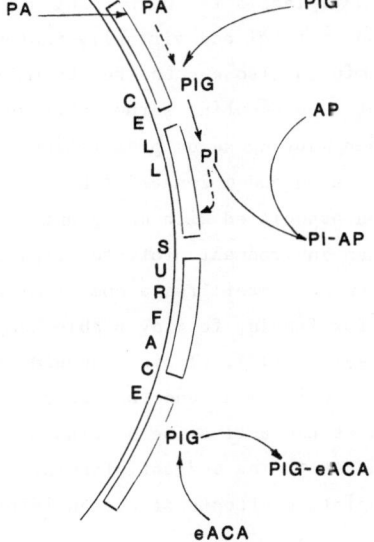

concentrations (9,10). In fact this series of antifibrinolytic agents exert
their antifibrinolytic activities at concentrations much lower than those needed
to directly inhibit the proteolytic activity of the active centre.

It is currently accepted that fibrin bound plasminogen is converted to
plasmin in situ by fibrin adsorbed plasminogen activator. The residues of the
plasmin heavy chain necessary for the rapid action of α-2-antiplasmin are masked
until plasmin is released from the fibrin by enzyme digestion (5). Following
fibrin digestion plasmin is immediately inhibited and under normal circumstances
is never detected as a free enzyme in plasma. This model is presented
schematically in Figure 1.

The Cancer Cell and the Molecular Mechanism of Fibrinolysis

The foregoing description of the mechanism of fibrinolysis shows the
importance of the regulatory site(s) which confines both plasminogen and plasmin
to the surface of fibrin and which mediate the rapid interaction with
α-2-antiplasmin. So far, this model has only been applied to the mechanism of
vascular fibrinolysis and the significance of these interactions to the malignant cell is presently speculative. However if plasmin formation is of any
importance to the malignant cell then the inhibitory effect of α-2-antiplasmin
will be of equal importance.

In vivo tumors are bathed with the extravascular fluid, the contents of
which reflect the plasma protein concentrations. From metabolic studies in
normal subjects (11,12) with radiolabelled plasminogen, fibrinogen and
α-2-antiplasmin, it has been found that the extravascular fraction of these
proteins are 35%, 51% and 48% respectively, showing that there is ample extravascular antiplasmin to inhibit any activated extravascular plasminogen unless
activation is total and virtually instantaneous. This difficulty in generating
free plasmin is also encountered by malignant cells in culture. The plasminogen
content of supplementing serum is frequently reduced by loss of fibrin bound
plasminogen during serum preparation, whereas the concentrations of
α-2-antiplasmin and α-2-macroglobulin are usually unaltered. The plasminogen
activation associated with malignant transformation and increased mobility must
occur in an environment protected from the inhibitory action of α-2-antiplasmin.
Plasminogen activator from a number of malignant human cell lines display high
affinity for fibrin, forming stable complexes similar to those that occur in the
vascular system (13). It is proposed therefore that the cell surface offers this
protective environment and that some cell surface component is present which
co-ordinates the activation of plasminogen by interacting with the regulatory
sites, and excluding α-2-antiplasmin. Such a component would be sensitive to
the dissociating effects of the antifibrinolytic lysine analogues and may be

fibrin(ogen) or some fibrin(ogen) derivative or could be related to fibronectin. These relationships are illustrated in Fig. 2.

References

(1) Donati, M.B. and Poggi, A. (1980). Malignancy and Haemostasis. Brit.J. Haematol., 44, 173-182.

(2) Ossowski, L., Quigley, J.P., Kellerman, G.M. and Reich, E. (1973). Fibrinolysis associated with oncogenic transformation. Requirement of plasminogen for correlated changes in cellular morphology, colony formation in agar and cell migration. J.Expt.Med., 138, 1056-

(3) Goldberg, A.R., Wolf, B.A. and Lefebure, P.A. (1975). Plasminogen activators of transformed and normal cells. In Proteases and Biological Control (Ed. Reich, Rifkin and Shaw), p. 857-868. Cold Spring Harbour Laboratory. Vol. 2.

(4) Yamada, K.M. and Olden, K. (1978). Fibronectins - adhesive glycoproteins of cell surface and blood. Nature, 275, 179-184.

(5) Wiman, B. and Collen, D. (1978). Molecular mechanism of physiological fibrinolysis. Nature, 272, 549-550.

(6) Wiman, B. and Collen, D. (1978). On the kinetics of the reaction between human antiplasmin and plasmin. Eur.J.Biochem., 84, 573-578.

(7) Cederholm-Williams, S.A., De Cock, F., Lijnen, R. and Collen, D. (1979). Kinetics of the reactions between streptokinase, plasmin and α-2-antiplasmin. Eur.J.Biochem., 100, 125-132.

(8) Wiman, B., Boman, L. and Collen, D. (1978). On the kinetics of the reaction between human antiplasmin and a low molecular weight form of plasmin. Eur.J.Biochem., 87, 143-146.

(9) Cederholm-Williams, S.A. (1977). The binding of plasminogen (mol. wt. 84,000) and plasmin to fibrin. Thrombosis Research, 11, 421-423.

(10) Cederholm-Williams, S.A. and Swain, A. (1979). The effect of fibrinogen degradation products and some lysine analogues on the dissociation of plasmin(ogen)-fibrin complexes. Thrombosis Research, 16, 705-713.

(11) Cederholm-Williams, S.A. and Dornan, T. (1980). Metabolism of plasminogen and fibrinogen in patients with diabetic retinopathy. Fifth International Conference on Synthetic Fibrinolytic Thrombolytic Agents. Ed. J. Davison (in press).

(12) Collen, D. and Wiman, B. (1979). Turnover of antiplasmin, the fast-acting plasmin inhibitor in plasma. Blood, 53, 313-324.

(13) Lloyd, D.A., Cederholm-Williams, S.A. and Sharp, A.A. (1980). Interaction of plasminogen activator with fibrin. Fifth International Conference on Synthetic Fibrinolytic Thrombolytic Agents. Ed. J. Davison, (in press).

FIBRINOLYSIS AND ANTICOAGULATION IN COLO-RECTAL CANCER - THE WAY AHEAD

H. White, J. Griffiths and A. Salsbury

There have been many studies of the role of fibrinolysis and anti-coagulation in the dissemination and development of metastatic deposit: in experimental tumours. These have mostly been in animals. Despite the abundance of laboratory work, the results have been somewhat conflicting and little can be said except that in some systems, parameters of coagulation and fibrinolysis appear to be one of the many influences on the release, transport and lodgement of cells - and perhaps the growth of micrometastases (Woods 1974). The role of fibrin which forms a primitive stroma and platelet aggregation appear to be of prime importance and a number of anticoagulants and fibrin-olytic agents have experimentally been shown to retard tumour growth and decrease or even inhibit the development of metastases (Hilgard 1976).

Only a few clinical studies have been undertaken to test the theories which have grown out of the experimental work. Michaels (1964) published a retrospective survey of patients receiving long-tern anticoagulants following pulmonary embolism. This suggested that, although the incidence of cancer in the anticoagulated group was identical with that found in the general population, the death-rate from cancer was only 12.5% of that expected. A trial by Thornes (1975) using warfarin in addition to chemotherapy for recurrent tumours of various types of histology (but mainly leukaemia and Hodgkin's disease) showed that the two-year survival in the treatment group was 40.6% as opposed to 17.8% in the control group.

A controlled trial reported by Clery et al (1972) showed an increased survival in patients undergoing resection for colorectal cancer.

Our group has, for many years been interested in the changes observed in the parameters of coagulation and fibrinolysis in patients with malignant disease and particularly colorectal cancer.

Observations by Newstead et al (1976) in patients undergoing resection for colorectal cancer have shown increased fibrinolysis in the blood draining tumours. Circulating malignant cells have been demonstrated by Salsbury et al (1973) both in the blood draining a tumour and in the peripheral circulation. We have now studied a group of 62 patients undergoing resection for colorectal cancer over a ten year period (White et al 1976). The survival of those patients in whom cells were present at the time of resection was analysed and found to be longer than those in whom no cells were present.

TEN-YEAR SURVIVAL

Cells	No. patients (Dukes' Classification)		Survival	
	Dead	Alive	Overall	Corrected
Absent 30 *	A = 1 B = 5 }22 C = 16	A = 2 B = 4 } 8 C = 2	27%	30%
Present 32 **	A = 0 B = 5 }14 C = 9	A = 4 B = 8 }18 C = 6	56%	58%

*   3 patients died of other causes
** 1 patient died of other causes

In this small group the level of significance was not high with the increase in survival of patients with cells at 10 years over those in whom cells were absent only being significant at the 5% level.

Unfortunately, in the early studies, parameters of coagulation were not measured. However, it is known that following surgery there is an increase in fibrinolytic activity and in the light of our subsequent work we must assume that there was indeed such an increase at least in those patients in whom circulating cells were demonstrated.

A pilot study was, therefore, initiated 5 years ago to
measure the changes in fibrinolytic activity which occurred after
surgery and whether a state of increased fibrinolytic activity
could safely be induced by the administration of urokinase during
operation and for the 6 hours following the end of surgery. We
felt that as we had been able to demonstrate the cells during the
period of natural fibrinolytic activity that accompanies the trauma
of surgery, prolonged artificial increase in fibrinolysis might
lead to cells being kept in the circulation for a long time and
this was found to be the case. There are theoretical reasons for
thinking that this might be of benefit and support comes from the
experimental work of Cliffton and Agostino (1962) who showed that
if cells are kept circulating they die and do not implant. If these
observations hold in the clinical situation as well as in experimenta
systems, they could to some extent explain the surprising increase
in survival at 10 years observed in our patients with circulating
malignant cells demonstrated at the time of surgery.

In order to produce a small but safe increase in fibrinolytic
activity during the operative and immediately post-operative period
sufficient for malignant cells generally to be found for some
6 hours after surgery 50,000 Plough units of urokinase were given
over 5 hours. No complications were observed and increased fibrinolytic activity was observed in 17 of the 22 patients studied. These
patients had an increase in fibrin degradation products (F.D.P.)
over 10 units and a reduction in the euglobulin lysis time below
20 minutes.

With induced fibrinolysis we were able to demonstrate cells in
the post-operative period in 11 of the 17 patients in whom fibrinolytic activity was increased but no cells were found unless there
was such an increase.

The patients were followed for three years and although the
numbers are too small for statistical analysis, no increase in
survival could be detected in this small group followed for such

a short period.

THREE-YEAR SURVIVAL

Cells	No. patients (Dukes' Classification)	
	Dead	Alive
Absent 11 ○	A = 0 B = 3 } 4 C = 1	A = 1 B = 4 } 7 C = 2*
Present 11 ▲	A = 0 B = 2 } 5 C = 3	A = 1 B = 5* } 6 C = 0

○ 3 patients died of other causes
▲ 2 patients died of other causes
* Alive but recurrent disease in
one patient

What can we conclude from our first series of patients studied
for 10 years in whom there appeared to be an increased survival
when circulating malignant cells were present and our recent series
followed for 3 years in which we have demonstrated that circulating
malignant cells can appear in relation to increased fibrinolytic
activity manipulated by the infusion of urokinase?

We feel that the presence of cells does not necessarily mean
that the prognosis is worse. Indeed from the experimental evidence
and our clinical results there is some reason to believe that
circulating malignant cells associated with increased fibrinolytic
activity may lead to an improved survival. Clearly this is only
one of the many factors which influence the development of metastases
in patients undergoing resection for colorectal cancer. However,
a controlled prospective trial is without doubt required and this
has now been started in which the effect of urokinase and post-
operative warfarin on long term survival in patients undergoing

resection will be studied. The protocol has a 2 x 2 factorial design, the patients being pre-operatively randomised to either urokinase treatment which immediately follows surgery for 5 hours or a control group. After pathological staging the patients are further randomised to long term warfarin treatment or a further control group. The main study is being limited to Dukes B & C patients. We hope for an answer to the tantalising questions posed by the experimental work on anticoagulants and fibrinolytic agents and previous clinical trials. It is only by large and rigidly controlled prospective studies that worthwhile information can be obtained and this, rather than small and somewhat questionable pilot studies, must be the way ahead.

REFERENCES

Clery, A.P., Hogan, B.L., Holland, P.D.J., Widdess, J.D.H., Ryan, M., Doyle, J.S., Bourke, G.J. and Thornes, R.D., 1972. J. Irish Coll. Phys. Surg. 1: 91-95
Cliffton, E.E. and Agostino, D., 1962. Cancer 15: 276
Hilgard, P. and Thornes, R.D., 1976. Europ. J. Cancer 12: 755
Michaels, L., 1964. Lancet 2: 832-35
Newstead, G.L., Griffiths, J.D. and Salsbury, A.J. 1976. Surg. Gynecol. and Obstet. 143: 61
Salsbury, A.J., White, C., Tsozakidis, P., McKinna, J.A., and Griffiths, J.D., 1973. Surg. Gynecol. and Obstet. 136: 733
Thornes, R.D., 1975. Cancer 35: 91
White, H., Griffiths, J.D. and Salsbury, A.J. 1976. Proc. Roy. Soc. Med. 69: 467
Wood, S. Jr., 1974. J. Med. 5: 7

STUDIES ON FACTORS INFLUENCING THE LODGEMENT OF CIRCULATING TUMOUR CELLS

G. Skolnik, M. Alpsten and L. Ivarsson

Many surgeons have observed on some occasion how surgical trauma undoubtedly has stimulated the formation of metastases in patients suffering from malignant diseases. Several experimental studies (Agostino and Cliffton,1965, Fisher et al., 1967, Ivarsson, 1976) have also shown that different kinds of trauma stimulate the formation of metastases after intravenous tumour cell injection. The mechanisms responsible for this effect of trauma have, however, not yet been fully clarified. Several post-traumatic reactions have been considered, such as disturbed microcirculation (Fisher et al.,1967, Rudenstam,1968), intravascular coagulation (Agostino and Cliffton,1965, Rudenstam,1968), increased microthrombus formation (Ivarsson, 1976) and damage to the vascular endothelium, which all can be supposed to cause an increased or rather a prolonged lodgement of circulating tumour cells.

It seems to have been clearly demonstrated that tumour cells adhering to the vascular endothelium as a rule must be surrounded by a micro-thrombus before they can penetrate the vascular endothelium (Wood Jr,1958) This microthrombus has been shown by several investigators (Wood Jr.1958, Warren and Vales, 1972) to be built up mainly of platelets and a fibrin-like material.

We have found that the formation of metastases after intravenous tumour cell injection and the stimulating effect of trauma on metasta-sis formation are depending on a platelet reaction, as thrombocyto-penia inhibits the formation of metastases and neutralizes the stimu-lating effect of trauma on metastasis formation (Gasic et al., 1973, Ivarsson, 1976). When studying the effect of heparin treatment and defibrinogenation we found an inhibiting effect on the formation of metastases. Treatment with high molecular weight dextran (dextran 1000), a dextran fraction causing microcirculatory disturbances, stimulated metastasis formation (Ivarsson and Rudenstam, 1975, Ivarsson, 1976).

Treatment with low molecular weight dextran (dextran 40), a dextran fraction which has antithrombotic properties and normalizes a disturbed microcirculation, did not influence the formation of metastases when given alone. But, when combined with trauma, low molecular weight dextran caused a further increase of the metastasis formation (Ivarsson and Rudenstam, 1975).

On the basis of these results we suggested that trauma caused increased metastasis formation because of an increased lodgement of
circulating tumour cells due to a stimulation of the microthrombus
formation (Ivarsson, 1976). The effect of heparin treatment, thrombocytopenia and defibrinogenation could be explained by an inhibition
of the microthrombus formation followed by a decreased lodgement of
tumour cells.

The effect of dextran 1000 could not be explained by an influence
on the microthrombus formation, as the effect was unaffected when
dextran 1000 was combined with heparin treatment or thrombocytopenia,
but was suggested to depend on disturbed microcirculation(Ivarsson,1976).
The combined effect of trauma and low molecular weight dextran seemed
more difficult to explain.

To confirm our theory concerning changes in the lodgement of circulating tumour cells as a mechanism causing alterations of the formation
of metastases, we have studied the lodgement of intravenously injected
radioactively labelled tumour cells.

We injected tumour cells from a syngeneic methylcholantren induced
fibrosarcoma into dextran non-sensitive Wistar rats. The cells were
kept in culture for 48 hours and were labelled with 125-iodine-2-deoxy-
uridine during the later half of the incubation period (Fidler, 1970).
The cells were then injected into the experimental animals as soon as
possible after harvesting. As a rule, the animals were sacrificed
4 hours after tumour cell injection. The lungs were removed and the
amount of 125-iodine in the lungs and in the injected number of tumour
cells was determined as counts per minute. The number of tumour cells
in the lungs could then be calculated.

Trauma and dextran 1000 caused, as expected, a significantly increased lodgement of tumour cells, while dextran 40 had no significant
effect neither when given alone nor when combined with trauma. Our
conclusion from this is that the mechanism responsible for the unexpected stimulating effect of dextran 40 on metastasis formation in combination with trauma is not an increased tumour cell lodgement(Skolnik
et al., 1980 a). Another explanation must be looked for. It might for
example be a result of the flow promoting properties of dextran 40,
which might cause a prolonged survival of circulating tumour cells.

Heparin treatment caused a marked reduction of the number of lodged
tumour cells in the lungs and so did even induced thrombocytopenia.
These results are completely in accordance with the results of our

earlier studies on the formation of metastases. Defibrinogenation, however, did not cause a significant decrease of tumour cell lodgement which had been expected from the earlier results on metastasis formation. There is reason to believe that defibrinogenation has a rather weak inhibiting effect on the microthrombus formation, as fibrin seems to be a small or unimportant part of the microthrombus.

As our theory is that the stimulating effect of trauma on tumour cell lodgement depends mainly on increased platelet adhesiveness and increased microthrombus formation, the logical next step seemed to be to study the effect of thrombocytopenia on the tumour cell lodgement in traumatized animals. When combined with thrombocytopenia, the stimulating effect of trauma on tumour cell lodgement was completely neutralized and we registered a decreased tumour cell lodgement when compared to control. Trauma, however, still had a stimulating effect on tumour cell lodgement in thrombocytopenic animals, as registered both 4 and 8 hours after tumour cell injection (Skolnik et al.,1980 b). This indicates that as long as there are platelets present, the trauma influenced tumour cell lodgement can not be completely inhibited.

	Effect on metastasis formation	Effect on tumour cell lodgement
Trauma	+	+
Dextran 1000	+	+
Dextran 40	0	0
Trauma + Dextran 40	++	+
Heparin	−	−
Thrombocytopenia	−	−
Defibrinogenation	−	0
Trauma + Thrombocytopenia	0	−

+=increased   − = decreased   0 = no effect

These studies confirm that the increased formation of metastases observed after trauma and infusion of high molecular weight dextran and the decreased formation of metastases observed after heparin treatment and induced thrombocytopenia is well correlated to an increased respectively decreased lodgement of circulating tumour cells.

On the other hand, it is evident that the enhancing effect of dextran 40
on metastasis formation in traumatized animals does not depend on
changes in tumour cell lodgement. Other explanations must be looked
for this effect of low molecular weight dextran in combination with
trauma.

REFERENCES

Agostino, D. and Cliffton, E.E., 1965. Trauma as a cause of localization
    of blood-borne metastases: Preventive effect ofheparin and fibrino-
    lysis. Ann. Surg. 161: 97-102.
Fidler, I.J., 1970. Metastasis: Quantitative analysis of distribution
    and fate of tumour emboli labelled with ^{125}I-5-iodo-2-deoxyuridine.
    J. Nat. Cancer Inst. 45:773-782
Fisher, B., Fisher, E.R. and Feduzka, N., 1967. Trauma and the localiza-
    tion of tumour cells. Cancer 20:23-30
Gasic, J.G., Gasic, T.B., Galanti, N., Johnson, T., Murphy, S., 1973.
    Platelet-tumour cell interactions in mice. The role of platelets in
    the spread of malignant disease. Int. J. Cancer 11:704-717
Ivarsson, L., 1976. Pulmonary metastasis formation after trauma. An
    experimental study on the relevance of rheological disturbances
    of blood. Acta Chir. Scand. Suppl. 463.
Ivarsson, L. and Rudenstam, C. M., 1975. Dextrans and the formation
    of pulmonary metastases after intravenous tumour cell injection in
    rats non-sensitive to dextran. Eur. Surg. Res. 7:326-340.
Rudenstam, C.M., 1968. Experimental studies on trauma and metastasis
    formation. Acta Chir. Scand. Suppl. 391.
Skolnik, G., Alpsten, M. and Ivarsson, L., 1980a.The influence of
    trauma, dextran 1000 and dextran 40 on the lodgement of circulating
    tumour cells. Accepted for publ. in J. Cancer Res. and Clin. Oncology.
Skolnik, G., Alpsten, M. and Ivarsson, L., 1980b Studies on mechanisms
    involved in metastasis formation from circulating tumour cells.
    Factors influencing tumour cell lodgement during normal and post-
    traumatic conditions. Accepted for publ. in J. Cancer Res. and
    Clin. Oncology.
Warren, B.A. and Vales, O., 1972. The adhesion of thromboplastic tumour
    emboli to vessel walls in vivo. Br. J. Cancer 53:301-322.
Wood J:r, S., 1958. Pathogenesis of metastasis formation observed in
    vivo in the rabbit ear chamber. AMA Arch. Path. 66:550-569

CRITICAL ANALYSIS OF EXPERIMENTAL MODELS FOR THE ANTIMETASTATIC EFFECTS OF ANTICOAGULANTS

B. Maat and P. Hilgard

It is well established that anticoagulant drugs have antimetastatic action in some experimental tumour models. Many investigations have shown a significant reduction in the number of secondary tumour deposits in anticoagulated animals (Hilgard and Thornes, 1976). Most of the evidence was derived from experiments in which tumour cells were injected intravenously and the animals subsequently monitored for tumour deposits in the lungs. Reviewing the available literature, it becomes apparent that the number of lung colonies can be reduced by a variety of different anticoagulant drugs such as heparin, ancrod, coumarin-derivatives and others. One might question whether this type of intrapulmonary tumour should be regarded as a true representation of spontaneous metastases. The intravenous injection of tumour cells into an experimental animal does not differ substantially from an intrapulmonary transplantation and probably has little in common with the pathophysiology of blood-borne metastases originating from a solid primary tumour. A more realistic approach to screening for the antimetastatic effects of drugs would be to measure their effects on spontaneous lung metastases derived from transplanted solid tumours. A review of the current literature on this topic reveals that only coumarin derivatives consistently bring about a reduction in spontaneous metastases; all other drugs give variable results (Table 1.).

TABLE 1.

Effects of different anticoagulants on spontaneous animal tumour metastases. Summary of the literature from 1956-1980 (total of 25 publications).

drug	Number of papers demonstrating effect on metastases		
	decrease	no effect	increase
Heparin	3	2	4
Coumarins	12	–	–
Ancrod + Batroxobin	1	3	2

To clarify this rather confusing situation, we have performed experiments with both coumarin and non-coumarin anticoagulants to investigate whether drugs capable of producing a clear antitumour effect in i.v. tumour systems also reduce spontaneous metastases in a similar fashion.

Two tumour models were used throughout the study: the Lewis lung (3LL) carcinoma and the B16 melanoma. Subcutaneously growing tumours were produced by injection of concentrated cell suspensions containing one million viable cells, into the footpads of 12-week-old male C57BL/Rij mice.

Ancrod (Arvin®, Knoll A.G., Ludwigshafen) was administrated s.c. in a dose of 220 U.kg^{-1} body weight at 24-hour intervals during the course of the experiment. This resulted in a stable state of anticoagulation, which was monitored by determining plasma fibrinogen levels and whole blood clotting times.

Heparin was given s.c. in a dose of 1000 USP-units per kg body weight at 12-hour intervals. The dose was corrected daily according to the whole blood clotting time records; it was attempted to maintain this at least **twice** normal (8-10 min) throughout therapy.

Phenprocoumon was administered intraperitoneally in an initial dose of 2.5 mg/kg^{-1} body weight. A steady state of anticoagulation was then achieved by adding the drug to the drinking water in concentrations ranging from 2-5 mg/1^{-1}. The degree of anticoagulation was monitored by the Thrombotest method (Nyegaard, Oslo), as described earlier (Hilgard and Maat, 1979).

Results are given in Table 2; no significant differences were observed in ancrod and heparin treated animals, only phenprocoumon produced a significant decrease in metastases.

TABLE 2.

Effect of continued treatment with different anticoagulants on spontaneous lung metastases in tumour bearing mice.

tumour	anticoagulant	no of animals	no of metastases (av. ± s.e.)	significance
Lewis lung exp. I	ancrod	15	6.6 ± 0.1	N.S.
	contr.	14	7.1 ± 1.2	
Lewis lung exp. II	ancrod	16	3.2 ± 0.6	N.S.
	contr.	16	2.7 ± 0.5	
B-16 exp. I	ancrod	15	0.7 ± 0.2	N.S.
	contr.	16	0.9 ± 0.4	
B-16 exp. II	ancrod	14	4.4 ± 1.1	N.S.
	contr.	15	4.1 ± 0.8	
Lewis lung	heparin	18	20.8 ± 5.5	N.S.
	contr.	15	22.7 ± 7.7	
B-16	heparin	13	10.9 ± 1.4	N.S.
	contr.	15	12.2 ± 1.3	
Lewis lung	phenprocoumon	30	1.1 ± 0.2	$p < 0.005$
	contr.	30	7.3 ± 0.5	
B-16	phenprocoumon	17	1.2 ± 0.3	$p < 0.005$
	contr.	17	6.9 ± 0.6	

Combining the data obtained from the literature and the present experimental results, we arrive at the following summary (Table 3.).

TABLE 3.
The effect of various anticoagulants on lung tumour colonies/metastases.
(↓ = decrease;   - = no effect)

tumour	heparin	ancrod	coumarins
i.v.	↓	↓	↓
s.c.	-	-	↓

The explanation of the mechanism of action of these drugs with respect to their supposed antimetastatic properties now needs consideration. From a fundamental point of view, it is important to establish whether drugs which affect the coagulability of the blood also influence the development of metastases. The model of i.v. introduced tumour cells has long been used for studies on this topic and many anticoagulants are now considered as having antimetastatic properties; however, it has not been possible to prove that these drug-induced effects are directly related to the alterations in blood coagulability.

To assess the significance of experimental results and their possible future application in human pathology, the study model requires careful consideration. An i.v. injection of up to one million tumour cells within thirty seconds into an animal weighing approximately 20 g , is a highly artificial situation. In addition, when tumour cells are introduced to the circulatory system either as a result of injection or a surgical procedure, careful account must be taken of their distribution within the blood vessel. The extensive studies of Salsbury (1975) have shown that the relevance of circulating tumour cells in relation to the formation of metastases is disputable. With respect to the effect of anticoagulants on tumour dissemination, the validity of the concept of whether fibrin formation is of pathogenic importance during the initial phase of tumour cell lodgement requires re-evaluation. Many investigators have studied the role of activation of blood coagulation in the formation of metastases; their results, however, are largely contradictory. The description of thrombotic material around intravascular tumour cell emboli by some investigators was based on morphological observations in lung capillaries following the i.v. injection of a tumour cell suspension. In contrast, when blood-borne cancer cells originating from primary solid tumours were studied, the presence of fibrin in association with intravascular cancer cells was a rare finding (see Table 4.).

TABLE 4.

Literature review of studies concerned with the possible presence of fibrin
around circulating tumour cells at the stage of adherence.

author in favour of presence of fibrin	way of investigation[*]	source of tumour cells
Warren and Gates (1936)	LM	i.v.
Wood (1958)	LM	intra-arterial
Wood (1961)	LM	i.v.
Jones et al. (1971)	LM + IF + EM	i.v.
Chew et al. (1974)	LM + IF + EM	i.v.
Hilgard and Gordon-Smith (1974)	EM	i.v.
Chew and Wallace (1976)	LM + EM	i.v.
in favour of absence of fibrin		
Baserga and Safiotti (1955)	LM	s.c.
Ludatscher (1967)	LM + EM	s.c.
Jones et al. (1971)	LM + EM	i.v.
Cotmore and Carter (1973)	LM + EM	s.c.
Sindelar et al. (1975)	LM + EM	i.v.
Warren et al (1977)	scanning EM	primary tumour

[*]LM = light microscopy; EM = electron microscopy; IF= immunofluorescence
i.v. = intravenous; s.c. = subcutaneous

Thus, in studies on the role of blood coagulability in the development of
metastases, the experimental model using i.v. introduced tumour cells apparently
represents an entirely different situation from those studies where spontaneously
metastasising transplantable tumours are used. The present study provides conclusive evidence that the capacity of circulating malignant cells to form spontaneous
metastases was not influenced by most drugs having anticoagulant properties, with
the exception of the coumarin dervatives. Therefore, in investigations where the
effect of anticoagulants on metastases is studied, the choice of the experimental
model is crucial. Results of experiments where i.v. introduced tumour cells are
used cannot be extrapolated to those studies where spontaneously metastasising
solid tumours are employed, although both approaches are still considered to be
experimental models for the haematogeous spread of cancer.

Furthermore, the experimental data presented here once again confirm that
coumarin-derivatives have unique and exceptional properties as antimetastatic
drugs. As we have previously suggested, in i.v. studies, they exert their action
independently of the clotting mechanism (Hilgard and Maat, 1979) and, in spontaneously metastasising tumour systems among diverse anticoagulant drugs, only
coumarin-derivatives are active antimetastatic agents, even in an adjuvant
situation (Table 5.).

TABLE 5.

The antimetastatic effect of phenprocoumon (phen.) administration after amputation of the tumour bearing leg. (Results of 3 experiments, groups of 15 mice).

day of amputation	average number of metastases ± s.e. phen.	contr.	sign.
10	1.5 ± 0.5	3.7 ± 1.2	$p = 0.06$
14	2.9 ± 1.1	4.6 ± 1.1	$p = 0.1$
14	0.6 ± 0.2	1.5 ± 0.4	$p < 0.05$
15	2.1 ± 0.6	8.1 ± 2.3	$p < 0.05$
16	8.8 ± 1.3	16.2 ± 2.2	$p < 0.005$
19	8.8 ± 1.3	15.1 ± 3.4	$p < 0.05$

It is therefore apparent that coumarin-derivatives interfere with malignant tumour growth, but the exact mechanism is still not sufficiently understood. A chronological analysis of the mechanism of the antimetastatic effect clearly reveals that clotting factors can be completely excluded (Table 6).

TABLE 6.

Analysis of the mechanism of the phenprocoumon induced antimetastatic effect.

treatment	lung metastases	clotting capacity
Phenprocoumon	↓	impaired
Phenprocoumon + vit. K	=	normal
vit. K deficiency (diet)	↓	impaired
Phenprocoumon + deprived clotting factors	↓	normal
Phenprocoumon + carrageenan / silica	=	impaired

Among the postulated mechanisms of drug action are the interference with vitamin K dependent protein synthesis (Stenflo, 1976) and nonspecific stimulation of macrophages (Maat, 1980), as suggested by studies using macrophage inhibitors (Tables 7 and 8).

TABLE 7.

Effect of carrageenan on the reduction in spontaneous metastases induced by vitamin K-deficiency (Lewis lung carcinoma)

treatment	number of metastases (av ± s.e.)	significance
Controls (normal diet)	8.8 ± 2.8	$p < 0.05$
Vit. K def. diet	1.6 ± 0.4	$p < 0.05$
Vit. K def. diet + carrageenan	12.3 ± 3.7	

TABLE 8.

Average number of lung metastases (± s.e.) in tumour bearing mice treated with carrageenan (carr), Silica (Si) and/or Warfarin (Warf).

Treatment	No. of animals	No. of metastases
1. Control.	15	5.7 + 0.9
2. Carr	13	10.0 + 1.3
3. Warf + Carr	14	8.0 + 0.9
4. Si	14	6.2 + 1.1
5. Warf + Si	12	6.2 + 1.2
6. Warf	15	1.1 + 0.3

Significance : 1-2 $P < 0.05$ 1-6 $p < 0.05$ 3-6 $p < 0.01$ 5-6 $p < 0.05$
1-4 N.S. 2-3 N.S. 4-5 N.S.

What can be expected from the therapeutic effectiveness of anticoagulants in human tumour therapy on the basis of the relevant literature and the present experimental data ? We may not expect much effect from heparin and defibrinating agents but may do so for the coumarins. In a few clinical studies, anticoagulants have been used in adjuvant therapy in the management of cancer patients (Table 9).

These studies reveal that the therapeutic effectiveness of heparin has never been consistently demonstrated and this drug is widely being considered as ineffective in controlling human malignant disease. On the other hand, anticoagulants of the coumarin type have proven effectiveness in a variety of human cancers. On the basis of the given literature and the results of the present study, we suggest that spontaneously metastasising tumours represent a more valid approach to the study of coagulation factors in tumour dissemination. The discrepancy between therapeutic results obtained in lung colony assays and those obtained under clinical conditions casts serious doubts on the relevance of this experimental approach to the screening of antimetastatic drugs. The evaluation of anticoagulants for their potential value in tumour therapy should not be discouraged, provided that the investigations are pursued by using the appropriate experimental models.

In conclusion we feel that:
1. Results from studies with i.v. introduced tumour cells cannot be extrapolated to spontaneously metastasising tumours.
2. Spontaneously metastasising tumours represent the preferable model for the study of antimetastatic effects of anticoagulants.
3. There is little evidence supporting the concept of the pathogenic role of fibrin formation in the establishment of spontaneous metastases from blood-borne tumour cells.
4. Coumarin-derivatives are potent antimetastatic drugs; their mode of action appears to be independent of their anticoagulant activity.

TABLE 9.

Anticoagulation in the treatment of cancer. Clinical studies with heparin and warfarin.

author	tumour	drug	number of of patients	effect
Elias et al. 1972, 1973, 1974	inoper. lung	heparin + combi chemo	4 (no controls)	tumour regression in non-responders
Elias et al. 1975, 1976	inoper. lung metas.	heparin + combi chemo	2 x 14	chemo: progression after 2.5 courses hep. + chemo: 7/14 $>$ 50% regression after 2.2 courses
Elias et al. 1976	inoper. lung metas.	heparin + cyclo	19 (pilot study no controls)	1/19: part. response 18/19: no response
Rohwedder + Sagastume 1977	inoper. lung	heparin + combi chemo	16 (no controls)	3/16: part. response 13/16: no response
Groppe et al. 1977	metast. lung	heparin + combi chemo	21 (randomised)	no benefit of heparin survival time equal
Thornes 1975	miscell. (recurrent)	warfarin + chemo	2 x 64	2y. surv. rate chemo 11 (18%) chemo + warf 26 (41%) $p < 0.01$
Hoover et al. 1978	osteosa.	warfarin	30	5y. surv. rate amp. 14% amp. + warf 56%
Zacharski 1979	oat cell	warfarin + chemo	45	2 x increase median surv.

REFERENCES

Hilgard, P. and Thornes, R.D., 1976. Anticoagulants in the treatment of cancer. Eur. J. Cancer, 12: 755-762.

Hilgard, P. and Maat, B., 1979. The mechanism of lung tumour colony reduction caused by coumarin anticoagulation. Eur. J. Cancer, 15: 183-187.

Maat, B., 1980. Selective macrophage inhibition abolishes warfarin-induced reduction of metastases. Br. J. Cancer, 41: 313-316.

Stenflo, J., 1976. A new vitamin K-dependent protein purification from bovine plasma and preliminary characterization. J. Biol. Chem., 251: 355-363.

Complete references of quoted publications (Tables 4 and 9) can be obtained from the authors.

EFFECT OF FIBRINOLYSIS INHIBITION ON THE GROWTH AND HEMATOGENOUS DISSEMINATION OF CANCER

K. Tanaka, M. Kinjo, A. Iwakawa, H. Ogawa and N. Tanaka

INTRODUCTION

The coagulation-fibrinolysis system is considered to be an important factor in the growth and spread of tumors (Kodama, 1974; Kinjo, 1978). At the advancing border of the tumors, deposition of fibrin has been clearly demonstrated and was shown to be more prominent in tumors with high thromboplastic activity than in those with low activity (Kodama, 1978). On the other hand, a varying degree of fibrinolytic activity was found in cancer cells and fibrinolytic activity was also observed in small blood vessels at the advancing border of tumors (Tanaka, 1977). Fibrinolysis is considered to be related to resolution of fibrin depositing around the primary tumor and also around the arrested tumor cells in the vessels of target organs of hematogenous metastasis. Inhibition of fibrinolysis may lead to more prominent deposition of fibrin around the tumor and promote the development of a stromal reaction by the host against malignant growth and may also inhibit the release of cancer cells into the vessels. The present experiments were planned to elucidate the role of the coagulation-fibrinolysis system in the growth and spread of tumors and to examine the clinical applicability of antifibrinolytic agents.

MATERIALS

Tumor cells: Lewis lung carcinoma (3LL), Ehrlich carcinoma, QG56 (cell line established from human lung cancer) and NKPP1 (cell line established from human renal pelvic cancer). Animals: C57BL/6, BDF$_1$, SLC-ddy mice and nu-nu mice. Chemicals: trans-4 aminomethyl cyclohexane-1-carboxilic acid (t-AMCHA, Daiichi Pharmaceutical Co. Ltd., Tokyo); urokinase (UK, Mochida Pharmaceutical Co., Ltd., Tokyo); 5-fluorouracil (5-FU); cyclophosphamide (CY). Other chemicals were analytical grades.

METHODS

Lewis lung carcinoma cells were obtained as follows: Solid tumors 7 to 10 days after implantation were minced, disaggregated with trypsin and EDTA for 15 min., filtered with a stainless steel mesh, resuspended with fetal calf serum and washed twice with Hanks' balanced salt solution (HBSS). The tumor cells (1×10^6 to 5×10^5) were suspended in HBSS. Ehrlich carcinoma cells were harvested from mice which had been transplanted intraperitoneally 7 days prior to the experiments, and the cell number adjusted to $5 \times 10^5/0.2$ml. QG56 and NKPP1 obtained from nude mice were cut into small pieces, $2 \times 2 \times 2$mm, and were used for the experiments. Experimental designs were as follows. The tumor cells, $5 \times 10^5/0.2$ml, of 3LL and Ehrlich carcinoma were injected subcutaneously into BDF_1 and SLC-ddy mice respectively. The mice with tumors were divided into an untreated group and a group treated with 6-AMCHA, 1g/kg/day, per os. For human cancer, the cubes of QG56 and NKPP1 were subcutaneously trans- planted and the recipients divided into control and t-AMCHA-treated groups. Every group was evaluated for the size of the primary tumors and number of metastatic nodules in the lungs. To observe the effect of t-AMCHA on release of the tumor cells from the primary tumor, 5×10^5 cells of 3LL were injected subcutaneously into the foot pad. From one day before the 12 days after the tumor inoculation, 500mg/kg of t-AMCHA was administered orally twice a day. Some groups were given t-AMCHA-containing food. Experiments with UK treatment were also performed. Tumor bearing legs were amputated 10 to 12 days after the inoculation and mice were killed 18 to 25 days after the inoculation. The combined effects of t-AMCHA with 5-FU and CY on growth and metastasis were also studied. The influence of t-AMCHA or UK on the distribution of CY or 5-FU was studied using radiolabelled compounds. Primary tumors were also observed by light, immunofluorescent and electron microscopy to estimate fibrin deposition on a morphological basis.

RESULTS

1. Effects of t-AMCHA on the growth of tumor: The size of the tumors treated with t-AMCHA was significantly smaller than untreated controls in the experiment using 3LL and Ehrlich carcinoma (Table 1). Experiments with QG56 also showed significant inhibition of tumor growth

TABLE 1.
Effect of t-AMCHA on solid tumors[1]

| Tumor | Treatment | Tumor weight | | No. of pulmonary |
		Mean±SE(g)	T/C(%)	metastasis
Lewis lung carcinoma	Control	4.65±0.40	100	13.3±2.0
	t-AMCHA 1g/kg/day	3.80±0.40*	82	4.8±1.1*
Ehrlich carcinoma	Contral	5.51±1.19	100	0/10
	t-AMCHA 3g/kg/day	4.43±0.63	80	0/10

1) 18th day after s.c. inoculation of 5x10 cells of Lewis lung carcinoma/mouse
   35th day after s.c. inoculation of 5x10 cells of Ehrlich carcinoma/mouse

2. Effects of t-AMCHA and UK on metastasis: Pulmonary metastatic nodules were considerably decreased in the group treated with t-AMCHA, but increased in the group receiving UK trectment compared with untreated controls (Tables 1 and 2). When the 3LL cells were injected intravenously, a considerable increase in the number of pulmonary metastatic nodules was found in the group treated with t-AMCHA. No cytotoxic effect of t-AMCHA was noted in in vitro experiments with cultured human lung cancer cells.

TABLE 2
Influence of fibrinolysis inhibition and acceleration on cell release from primary tumors

Treatment[1]	No. of animals	Occurence of pulmonary mets.(%)	No. of pulmonary mets.[2]
Control	12	10/12 (83.3)	11.25±2.88
t-AMCHA	14	11/14 (78.6)	3.14±0.75*[3]
UK 500U/kg	12	12/12 (100.0)	34.41±3.48***
UK 10,000U/kg	12	12/12 (100.0)	38.42±2.61***

1) t-AMCHA was administered during the experiment and mean dosage/day was 3g/kg. UK was intravenously injected twice a day. Foot amputation on day 12. 2) mean ± S.E.
3) statistical significance by t-test vs. control. * : $p<0.05$,   *** : $P<0.001$.

3. Combined effects of t-AMCHA with CY and 5 FU: Administration of t-AMCHA tended to inhibit the tumor (Ehrlich carcinoma) growth when CY was administered simultaneously. Similar phenomena were also shown when 5-FU was administered to 3LL during t-AMCHA treatment (Table 3 & 4).

TABLE 3
Combined effect of t-AMCHA with cyclophosphamide(CY) on tumor growth of Ehrlich carcinoma 35 days after inoculation.

Treatment	No. of animals	Tumor weight(g)[1]	T/CY[2]
Control	10	5.51±1.19	
CY	10	0.31±0.17	100
t-AMCHA(-1d→)+CY	10	0.22±0.14	73
CY+t-AMCHA(8d→)	10	0.02±0.01	7
UK+CY	10	0.35±0.20	113

1) mean value±S.E.
2) mean tumor weight of treatment group/that of CY treated group; percentage.

4. Effects of t-AMCHA and UK on the distribution of CY or 5FU: Treatment with t-AMCHA showed no remarkable effects on the distribution of C^{14}-CY or C^{14}-5FU (Table 5 & 6).

5. Pathological observations: In immunofluorescent studies of fibrinogen, specific fluorescence surrounded each tumor cell. Electron microscopically, capillary endothelial cells were dissociated and tumor cells invaded capillary wall by digitation. Much fibrin was deposited around tumor cells invading the endothelial cells in groups treated with t-AMCHA, while little fibrin was found in untreated control or UK-treated groups.

TABLE 4
Combined effect of t-AMCHA with 5-FU on pulmonary metastasis of Lewis lung carcinoma 21 days after inoculation

Treatment	No. of animals	Positive rates	Metastatic foci[1] total No. (No. of large foci)	
Control	5	5/5	37.2±3.1	(20.6±4.3)
5-FU	5	3/5	1.6±0.7	(0.2±0.2)
5-FU+t-AMCHA(9d→)	5	3/5	2.4±1.4	(0)
t-AMCHA(-1d→)+5-FU	5	2/5	0.6±0.4	(0)
UK+5-FU	5	4/5	1.8±0.6	(0)
UK+5-FU+t-AMCHA(9d→)	5	3/5	0.8±0.4	(0)

1) mean value ± S.E.

TABLE 5

Tissue distribution of radioactivity after the injection of [14]c-Cyclophosphamide (CY) intraperitoneally in Ehrlich carcinoma bearing mice

Time after inoculation	1 week			5 weeks	
Tissues \ Treatment	μg/ml Whole blood	μg/g Cancer	μg/g Liver	μg/ml Whole blood	μg/g Cancer
CY	42.78±3.74	29.37±2.86	63.73±4.75	48.29±3.93	31.73±2.77
t-AMCHA[1]+CY	36.43±2.86	27.95±1.57[4] [1]	60.84±6.28[4] [2]	48.53±2.21	31.80±4.09
UK 200u/kg[2] +CY	39.54±1.94	32.96±2.14	66.88±4.25		
UK10,000u/kg[2] +CY	38.64±1.91	32.30±3.91	64.06±5.21	59.39±8.26	28.16±5.64
UK10,000u/kg[3] +CY	43.80±3.74	37.94±3.51*	74.65±3.70		

1) Feed containing 2.5% t-AMCHA during the experiment
2) UK was intravenously injected 0.5hr. before dosing of CY
3) UK was intravenously injected immediately before dosing of CY
4)-1 t-AMCHA concn. 15 65±3.60 μg/g of cancer
 -2 t-AMCHA concn. 39.93±3.25 μg/g of liver

DISCUSSION

The process of metastasis is closely related to coagulation and fibrinolysis beginning with the release of cells from the primary tumor. The processes following intravasation of tumor cells have been studied by many investigators using intravenous injection of tumor cells.

TABLE 6

Tissue distribution of radioactivity after the injection of C[14]-5-FU intraperitoneally in Lewis lung carcinoma bearing mice 10 days after inoculation

Treatment	TISSUE		
	Whole blood μg/ml	Cancer μg/g	Liver μg/g
5-FU[1]	46.79 ± 1.52	50.18±3.89	42.94±1.95
t-AMCHA[2] +5-FU	42.66 ± 1.18	43.79±1.83	38.68±1.38
UK10,000U/kg[3] +5-FU	49.35 ± 4.92	44.24±2.24	43.84±5.82

1) 40mg/kg of 5-FU was intraperitoneally injected on day 8, 9, and 10.
2) 2.5% of t-AMCHA in feed during the experiment.
3) UK was intravenously injected immediately before dosing of 5-FU.

On the other hand, few reports have been concerned with release of cells from the primary tumor. The present study was concerned with growth and intravasation of tumor cells in the development of metastasis. Peterson (1968) showed an inhibitory effect of anti-fibrinolysis with t-AMCHA on tumor growth and metastases of mammary carcinoma in syngeneic mice. In addition, Tanaka et al (1977) observed that administration of urokinase to rabbits with V_2 carcinoma enhanced tumor growth and metastasis, and concluded that thrombi associated with vascular invasion of tumor cells inhibited their release from the primary tumor. In the present study, anti-fibrinolytic treatment with t-AMCHA inhibited the growth of the primary tumor and prevented pulmonary metastases. On the other hand, UK treatment enhanced metastasis formation. Electron micro-scopy revealed fibrin around the tumor cells which were passing through the vessel wall when t-AMCHA was administered.   It was also shown that t-AMCHA did not change the distribution pattern of simul-taneously administered antitumor drugs such as 5-FU or CY. No cytotoxic effect of t-AMCHA was observed in _in vitro_ experiments with cultured human cancer cells. From these facts, t-AMCHA is thought to be a suitable agent in preventing growth and metastasis of tumors by means of antifibrinolysis.

REFERENCES

Kinjo, M., 1978. Lodgement and extravasation of tumor cells in blood-borne metastasis: An electron microscope study. Br.J.Cancer, 38:293-301.

Kodama, Y., 1974. Experimental studies on significance of coagulation-fibrinolysis system in growth and metastasis formation of rabbit V2 and V7 carcinomas. Fukuoka Acta Med., 65:941-966. (in Japanese)

Peterson, H.I., 1968. Experimental studies of fibrinolysis in growth and spread of tumor. Acta Chir. Scand., Suppl., 394:2-42.

Tanaka, K., Kohga, S., Kinjo, M. and Kodama, Y., 1977. Tumor metastasis and thrombosis, with special reference to thromboplastic and fibrinolytic activities of tumor cells. GANN Monograph on Cancer Res. 20:97-119.

MECHANISMS BEHIND THE INHIBITING EFFECT OF TRANEXAMIC ACID ON TUMOUR GROWTH AND SPREAD

H. Peterson and A. Sundbeck

INTRODUCTION

An inhibiting effect of antifibrinolytic drugs on tumour growth and spread has been found in several experimental studies (Rudenstam, 1967; Peterson, 1968; Hagmar, 1970; Verloes et al., 1978). Similar observations have also recently been reported in clinical studies with tranexamic acid – Cyklokapron[R], Kabi, Sweden – (Åstedt et al., 1977 a,b; Bramsen, 1978). In early experimental studies a significant inhibition of the growth rate and spontaneous pulmonary metastasis formation of transplantable mouse tumours was found after administration of tranexamic acid (Peterson, 1968). The inhibiting effect on spontaneous metastases by tranexamic acid was at variance with many previous studies in which an enhancing effect of antifibrinolytic drugs on the metastasis formation from intra-venously injected tumour cells had been reported (see Peterson, 1977). One explanation of the inhibiting effect of tranexamic acid on spontaneous metastases was a pronounced inhibition of tumour cell shedding from the primary tumour overshadowing an enhancing effect of tranexamic acid on tumour cell lodgement in the lungs.

The inhibiting effect of antifibrinolytic drugs on tumour growth was explained by different mechanisms. Thus, localization of fibrin to tumour tissue, as reported by O'Meara (1958) and primarily suggested to be a stroma for invasive growth, was later supposed to be part of a mechanism to delimit invasive tumour growth by "encapsulating" the tumour. Such a fibrin capsule might then be protected by induced antifibrinolysis (Peterson, 1968; Åstedt et al., 1977 a,b; Bramsen, 1978). However, in a series of experimental studies on tumour uptake of intravenously in-jected labelled fibrinogen, no evidence for a concentration of fibrinogen, transformed to fibrin, was found in tumour. On the other hand, a diffu-sion of labelled fibrinogen into tumour tissue was found, based on a high tumour capillary permeability for large protein molecules (see Peterson, 1977). In recent studies a direct influence of tranexamic acid on tumour cell growth in culture was found only with very high concentrations of the drug added to the substrate (Sundbeck, 1980).

Thus, the mechanisms behind the influence of tranexamic acid on tumour growth and spread are still not clarified and the aim of the studies

reported in this presentation was to further investigate possible mechanisms. This seemed to be of importance based on the possibility of tranexamic acid being used in tumour therapy.

TRANEXAMIC ACID AND PERI-OPERATIVE TUMOUR SPREAD

Based on the hypothesis that tranexamic acid might significantly inhibit the shedding of cells from tumours, the influence of tranexamic
acid on peri-operative intravascular tumour cell shedding was studied
(Peterson & Risberg, 1976). A standardized operative procedure with
total removal or biopsy of a sarcoma, transplanted intramuscularly into
one hindleg of inbred rats, was used. During this procedure, blood drained
through the lower caval vein from the operative area was collected and
injected intramuscularly into recipient animals. The outgrowth of secondary tumours in these animals was recorded and suggested to reflect the
per-operative shedding of tumour cells into blood in the operative area.
By this technique no influence of tranexamic acid on tumour cell shedding
was found. On the other hand, the shedding of cells from "large" tumours
was significantly higher than the shedding of cells from "small" tumours
during tumour biopsy. This suggested that an inhibiting influence on
spontaneous tumour metastases by tranexamic acid is not explained by a
direct effect on tumour cell shedding, but does probably follow a decreased
tumour growth rate.

TRANEXAMIC ACID AND TUMOUR GROWTH

Some possible mechanisms behind the inhibiting effect of tranexamic
acid on tumour growth rate, including an influence on tumour blood flow
or on tumour angiogenesis, were studied.

Influence of tranexamic acid on tumour blood flow.

This aspect was earlier studied by local Xenon-clearance technique in
two transplantable mouse tumours, based on observations of microthrombus
formation in tumour vessels (Peterson et al., 1969). No significant influence of tranexamic acid on local tumour blood flow was found. However,
a wide spread of local flow values were recorded based on the heterogen-
ous intra-tumour blood flow distribution (see Peterson, 1979) and this
complicated conclusions to be drawn from the results of this study.

The influence of tranexamic acid on the intra-tumour blood flow distribution studied by intra-tumour uptake of ^{86}Rb according to Sapirstein
(see Appelgren, 1979) has now been investigated (Sundbeck, 1980). In
these studies the intra-tumour distribution of ^{86}Rb, by the technique

used reflecting the intra-tumour distribution of cardiac output (presented as % of given amount of ^{86}Rb / gram tissue), showed a change towards
lower ^{86}Rb (tumour blood flow) values in animals given tranexamic acid.
This change was, however, not statistically significant ($p < 0.10 > 0.05$).
A cumulative frequency distribution diagram of the results is presented
in Fig. 1.

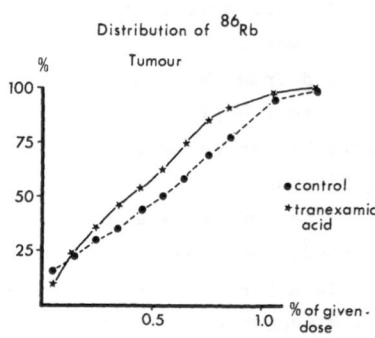

Fig. 1. Intra-tumour blood flow distribution recorded as percentual uptake of intravenously injected ^{86}Rb/gram tissue. Cumulative frequency
distribution diagram, which shows the tendency towards lower values
(lower blood flow) in animals given tranexamic acid.

Influence of tranexamic acid on tumour vascularization.

The vascularization of tumours (tumour angiogenesis) has been the
focus for many studies during the last years (see Warren, 1979). A
tumour angiogenesis factor has been isolated. Fibrin has been suggested
to be a stroma for tumour vascularization and even if no active localization of fibrin in tumours was found in our studies (Peterson, 1977),
these observations directed our interest at a possible influence of tranexamic acid on tumour angiogenesis.

A transplantable rat sarcoma was studied, inplanted into the tibialis anterior muscle of one hindleg of rats. Control animals and animals given
tranexamic acid intraperitonally in a dose of 200 mg/100 gram B.W. once
daily were studied by microangiography 5 days after tumour transplantation.

The technique was previously described by Kjartansson (1976) and included ink perfusion and subsequent Spalteholz preparation. Some sections are shown in Fig. 2. In control tumours numerous vascular connections were found between tumour and muscle, and a rather prominent "vascular reaction" was also found in muscle. In tranexamic acid treated tumours a sparse vascular reaction was found in muscle and a rather marked limitation between tumour and muscle.

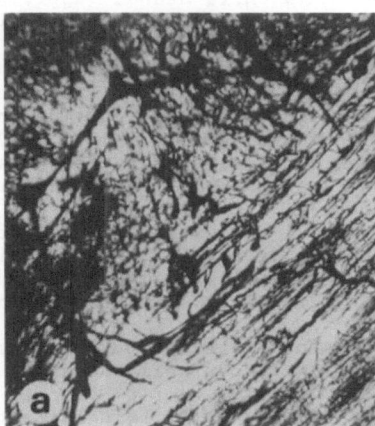 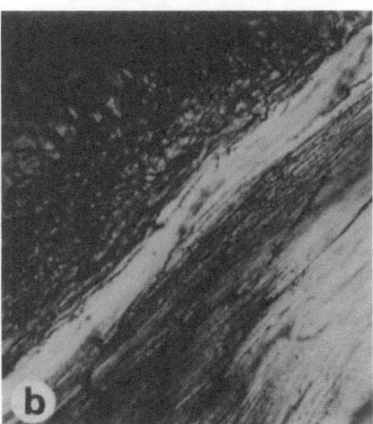

Fig. 2. Microangiographic specimens from intramuscularly transplanted control tumour and tumour from animal given tranexamic acid. Note the frequent vascular connections between tumour and muscle in the control specimen compared with the more marked limitation between tumour and muscle in tumour from animal given tranexamic acid. Control to the left.

CONCLUSIONS

An inhibiting effect of tranexamic acid on spontaneous metastasis formation is probably not explained by a direct effect on tumour cell shedding but by an inhibition of primary tumour growth followed by decreased metastasis formation. The direct influence of tranexamic acid on tumour growth might be explained by an inhibition of tumour angiogenesis. Thus, an inhibited vascularization of tumour might be followed by a decreased metastasis formation.

REFERENCES

Appelgren, L., 1979. Methods of recording tumour blood flow. In: Tumor
    Blood Circulation. Ed. H.-I. Peterson. CRC Press, Inc., Boca Raton.
Åstedt, B., Glifberg, I., Mattsson, W. & Tropé, C., 1977. Arrest of growth
    of ovarian tumour by AMCA. JAMA. 238: 154-157.
Åstedt, B., Mattsson, W. & Tropé, C., 1977. Treatment of advanced breast
    cancer with chemotherapeutics and inhibitor of coagulation and fibri-
    nolysis. Acta Med. Scand. 201: 491-495.
Bramsen, T., 1978. Effect of tranexamic acid on chorioidal melanoma. Acta
    ophthalmologica 56: 264-270.
Hagmar, B., 1970. Experimental tumour metastases and blood coagulability.
    Acta Pathol. Microbiol. Scand. Suppl. 211.
Kjartansson, I., 1976. Tumour circulation. Acta Chir. Scand. Suppl. 471.
O'Meara, R.A.Q., 1968. Fibrin formation and tumour growth. Thromb. Diath.
    Haemorrh. Suppl. 28, 137.
Peterson, H.-I., 1968. Experimental studies on fibrinolysis in growth and
    spread of tumour. Acta Chir. Scand. Suppl. 394.
Peterson, H.-I., 1977. Fibrinolysis and antifibrinolytic drugs in the
    growth and spread of tumours. Cancer Treatment Reviews. 4: 213-217.
Peterson, H.-I., 1979. Tumor Blood Circulation. Angiogenesis, Vascular
    Morphology and Blood Flow of Experimental and Human Tumors. CRC Press,
    Inc., Boca Raton.
Peterson, H.-I., Appelgren, K.L., Rudenstam, C.-M. & Lewis, D.H., 1969.
    Studies on the circulation of experimental tumours. I. Effect of in-
    duced fibrinolysis and antifibrinolysis on capillary blood flow and
    the capillary transport function of two experimental tumours in the
    mouse. Europ. J. Cancer 5: 91-97.
Peterson, H.-I. & Risberg, B., 1976. Experimental studies on the effect
    of induced antifibrinolysis on peroperative tumour cell shedding. Z.
    Krebsforsch. 86: 121-125.
Rudenstam, C.-M., 1967. Effect of fibrinolytic and antifibrinolytic thera-
    py on the dissemination of experimental tumours. Bibl. anat. 9: 418-
    424.
Sundbeck, A., 1980. Tumour growth inhibition by tranexamic acid. To be
    publ. as suppl. to Acta Chir. Scand.
Verloes, R., Atassi, G., Dumont, P. & Kanarek, L., 1978. Tumour growth
    inhibition by trypsin inhibitor or urokinase inhibitors. Europ. J.
    Cancer 14: 23-31.
Warren, B.A., 1979. Tumor angiogenesis. In: Tumor Blood Circulation. Ed.
    H.-I. Peterson. CRC Press, Inc., Boca Raton.

THE INHIBITORY EFFECT OF SULFATED POLYSACCHARIDES, ANCROD OR TRANEXAMIC ACID ON PULMONARY METASTASES IN ANIMALS

T. Yamashita, Y. Higuchi and E. Tsubura

The pathogenesis of tumor metastasis is a complicated process which depends on the interaction of tumor cells with their host. Various host factors such as hemodynamics, blood coagulation, fibrinolysis, platelet systems or host defense mechanism may contribute to the metastasis formation. Many observations have pointed out an association between metastasis and blood coagulation, notably the frequent ocurrence of thrombi around embolic tumor cells and further intravascular coagulation. At an early stage of blood-borne metastasis, intravascular coagulation is the most important mechanism for the attachment of tumor cells to the capillary endothelium. In order to inhibit blood-borne metastases, we attempted to find more reliable antimetastatic agents through experimental models of blood-borne pulmonary metastases in rats or mice. The inhibitory effect of several sulfated polysaccharides, ancrod or tranexamic acid on metastases were examined, and their inhibitory mechanism is discussed from the viewpoint of the blood coagulation-fibrinolysis system.

Inhibition of Pulmonary Metastases by Sulfated Polysaccharides in Rats The sulfated polysaccharides tested were xylan sulfate $(3-4 \times 10^3 \text{Mw}$, S content:18%, XS), dextran sulfate $(6-7 \times 10^3$, S:18%, DS), chondroitin polysulfate $(6-7 \times 10^3$, S:15%, CPS), chondroitin sulfate $(30-40 \times 10^3$, S:6%, CSN) and glucose polysulfate (ca 360, S:18%, GPS). We screened the antimetastatic effect of these compounds on intravenously induced pulmonary metastases in rats. The animals used were 8 to 10-week-old female Donryu strain rats, weighing about 100g. The tumor used was rat ascites hepatoma AH-109A. The anticoagulative and fibrinolytic activities of sulafated polysaccharides reached a maximum in the plasma 1 hr. after intraperitoneal injection.

The inhibitory effect of these compounds were evaluated 2 weeks after tumor inoculation by counting the numbers of metastatic nodules on the pulmonary surface. A dose of 100 mg/kg of XS and DS strongly inhibited the development of pulmonary metastases; CPS was less inhibitory, and CSN and GPS were not inhibitory. The inhibition of pulmonary metastases by sulfated polysaccharides depended on dose and time of their injections (Tsubura et al., 1976). However, the

injections of XS once daily from third to seventh day after tumor
inoculation had no inhibitory effect. Therefore, these compounds
seemed to act at a very early stage of blood-borne metastases.

   *Correlation Between Antimetastatic and Anticoagulative, Fibrino-
lytic Activity of Sulfated Polysaccharides*   The coagulative activity of blood was measured by determining whole blood clotting time,
partial thromboplastin time, prothrombin time and thrombin time.
We examined the anticoagulative activities of three sulfated polysaccharides, XS, CPS and CSN having strong, weak, and no inhibitory
effect on metastases, respectively. The anticoagulative activity of
XS was most potent and closely dose-dependent. The anticoagulative
activity of CPS was less than that of XS. CSN had no detectable
effect. These results indicate that the antimetastatic activity of
sulfated polysaccharides can be correlated with their anticoagulative
activity.

   We then investigated the effect of the 3 compounds on blood
coagulation factors. The surface contact factors, factor XII (Hage-
man factor) and factor XI (plasma thromboplastin antecedent) were
markedly inactivated in the plasma from the rats injected with XS.
Moderate inactivation of factors II, V, VII, VIII, IX and X were
also noted. On the other hand, marked inactivation of factor XI and
XII, and moderate inactivation of factor VIII were noted in the plasm.
of rats injected with CPS. CSN did not cause any inactivation. These
results indicate that the inactivation of the intrinsic coagulation
factor, particularly the surface contact factors was also closely
related to the inhibition of blood-borne metastases.

   The time course of changes in fibrinolytic activity in the blood
of rats after injection of these compounds was measured as the euglobulin clot-lysis time and fibrinolysis on a fibrin plate. XS had the
strongest fibrinolytic activty of three compounds. CPS prolonged only
the euglobulin clot-lysis time. CSN did not show any activity.

   *Effect of XS on Pulmonary Metastases and Survival of Rats Bearin₍
Different Tumor Strains*   Biological characteristics of tumor strain:
play an important role in determining metastases. Three types of ascites hepatomas, AH-109A, AH-130 or AH-100B having different cell deformability were used. AH-109A cells are highly deformable; AH-100B are
slightly deformable, and AH-130 are moderatedly deformable (Sato and
Suzuki, 1976). The inhibition of pulmonary metastases by XS was almos·
similar, but the survuval in rats was quite different in each strain.
Marked prolongation of survival was observed in XS-treated rats bearing ascites hepatomas, AH-100B or AH-130. On the other hand,

the rats bearing AH-109A did not survive longer than the controls. AH-100B with low deformability were easily trapped in the pulmonary capillaries. The escaped cells from the lung tended to die in post-pulmonary circulation. On the other hand, AH-109A cells being highly deformable, survived better in the postpulmonary circulation. This evidence resulted in longer survival in XS-treated rats bearing AH-100B or AH-130 (Tsubura et al., 1977).

Combined Effect of XS and Cyclophosphamide on Pulmonary Metastases We attempted combined anticancer chemotherapy with cyclophosphamide (CY) against intravenously induced pulmonary metastases to study adjuvant chemotherapeutic usefulness of XS. A dose of 100 mg/kg of XS was injected intraperitoneally into C57BL/6 mice 1 hr. before Lewis lung tumor (3LL) inoculation. 50 mg/kg of CY was injected intraperitoneally 3 days after tumor inoculation. Significant prolongation of survival was observed in mice treated with combined therapy, compared with that in mice received each treatment alone.

Subsequently, the inhibitory effect of XS on spontaneous pulmonary metastases was studied in mice implanted 3LL into foot pads. A dose of 30 mg/kg of XS was injected into mice twice a day from third to seventh day. Primary tumor was removed on eighth day after tumor implantation. We obtained the inhibitory effect of XS on spontaneous metastases as well as intravenously induced metastases.

Effects of Ancrod or Tranexamic Acid on Pulmonary Metastases For the purpose of investigating the role of fibrinogen on tumor growth and metastases, we studied the effect of defibrinogenation with snake venom enzyme, ancrod or antifibrinolysis with tranexamic acid (t-AMCHA) on 3LL in mice.

Significant reduction of intravenously induced pulmonary metastases was observed in mice with 200 NIH units/kg of ancrod once intraperitoneally 1 hr. before tumor inoculation. Plasma fibrinogen level decreased to the extent of a trace in the first 4 hr. and 55 mg/dl in 12 hr. after intraperitoneal injection of 200 units/kg. FDP level increased to 100 μg/ml in 1 hr. and declined to 2 μg/ml within 24 hr. The inhibition of spontaneous pulmonary metastases was also observed in mice treated with same dose of ancrod twice daily for the period after removal of primary tumor, day 15 to 22. Plasma fibrinogen level in mice bearing tumor tended to increase, and reached its highest level three days after surgical resection of primary tumor. We only observed a slight prolongation of survival with ancrod. However, 40% of mice treated by combined chemotherapy with CY and ancrod survived much longer than the others.

Tumor growth of 3LL in the foot pad was inhibited in mice injected 1.0g/kg of tranexamic acid for 12 days before removal of primary tumor. In this condition, reduction of pulmonary metastatic nodules was observed. However, no inhibitory effect was obtained on intravenously induced pulmonary metastases.

DISCUSSION

Intravascular thrombus formation around embolic tumor cells in metastatic sites have been confirmed by many investigators since Wood's microcinematographical observations (1958). Sato (1967) emphasized that changes in microcirculatory hemodynamics occurred after intravasation of tumor cells and that the tumor cells then became attached to injured endothelium, forming an extravascular tumor growth. From these morphological observations, it seems likely that intravascular coagulation is important at the early stage of tumor lodgement in capillary beds. It is thought that the mechanism of intravascular coagulation in an early stage of metastasi works as follows: 1) obstruction of blood flow by tumor cell emboli, 2) release of tissue thromboplastin from the injured endothelium, 3) activation of contact factors by tumor cells, and 4) activation of the extrinsic coagulation system or factor X by tumor cells.

Sulfated polysaccharides tested are acid polysaccharides, which are the socalled heparinoids and have O-sulfate groups. The difference in chemical properties of these compounds is due to difference in their chemical structure, molecular weight, sulfur content and polyanionic properties. The biological activities of these compounds have not been fully clarified but they seem to inhibit blood clotting at three stages of the coagulation mechanism, namely inhibition of thromboplastin generation, thrombin formation and antithrombin activity. Our important finding was that the inhibitory effect of these compounds on pulmonary metastases was well correlated with their anticoagulative and fibrinolytic activitie Another significant finding was that xylan sulfate showed the inhibitory effect on spontaneous pulmonary metastases. It might be useful in clinical medicine that combined therapy with xylan sulfate and cyclophosphamide prolonged the survival of mice with pulmonary metastases.

Our general conclusion is that the defibrinogenating agent ancrod inhibits metastatic growth in the lung after removal of primary tumor, and conversely the antifibrinolytic agent tranexamic acid inhibits pulmonary metastases based on a reduction of release of tumor cells due to inhibition of primary tumor.

CONCLUSION

The blood coagulation-fibrinolysis system might play a major role in the tumor cell attachment. We showed that intrinsic anticoagulants such as sulfated polysaccharides acted on the inhibition of tumor cell attachment due to the inactivation of surface contact factors in the blood clotting mechanism. The antifibrinolytic state in the host brought about the inhibition of development of pulmonary metastases based on regression of primary tumor, whereas the defibrinogenating state resulted in the inhibition of growth of metastatic foci.

REFERENCES

Sato, H., 1967. Cancer metastasis, from pathological studies on ascites tumors. Trans. Soc. Pathol. Jpn., 56: 9-36.
Sato, H. and Suzuki, M., 1976. Deformability and viability of tumor cells by transcapillary passage, with reference to organ affinity of metastasis in cancer. In Fundamental Aspects of Metastasis, edited by L. Weiss, pp. 311-317, North-Holland, Amsterdam.
Tsubura, E., Yamashita, T., Kobayashi, M. and Higuchi, Y., 1976. Effect of sulfated polysaccharides on blood-borne pulmonary metastasis in rats. Gann, 67: 849-856.
Tsubura, E., Yamashita, T. and Higuchi, Y., 1977. An inhibitory mechanism of blood-borne metastasis by sulfated polysaccharides. In Cancer Invasion and Metastasis: Biologic Mechanisms and Therapy, edited by S.B. Day et al., pp. 367-381, Raven Press, New York.
Wood, S., Jr., 1958. Pathogenesis of metastasis formation observed in vivo in the rabbit ear chamber. Arch. Pathol., 66: 550-568.

PROSTACYCLIN AS A MARKER FOR DIAGNOSING AND STAGING CARCINOMA OF THE PROSTATE

O. Khan, C.N. Hensby, H.D. Mitcheson and G. Williams

Introduction

Prostaglandins can increase tumour dissemination (Stein-Werblovsky, 1974). This clinical study was designed to determine the relationship between prostaglandins and prostatic disease.

Patients and Methods

Prostacyclin 6-oxo-PGF$_{1\alpha}$ levels were measured in 17 healthy volunteers, 17 patients with benign prostatic hyperplasia (B.P.H.) 7 patients with cancer of the prostate initially misdiagnosed as B.P.H., and 58 patients with confirmed cancer of the prostate. Of the 58 patients with known cancer 6 had stage T_{1-4} M_o disease (UICC, 1978) and were untreated, 24 had stage T_{1-4} M_o disease and had received treatment, 4 had stage T_{1-4} M_1 and were untreated and 24 had stage T_{1-4} M_1 and had received treatment.

Uncuffed venous blood samples were taken into cold lithium heparin tubes containing indomethacin, centrifuged immediately and the plasma stored at -20°C until assay.

Prostaglandin assay

Prostaglandins in tissue, plasma and urine were assayed using gas chromatography and mass spectrometry.

Statistics

Groups were compared using Student's t test for unrelated data.

Results

Seven prostanoids were identified in 13 specimens of prostate (Histopathology malignant in 7, benign in 6). The only prostanoid present in all 13 specimens was 6-oxo-PGF$_{1\alpha}$, a prostacyclin hydration product of PG I$_2$. 6-oxo-PGF$_{1\alpha}$ was thereafter selectively studied.

The mean level of 6-oxo-PGF$_{1\alpha}$ in healthy volunteers was 98.4 ± 4.24
pg/ml (Fig. 1). Patients with B.P.H. also had normal levels, mean of
107 ± 8.25 pg/ml. Patients treated T$_{1-4}$ M$_0$ prostatic cancer had
significantly increased levels with a mean of 182 ± 13.87 pg/ml (p < 0.01),
and there was a further increase in those with metastatic disease
(T$_{1-4}$ M$_1$), with a mean of 221 ± 10.21 pg/ml. The 7 patients with cancer
who were initially misdiagnosed as B.P.H. had abnormal levels (indicated
by ▲ in Fig. 1).

The level of 6-oxo-PGF$_{1\alpha}$ tended to be higher in untreated cancer patients
(Fig. 2, open circles = untreated patients).

In 6 cancer patients 6-oxo-PGF$_{1\alpha}$ was compared to the prostatic fraction
of serum acid phosphatase (tartrate labile fraction, T.L.F.). When these
patients had T$_{1-4}$ M$_0$ disease the T.L.F. was within normal limits but 5 of
the 6 had abnormal 6-oxo-PGF$_{1\alpha}$ levels (Fig. 3). After disease progression
to T$_{1-4}$ M$_1$ (Fig. 4), 3 of the 6 had elevated T.L.F. and all 6 had abnormal
6-oxo-PGF$_{1\alpha}$ which was significantly increased (p < 0.01).

Fig. 5 shows the progress of 12 patients with prostatic cancer. As the
disease progressed and bony metastases occurred (change from bone scan
negative to positive) the levels of 6-oxo-PGF$_{1\alpha}$ increased. Eight patients
treated with orchidectomy had a symptomatic response and their levels fell.
When the disease relapsed levels again increased.

Discussion

Prostaglandins may be associated with the spread of certain tumours,
(Stein-Werblovsky, 1974; Bennett et al, 1977). PG I$_2$, which can induce
bone resorption, is labile and readily breaks down to 6-oxo-PGF$_{1\alpha}$ and
this was the prostanoid present in all the specimens of prostatic tissue
that we examined.

Patients with benign disease had plasma levels of 6-oxo-PGF$_{1\alpha}$ within
the normal range, whereas those with prostatic cancer had increased
levels. Levels were higher in untreated patients and there was a further
increase with disease progression. Interestingly 7 patients initially
misdiagnosed as having B.P.H. had elevated levels, and all 7 were
subsequently found to have malignant change.

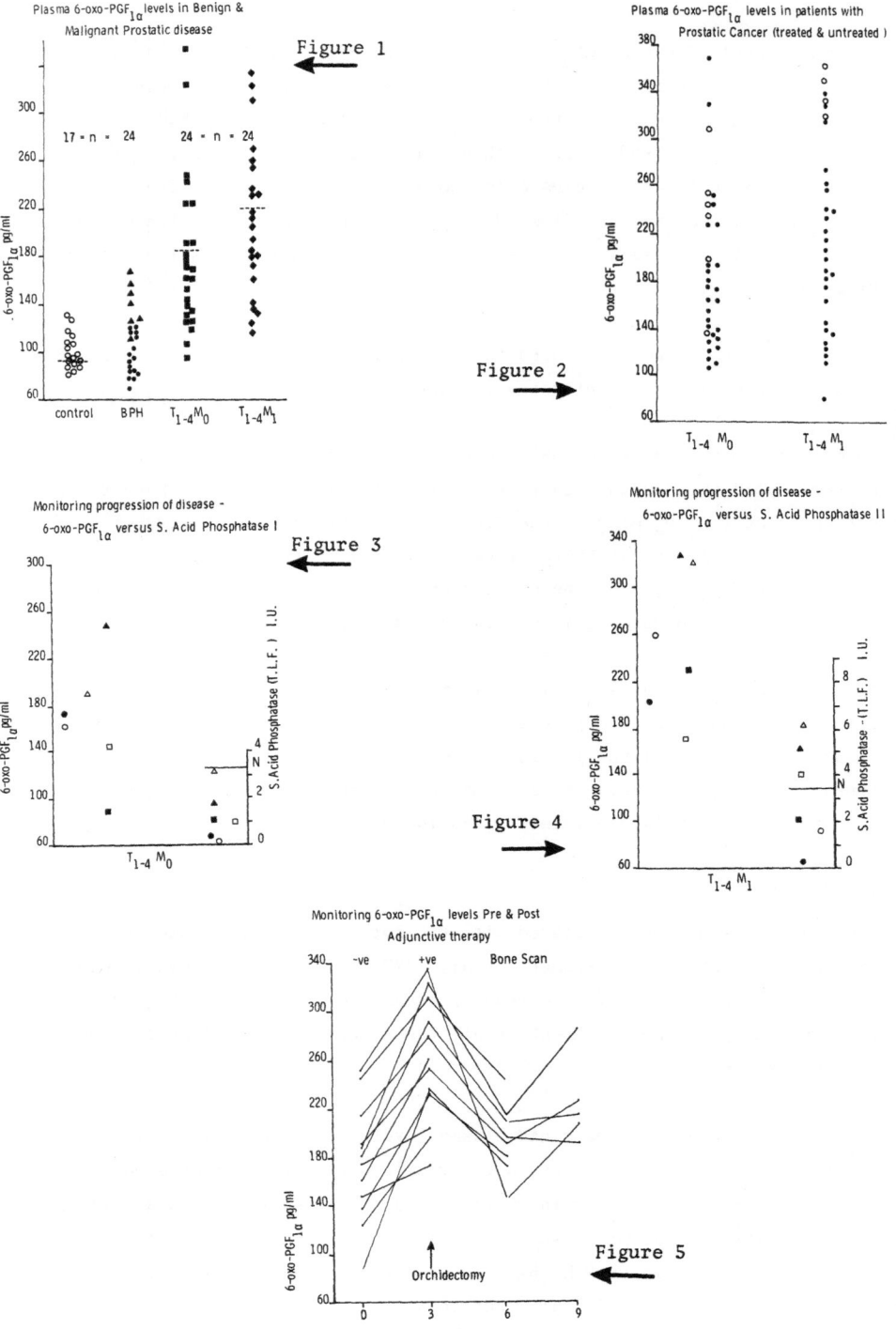

Plasma 6-oxo-PGF$_{1\alpha}$ levels in Benign & Malignant Prostatic disease

Figure 1

Plasma 6-oxo-PGF$_{1\alpha}$ levels in patients with Prostatic Cancer (treated & untreated)

Figure 2

Monitoring progression of disease – 6-oxo-PGF$_{1\alpha}$ versus S. Acid Phosphatase I

Figure 3

Monitoring progression of disease – 6-oxo-PGF$_{1\alpha}$ versus S. Acid Phosphatase II

Figure 4

Monitoring 6-oxo-PGF$_{1\alpha}$ levels Pre & Post Adjunctive therapy

Figure 5

The levels correlated well with clinical progession and response to
adjunctive therapy. Furthermore 6-oxo-PGF$_{1\alpha}$ was a more sensitive tumour
marker than the tartrate labile fraction of serum acid phosphatase.
We conclude that 6-oxo-PGF$_{1\alpha}$ is a sensitive and accurate tumour marker
for cancer of the prostate.

References

1. Stein-Werblovsky R.
   The Effect of Prostaglandin on Tumour Implantation
   Experientia. 30, p.p. 957-959, 1974.

2. U.I.C.C. (Union Internationale Contre le Cancer)
   T.N.M. Classification of Malignant Tumours
   Third Edition, Geneva, 1978.

3. Bennett A, McDonald A.M., Stamford I.F., Charlier E.M., Simpson J.S.,
   Zebro T.
   Prostaglandins and Breast Cancer
   Lancet ii, p.p. 624-626, 1977.

Acknowledgements

We wish to thank Professor C.T.Dollery and the Department of Clinical
Pharmacology for their co-operation with this study.

PROSTAGLANDINS AND METASTASIS

M.J. Tisdale

The prostaglandins are ubiquitous tissue hormones which are bio
synthesized from essential unsaturated fatty acids such as arachidon
acid in response to a variety of stimuli, and rapidly inactivated by
catabolic enzymes.   Many tumours particularly medullary carcinoma
of the thyroid and other amine peptide-secreting tumours produce
important quantities of prostaglandins which give rise to some of th
clinical symptoms such as attacks of flushing and diarrhoea (1).
Other carcinomas whether primary or secondary also produce prostaglandins (2).   The primary prostaglandins produced are of the E series
particularly PGE$_2$.   It is interesting to note that many of the
changes associated with prostaglandins are in fact diametrically
opposite to those that take place during tumour growth (2).

(a)   While PGE's promote morphological differentiation of malignant
      cells, dedifferentiation is a characteristic feature of maligna
      transformation.

(b)   Prostaglandins particularly of the E series inhibit tumour grow
      (3) and may actually act to restrain growth of some tumours
      since low doses of indomethacin, an inhibitor of the prosta-
      glandin synthetase complex, stimulate tumour growth.

Human malignant breast tumours synthesize more prostaglandins
than normal breast tissue from the same patient or benign neoplasms
(4).   Rolland et.al. (5) have recently been studying prostaglandin
production in human breast cancer and found that a high prostaglandi
production was associated with the presence of neoplastic cells in
tumour lymphatic and blood vessels and in axillary lymph nodes.   The
found that prostaglandin production by node metastases was always
higher than that by primary tumour sites.   The analysis of the strom
reaction and the presence of oedema and necrosis suggested that an
active prostaglandin synthesis occurred in lesions in which the tumo
cell surroundings presented characteristics of low resistance to
invasive growth of cancer cells.   Evidence was presented that prosta

glandin production occurs early in the natural course of breast
cancer and that prostaglandin production is elevated in tumours at
a time when active tumour invasion proceeds. By contrast prostaglandin production decreases later in the course of tumour development.

Bone metastases are associated with tumours having high levels
of prostaglandins (4). Also breast tumours from patients with bone
metastases contain and can synthesize more prostaglandins than those
from patients with no metastases. This suggests that some malignant
cells become established in bone by first releasing a prostaglandin
which causes bone resorption. Low concentrations of PGE and PGF lead
to resorption of bone tissue culture and osteolysis effected in vitro
by breast carcinomas can be inhibited by asprin (6), also an inhibitor
of prostaglandin synthetase. Bone resorption produced by a transplantable mouse fibrosarcoma has been shown to be due to production
of PGE_2 (7). Administration of indomethacin to tumour-bearing mice
lowers serum calcium and PGE_2 concentrations, reduces in parallel the
tumour content of bone-resorption-stimulating activity and PGE_2 and
diminishes tumour size. Inhibition of prostaglandin synthesis by
indomethacin reduces bone metastases in rats and rabbits.

Many observations point to an association between metastases and
blood coagulation notably the frequent occurrence of thrombi around
embolic tumour cells and further the intravascular coagulation and
other haematological disorders in many patients with disseminated
cancer. Cancer cells display a tendency to stick to the vascular
endothelium. Platelets may aggregate on such sticky cancer cells and
such a mass attaches more readily to the endothelium. Once tumour
cells are attached, the cross-section of the small vessels is diminished thus obstructing blood flow. Turbulence results behind the
obstruction. Thrombocytes and leucocytes are attracted to this turbulence and preferably aggregate there and within minutes they become
enmeshed in a fibrin clot.

A number of studies on metastasis have been conducted with the
B16 melanoma. Fitzpatrick and Stringfellow (8,9) have recently shown
that B16 malignant melanoma cell lines transform arachidonic acid and
its transient metabolite the prostaglandin endoperoxide PGH_2 into PGD_2.

The highly metastatic B16 F_{10} formed less PGD_2 compared with the moderately metastatic B16 F_1. Since platelet aggregation may be one factor involved in B16 metastasis and since PGD_2 inhibits platelet aggregation this prostaglandin could affect the outcome of platelet-tumour interactions which may contribute ultimately to metastases. This suggests that qualitative and quantitative aspects of arachidor acid metabolism may be one of the inherent biochemical properties of the tumour cell that can affect metastases. Thus B16 F_1 cells metastasize less easily because they release sufficient PGD_2 to resi the formation of platelet-tumour emboli which could arrest them in pulmonary capillary beds. Conversely B16 F_{10} cells may metastasize more easily because they release insufficient PGD_2 to resist the formation of platelet-tumour emboli. After treatment of the cells with indomethacin in vitro and subsequent injection into mice both B16 F_1 and B16 F_{10} metastasis increased noticeably and there was a normalisation of metastatic differences between the two cell lines (9). Injection of PGD_2 reversed and decreased indomethacin-enhancec metastasis threefold.

Recent results suggest that human platelet aggregation is controlled by the "reciprocal regulation" of cyclic AMP levels in th platelet by the endoperoxide-thromboxane A_2 (T x A_2) system which leads to inhibition of adenylate cyclase and the stimulation of adenylate cyclase by prostacyclin (PGI_2) (10). As PGI_2 is a potent inhibitor of platelet aggregation it could be used for the local vascular regulation of thrombolic events, particularly in the presence of a phosphodiesterase inhibitor such as dipyridamole or theophylline. Moncada and Korbut (11) have established that the action of the phosphodiesterase inhibitors is mainly dependent on the presence of circulating endogenous PGI_2. Low concentrations of circulating PGI_2 will gently stimulate the production of platelet cyclic AMP. A combination of a T x A_2 synthetase inhibitor such as imidazole (12) or 9,11-iminoepoxyprosta-5,13-dienoic acid (13) and a phosphodiesterase inhibitor would have a more effective anti-thrombotic action than a combination with asprin because it

would leave endoperoxides from platelets available for the vessel
wall to synthesize PGI_2.

Lipid peroxides and their methyl esters are strong and selective
inhibitors of the formation of PGI_2. Lipid peroxidation induced by
free radical formation is known to occur in several pathological
conditions and could occur during radiation therapy. In some
experimental systems irradiation of a transplanted tumour has enhanced its metastatic spread (14) and there is evidence that prior
irradiation of tissues such as the lungs, liver and kidneys may
render these tissues more susceptible to metastatic involvement when
tumour cells are subsequently injected (15). If such metastatic
spread occurs in humans after irradiation it could be due to an enhanced platelet aggregation and could be prevented by the administration of antioxidants such as vitamin E.

If prostaglandins and PGI_2 play a role in metastasis then diet
could have an effect. Eicosapentaenoic acid gives the trienoic
prostaglandins, the antiaggregating Δ^{17} prostacyclin (PGI_3) and
$T \times A_3$ which is not proaggregatory (16). Thus the use of this fatty
acid could afford a dietary protection against tumour spread.
Indeed it has been suggested that the low incidence of myocardial
infarction in Eskimos and their increased tendency to bleed could be
due to the high eicosapentaenoic acid and low arachidonic acid content
of their diet and consequently of their tissue lipids.

Another way in which prostaglandins may facilitate tumour cell
metastasis is by subversion of the immune system. PGE_2 is immunosuppressive and indomethacin and asprin which inhibit prostaglandin
synthetase block the immunosuppressive activity of tumour cells (17).
Administration of indomethacin to immunologically competent mice at
the time they were inoculated with Moloney sarcoma virus prevented
the development of tumours (18). The fact that indomethacin was
effective only in immunologically competent mice argues against
indomethacin being a toxic antitumour agent. Thus tumour cells
having developed a capacity for immunosuppression may have evolved
an efficient means of escaping immunosurveillance. If PGE_2 is an

important factor in subversion, indomethacin could be important because unlike certain other types of anti-inflammatory drugs it is not immunosuppressive. Cyclic nucleotides appear to be the mediators of this inhibition of immune cell activity (19).

Metastasis is often associated with destruction of connective tissue. The production of collagenase by endotoxin-stimulated macrophages is significantly inhibited by indomethacin. Wahl et al. (2) suggested that prostaglandins mediate collagenase production since inhibition of collagenase production by indomethacin was overcome by the addition of 10nM exogenous PGE_2 and higher PGE_2 concentrations increased the enzyme production to three-times that achieved by endotoxin. There may similarly be a correlation between the increase collagenolytic activity of invasive breast tumours and the increased prostaglandin production.

REFERENCES

1. Werblowsky, R.S. (1974) Oncology 30, 169-176.
2. Karim, S.M.M. and Rao,B. (1976) in Prostaglandins: Physiological, pharmacological and physical aspects (Ed.Karim, S.M.M.) p.303.
3. Santoro, M.G., Philpott, G.W. and Jaffe, B.M. (1977) Cancer Res. 37, 3774-3779.
4. Bennett, A., McDonald, A.M., Simpson, J.S. and Stamford, I.F. (1975) Lancet, 1218.
5. Rolland, P.H., Martin, P.M. and Jacquemier, J. (1979) Medical Oncology p.41.
6. Dowsett, M., Easty, G.C., Powles, T.J., Easty, D.M. and Neville, A.M. (1976). Prostaglandins 11, 447-463.
7. Tashjian, A.H., Voelkel, E.F., Goldhaber, P. and Levine, L. (1974) Fed. Proc. 33, 81-86.
8. Fitzpatrick, F.A. and Stringfellow, D.A. (1979) Proc. Natl. Acad. Sci. U.S.A. 76, 1765-1769.
9. Stringfellow, D.A. and Fitzpatrick, F.A. (1979) Nature 282, 76-78
10. Gorman, R.R. (1979) Fed. Proc. 38, 83-88.
11. Moncada, S. and Korbut, R. (1978) Lancet 1, 1286.

12. Needleman, P., Raz, A., Ferrendelli, J.A. and Minkes, M.
    (1977) Proc. Natl. Acad. Sci. USA 74, 1716-1720.

13. Fitzpatrick, F., Gorman, R., Bundy, G., Honohan, T., McGuire,
    J. and Sun, F. (1979) Biochim. Biophys. Acta 573, 238-244.

14. van den Brenk, H.A.S. and Sharpington, C. (1971) Br. J. Cancer
    25, 812.

15. van den Brenk, H.A.S. and Kelly, H. (1973) Br. J. Cancer 28,349.

16. Needleman, P., Raz, A., Minkes, M.S., Ferrendelli, J.A. and
    Sprecher, H. (1979) Proc. Natl. Acad. Sci. USA 76, 966-948.

17. Plescia, O.J., Smith, A.H. and Grinwich, K. (1975) Proc. Natl.
    Acad. Sci. USA 72, 1848-1851.

18. Strausser, H. and Humes, J. (1975) Int. J. Cancer, 17.

19. Bourne, H.R., Lichtenstein, L.M., Melmon, K.L., Henney, C.S.,
    Weinstein, Y. and Shearer, G.M. (1974). Science 184, 19-28.

20. Wahl, L.M., Olsen, C.E., Sandberg, A.L. and Mergenhagen, S.E.
    (1977) Proc. Natl. Acad. Sci. USA 74, 4955-4958.

THE APPLICATION OF A DEFIBRINOGENATING SNAKE VENOM ENZYME IN EXPERIMENTAL TUMOR METASTASIS

F.S. Markland, K.M. Hwang, S.S. Bajwa and G.B. Patkos

INTRODUCTION

The thrombin like enzyme (crotalase) has been purified from the venom of the eastern diamond-back rattlesnake (Crotalus adamanteus) (Markland and Damus, 1971). Crotalase is a single chain glycoprotein with a molecular weight of 33,000. The enzyme clots purified fibrinogen, plasma, and plasma anticoagulated with EDTA, citrate or heparin (Markland and Pirkle, 1977a). In contrast to thrombin, crotalase cleaves only fibrinopeptides A from fibrinogen (Markland and Pirkle, 1977b). In vivo studies have shown that when purified crotalase is infused into animals a benign state of defibrinogenation results. There is no fibrin deposition in internal organs, disseminated intravascular coagulation does not occur, and there are minimal changes in clotting factors during defibrinogenation. Crotalase apparently attacks fibrinogen directly, forming soluble fibrin monomers or abnormal fibrin microclots which are rapidly removed by secondary activation of the fibrinolytic system and/or by the reticuloendothelial system. Separate studies have shown that crotalase neither activates the fibrinolytic system nor is fibrinolytic itself at the levels used for defibrinogenation (Damus et al., 1972).

Fibrin deposition has been implicated in the pathogenesis of tumor growth and metastasis formation. Several investigators have identified tumor specific procoagulants (Gordon et al., 1979; Pineo et al., 1973; and Curatolo et al., 1979). However, there are conflicting reports on the role of fibrin deposition (Chew and Wallace, 1976; Sindelar et al., 1975; and Laki, 1974), and the effects of fibrinolytic agents (Grossi et al., 1960; and Peterson et al., 1973) and anticoagulants (Hagmar, 1972; Hilgard and Thornes, 1976; Donati et al., 1978; De Wys et al., 1976; Brown, 1973; and Wood and Hilgard, 1973) on tumor growth and metastasis. This is in part due to the different experimental systems being studied and also, perhaps, to incomplete anticoagulation or defibrinogenation due to species specific responses to the various agents used.

In the present study we report the effect of the defibrinogenating snake venom enzyme, crotalase, on growth and metastasis formation of the B16 melanoma carried in C57BL/6J mice.

MATERIALS AND METHODS

Lyophilized venom of eastern diamond back rattlesnake was obtained from Dr. F.E. Russell, University of Southern California School of Medicine or from the Miami Serpentarium, Miami, Florida. Crotalase was purified by the method of Bajwa and Markland (1979). The purified enzyme was dialyzed against normal saline containing 4mM Tris-HCl buffer, pH 7.0, and was stored at minus 20°C until used. Defibrinogenation studies with C57BL/6J mice (weighing 18-20 g) were conducted by IV or IP administration of crotalase. Blood samples were withdrawn from the eye and fibrinogen content was estimated at varying time intervals after infusion of crotalase (Bajwa and Markland, 1978). The enzyme (doses ranging from 100-400 units per kg body weight) defibrinogenated mice after either IP or IV administration. C57BL/6J mice carrying B16 melanotic melanoma were obtained from the Southern Research Institute, Birmingham, Alabama, and were made available to us by Dr. T.A. Khwaja of the University of Southern California Cancer Center. The tumor was freshly isolated as a single cell suspension by the following procedure. The solid tumor was excised from tumor bearing C57BL/6J mice and rinsed with RPMI medium 1640. The tumor was then cut into small pieces and mechanically pressed on a metallic sieve which was immersed in RPMI medium. The cell suspension in a test tube was allowed to stand for about two minutes at room temperature to separate single cells from large cell aggregates. After pipetting off the cell suspension, it was centrifuged in an International Centrifuge at 1000 rpm for 5 minutes. The cells were resuspended in RPMI medium and the process was repeated. The tumor cells (4×10^4/ml) were finally suspended in normal saline containing 4mM Tris-HCl, pH 7.5, in the presence or absence of crotalase (32.5 unit/ml). The tumor cell suspension in a volume of 0.1 ml (2×10^3 cells, with or without crotalase) was injected subcutaneously into the inside portion of the thighs of C57BL/6J mice. Tumor growth was followed by measuring the length and width in perpendicular directions.

In vitro cytotoxic or cytostatic effect of crotalase on B16 melanoma was measured by both [^{3}H]-thymidine incorporation or direct cell count of B16 melanoma following exposure of tumor cells to enzyme at 32.5 unit/ml, the same enzyme concentration used in the in vivo experiments. The B16 melanoma cells were plated on Falcon tissue culture discs (35 x 10 mm) at a concentration of 2×10^4/ml in RPMI medium. Crotalase in buffered saline was then added to one culture, and after various periods of time of incubations the cells were pulsed with 1μCi/ml of [methyl-^{3}H] thymidine (20-30 Ci/mmol) for one hr. The cells were detached by trypsin-EDTA and an aliquot was used to count cell number; another aliquot was used to determine the incorporation of [^{3}H]-thymidine into DNA. [^{3}H]-Thymidine incorporation was measured by addition of 4 ml of ice-cold 10% TCA to 0.25 ml of either untreated or treated cells. Pellets were collected by centrifugation at 4°C and washed consecutively with 4 ml of ice-cold 5% TCA (twice) and 4 ml of absolute ethanol. The pellet was hydrolyzed by 1 ml of 10% TCA at 90°C for 30 minutes, and its radioactivity was determined with a Beckman liquid scintillation spectrometer. The cell number was counted by Coulter counter.

RESULTS

The effect of crotalase on the level of circulating fibrinogen in C57BL/6J mice was measured. Mice that received a single IV infusion of crotalase at doses between 100-400 units/kg were shown to have significantly lower fibrinogen levels than control untreated mice. At the highest dose of enzyme employed in this study (400 units/kg), the level of circulating fibrinogen in the treated mice dropped to less than 10% of control by 2 hr after infusion. Fibrinogen levels remained at this low level for at least 2 days. At a lower dose (100 units/kg), the rate of decrease in fibrinogen induced by crotalase was much slower and reached 10% of control levels 24 hr after infusion. This was followed by an increase in circulating fibrinogen levels. At 200 units/kg there appeared to be an intermediate effectiveness in suppressing fibrinogen levels. These studies indicated that there was a dose-response relationship of crotalase in bringing about defibrinogenation in mice. IP injection of crotalase at the same doses appeared less effective in defibrinogenating the mice and plasma fibrinogen levels varied widely.

The effect of crotalase on the growth of locally implanted B16 melanoma was measured. When 32.5 units/ml of crotalase was mixed with tumor cells and this mixture was then injected subcutaneously into C57BL/6J mice, the growth of the tumor after implantation was retarded significantly by crotalase pretreatment. On day 17 after implantation of 2×10^3 tumor cells alone, most mice (9/10) developed detectable tumor mass visually and the average tumor weight was 70 mg/mouse. By contrast only 50% of mice that received the mixture of B16 melanoma and crotalase formed local tumor and the average tumor mass was only 2 mg/mouse. By day 24, the average size of the tumor mass in control mice (90% of which had tumors) had reached 843 mg/mouse; the average size of tumor mass in crotalase treated mice had only reached 119 mg/mouse (50% of animals still remained free of tumor). It should also be noted that crotalase was neither cytotoxic nor cytostatic to B16 melanoma as measured both by the growth of tumor cells in vitro and by thymidine incorporation after various times of culture in the presence of absence of crotalase (Table 1).

TABLE 1

Cytostatic and Cytotoxic effect of Crotalase on B16 Melanoma In Vitro

Incubation Conditions[a]	Growth Parameter[a]	
	$[^3H]$-TdR incorporation (cpm/10^5 cells)	Cell number
0 Hr, Saline (S)	----------	2×10^4
Crotalase 32.5 unit/ml(C)	----------	2×10^4
6 hr, S	3760 ± 203	2×10^4
C	3450 ± 195	2×10^4
24 hr, S	6200 ± 405	2.8×10^4
C	6500 ± 512	3.0×10^4
52 hr, S	7405 ± 892	1.05×10^5
C	7708 ± 1040	1.01×10^5
78hr, S	----------	3.06×10^5
C	----------	3.12×10^5

[a] Procedures used are described in Materials and Methods.

The survival of tumor-bearing animals in both control and crotalase treated groups was also measured. Duplicate experiments showed that the median survival times in the control and crotalase-treated groups averaged 43 and 47 days, respectively. Therefore, crotalase has no significant effect on increasing the median survival time of mice carrying B16 melanoma. However, it is important to point out that only 10% of the animals injected with 2×10^3 tumor cells completely reject the tumor, whereas, 30% of the animals in the group injected with tumor cells pretreated with crotalase are capable of resisting the tumor challenge.

DISCUSSION

There is sufficient experimental evidence (as described above) to suggest that the coagulation and fibrinolytic mechanisms may be involved in the metastasis of malignant cells. In fact, Nicholson et al. (1976) have reported a direct fibrinolytic activity in B16 melanoma and more recently Wang et al. (1980) have shown that the more highly metastatic sublines of B16 melanoma had more fibrinolytic activity than did sublines with a lower incidence of metastasis. These differences in fibrinolytic activities of the tumor sublines were shown to be due to differences in their plasminogen activator production (Wang et al., 1980). The actual role of the fibrinogen-fibrin system in modulating the microenvironment for tumor growth and spread, however, remains to be established. The data presented here suggests that crotalase, an enzyme from rattlesnake venom that is effective in defibrinogenating C57BL/6J mice, is capable of significant inhibition of tumor growth of B16 melanoma in the syngeneic host. Interestingly, this enzyme does not have a direct cytotoxic or cytostatic effect on tumor cells in vitro, thereby suggesting that the inhibition of tumor growth may be mediated by the hosts' immunologic mechanism or by a non-specific inflammatory response at the site of injection. It is possible that crotalase pretreatment of tumor cells inhibits the fibrin-gel formation that has been reported to surround certain tumor cells and mask their immunologic identity (Dvorak et al., 1979). This action of crotalase could therefore create a more favorable condition for immunologic attack by macrophages or other effector cells. Alternatively, there could be a direct proteolytic (thrombin-like) action of crotalase on an exposed protein (s) on the B16 melanoma cell surface that is involved in tumor growth and metastasis. A significant observation is that there is an increased proportion of mice that have completely rejected the crotalase pretreated tumor and survived for several months. The mechanism of this tumor rejection is currently under investigation.

ACKNOWLEDGEMENT

This work was supported in part by the Department of Health, Education and Welfare, Research Grant HL22875 from the National Heart, Lung and Blood Institute.

146

REFERENCES

Bajwa, S.S. and Markland, F.S., 1978. Defibrinogenation studies with crotalase: possible clinical applications. Proc. Western Pharmacology Soc., 21: 461–469.

Bajwa, S.S. and Markland, F.S., 1979. A new method for purification of the thrombin-like enzyme from the venom of the eastern diamondback rattlesnake. Thrombosis Res., 16: 11–23.

Brown, J.M., 1973. A study of the mechanism by which anticoagulation with warfarin inhibits blood-borne metastases. Cancer Res., 33: 1217–1224.

Chew, E-C. and Wallace, A.C., 1976. Demonstration of fibrin in early stages of experimental metastases. Cancer Res., 36: 1904–1909.

Curatolo, L., Colucci, M., Cambini, A.L., Poggi, A., Morasca, L., Donati, M.B. and Semeraro, N., 1979. Evidence that cells from experimental tumours can activate coagulation factor X. Br. J. Cancer, 40: 228–233.

Damus, P.S., Markland, F.S. Davidson, T.M. and Shanley, J.D., 1972. A purified procoagulant enzyme from the venom of the eastern diamondback rattlesnake (Crotalus adamanteus): in vivo and in vitro studies. J. Lab. Clin. Med., 79: 906–923.

DeWys, W.D., Kwaan, H.C. and Bathina S., 1976. Effect of defibrination on tumor growth and response to chemotherapy. Cancer Res., 36: 3584–3587.

Donati, M.B., Mussoni, L., Poggi, A., DeGaetano, G. and Garattini S., 1978. Growth and metastasis of the Lewis lung carcinoma in mice defibrinated with batroxobin. Europ. J. Cancer, 14: 343–347.

Dvorak, H.F., Dvorak, A.M., Manseau, E.J., Wilberg, L. and Churchill, W.H., 1979. Fibrin gel investment associated with line 1 and line 10 solid tumor growth, angiogenesis, and fibroplasia in guinea pigs. Role of cellular immunity, myofibroblasts, microvascular damage, and infarction in line 1 tumor regression. J. Nat. Cancer Inst., 62: 1459–1472.

Gordon, S.G., Franks, J.J. and Lewis, B.J., 1979. Comparison of procoagulant activities in extracts of normal and malignant human tissue. J. Natl. Cancer Inst., 62: 773–776.

Grossi, C.E., Agostino, D. and Cliffton, E.E., 1960. The effect of human fibrinolysin on pulmonary metastases of Walker 256 carcinosarcoma. Cancer Res., 20: 605–609.

Hagmar, B., 1972. Defibrination and metastasis formation: effects of arvin on experimental metastases in mice. Europ. J.Cancer, 8: 17–28.

Hilgard, P. and Thornes, R.D., 1976. Anticoagulants in the treatment of cancer. Europ. J. Cancer, 12: 755–762.

Laki, K., 1974. Fibrinogen and metastases. J. Med., 5: 32–37.

Markland, F.S. and Damus, P.S., 1971. Purification and properties of a thrombin-like enzyme from the venom of Crotalus adamanteus (eastern diamondback rattlesnake). J. Biol. Chem., 246: 6460–6473.

Markland, F.S and Pirkle, H., 1977a. Biological activities and biochemical properties of thrombin-like enzymes from snake venoms. In: R.L. Lundblad, J.W. Fenton and K.A. Mann (Editors), Chemistry and Biology of thrombin. Ann Arbor Science Press, Ann Arbor, Michigan, pp. 71–90.

Markland, F.S. and Pirkle, H., 1977b. Thombin-like enzyme in the venom of the eastern diamondback rattlesnake (Crotalus adamantus). Thrombosis Res., 10: 487–494.

Nicolson, G.L., Winkelhake, J.L. and Nussey, A.C., 1976. An approach to studying the cellular properties associated with metastasis: some in vitro properties of tumor variants selected in vivo for enhanced metastasis. In: L. Weiss (Editor), Fundamental Aspects of Metastasis, North-Holland, Amsterdam, pp. 291–303.

Peterson, H-I., Kjartansson, I., Korsan-Bengtsen, K., Rudenstam, C-M, and Zettergren, L., 1973. Fibrinolysis in human malignant tumors. Acta. Chir. Scan., 139: 219–223.

Pineo, G.F., Regoeczi, E., Hatton, M.W.C. and Brain, M.C., 1973. The activation of coagulation by extracts of mucus: a possible pathway of intravascular coagulation accompanying adenocarcinoma. J. Lab. Clin. Med., 82: 255–266.

Sindelar, W.F., Tralka, T.S. and Ketcham, A.S., 1975. Electron microscopic observations on formation of pulmonary metastases. J. Surg. Res., 18: 137–161.

Wang, B.S., McLoughlin, G.A., Richie, J.P. and Mannick, J.A., 1980. Correlation of the production of plasminogen activator with tumor metastasis in B16 mouse melanoma cell lines. Cancer Res., 40: 288–292.

Wood, S., Jr. and Hilgard, P.H., 1973. Arvin-induced hypofibrinogenemia and metastasis formation from blood-borne cancer cells. Johns Hopkins Med. J., 133: 207–213.

EFFECT OF TICLOPIDINE ON BLOOD-BORNE METASTASIS

K. Tanaka, S. Kohga, H. Ogawa, M. Ishihara and N. Tanaka

INTRODUCTION

We have previously shown that thrombogenic tumor cells cause
marked thrombocytopenia and hypofibrinogenemia when injected intravenously and this phenomenon is thought to contribute to the early
phase of metastatic spread (Kohga, 1978; Tanaka et al.,1977;
Kohga and Tanaka, 1979; Kinjo, 1978). Several investigators have
tried to prevent metastasis using platelet aggregation inhibitors
(Gasic et al.,1972; Hilgard, 1973). However, no positive effects
have been found. In the present study, we examined the effectiveness of a new platelet aggregation inhibitor, 5-(2-chlorobenzyl)-4,
5,6,7-tetrahydrothieno(3,2-C) pyridine hydrochloride (Ticlopidine,
Parcor), against blood-borne metastasis of rat ascites hepatoma
AH130, B16 melanoma and Lewis lung carcinoma, to see whether it
had clinical potential.

MATERIALS

Tumors: Rat ascites hepatoma AH130 (Sasaki Institute, Tokyo), B16
melanoma and Lewis lung carcinoma.
Platelet aggregation inhibitors: Ticlopidine (Daiichi Pharmaceutical
Co., Tokyo) and acetylsalicylic acid (Sigma Chemical Co.).
Platelet aggregating agents: ADP (Sigma Chemical Co.), thrombin
(Parke-Davis Lab.) and tumor extract, obtained by centrifugation
(12,500xg for 30 min) of sonicated AH130 cells (5×10^7/ml) in
Hanks' balanced salt solution (HBSS).
Animals: Donryu rats and C57BL/6 mice.
Platelet rich plasma (PRP): Citrated heparinized blood of rats and
mice was used. Heparinized PRP was used in aggregation studies
with tumor cells and tumor extract. The platelet number was
adjusted to 5×10^5/μl by adding platelet poor plasma (PPP). PRP
for tests was prepared 3 hrs. after the p.o. administration of
100mg/kg of Ticlopidine. PRP consisting of platelets of Ticlopidine-

treated rats suspended in PPP of untreated rats was also prepared.

METHODS

Ex vivo experiments

Platelet aggregation was measured turbidimetrically with a Lumi aggregometer Model 400 (Chrono-Log Co., USA). Aggregation was induced by adding 50µl of an aggregating agent solution to 0.45ml of PRP. The agents were ADP (20µM in 10mM $CaCl_2$), thrombin (20 NIHu/ml for experiments in rats and 15 NIHu/ml in mice), tumor extract and viable cells (AH130 and B16 melanoma). Aggregation studies with AH130 were performed using PRP (platelets of Ticlopidine-treated rat in PPP of untreated rat) to elucidate the mode of action of Ticlopidine.

In vivo experiments

Effect of Ticlopidine and acetylsalicylic acid on blood-borne pulmonary metastasis of tumor cells was examined as follows; AH130 cells (1×10^7 in 0.2ml of HBSS), Lewis lung carcinoma (1×10^6 in 0.1ml of HBSS) and B16 melanoma (5×10^5, 1×10^6 and 2×10^5 in 0.1ml of HBSS) were prepared. AH130 was inoculated in the tail vein of Donryu rats; Lewis lung carcinoma and B16 melanoma were inoculated into C57BL/6 mice. Treatment with each drug was given 3 hrs. prior to tumor inoculation using a stomach tube. The lung colony assay was done 7 days after inoculation. In mice inoculated with Lewis lung carcinoma, lungs were first filled with Indian ink followed by fixation in 10% formalin and then the number of metastatic foci on the pleural surface were counted stereoscopically. In rats the number of metastatic foci were counted microscopically on the largest cross section passing through the hilus of the left lung.

RESULTS

Ex vivo experiments

Ticlopidine showed significant inhibitory effects on the platelet aggregation induced by ADP (Fig.1) and by thrombin (Fig.2). AH130 cells (viability more than 98%) caused platelet aggregation as shown in Fig.3, which was absent in PRP of rats after Ticlopidine treatment. Furthermore, aggregation of washed platelets

from rats receiving ticlopidine treatment was not observed on
adding AH130 (Fig.3). Ticlopidine effectively suppressed the platelet release reaction induced by tumor extract (Fig.4). Viable B16
melanoma cells also aggregated platelets of untreated mice, but did
not in PRP of mice which had ticlopidine treatment.

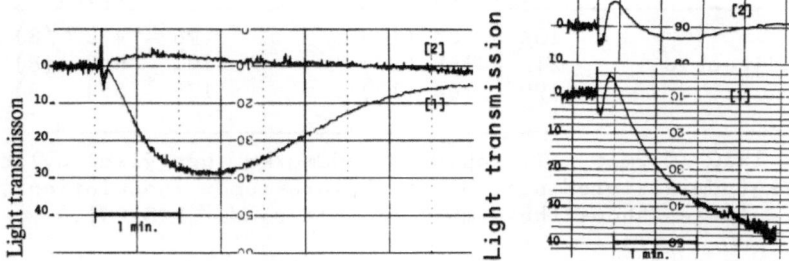

Fig. 1.   Inhibitory effect of ticlopidine on platelet aggregation
induced by ADP. (1) PRP of control B57Bl mice; (2) PRP of mice
administered ticlopidine 3 hrs. before blood-sampling.
Fig. 2.   Inhibitory effect of ticlopidine on platelet aggregation
induced by thrombin. (1) PRP of control mice; (2) PRP of ticlopidine-treated mice.

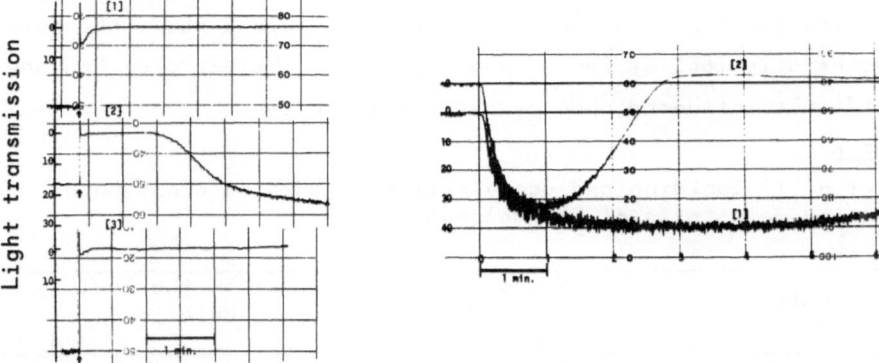

Fig. 3.   Inhibitory effect of ticlopidine on platelet aggregation
induced by AH130 cells. Addition of cells (arrow) is followed by
lag period and irreversible aggregation. (1) PRP of rat with
ticlopidine-treatment; (2) PRP of control rat; (3) platelets of
treated rat in PPP of untreated rat.
Fig. 4.   Inhibitory effect of ticlopidine on platelet aggregation
and release reaction induced by extract of AH130. (1) PRP of
control rat; (2) PRP of treated rat.

In vivo experiments

As shown in Table 1, the number of metastatic foci was smaller
in the ticlopidine-treated group ($p < 0.001$) than in controls. On
the other hand, pretreatment with acetylsalicylic acid tended to
increase the number of metastatic foci, but this was not significant.

TABLE 1

Effect of ticlopidine and acetylsalicylic acid on hematogenous
pulmonary metastasis of rat ascites hepatoma AH130*

Treatments**	No. of metastatic foci in the lung 7 days after inoculation	
	1st trial	2nd trial
Ticlopidine	$104 \pm 88^{\#}$ (10)	$96 \pm 4.3^{\#}$ (8)
Acetylsalicylic acid	217 ± 168 (10)	191 ± 8.3 (8)
Water	199 ± 164 (12)	175 ± 5.4 (8)

*AH130 cells: 1×10^7/0.2ml. **Ticlopidine: 100mg/kg, acetylsalicylic
acid: 150 mg/kg(administered p.o. 3 hrs. before tumor inoculation).
Number in parentheses shows the number of rats used. $\#$P<0.001.

The effect of ticlopidine and acetylsalicylic acid on pulmonary
metastasis of B16 melanoma is shown in Table 2. The number of
inoculated tumor cells varied in these three trials, however ticlo-
pidine-pretreatment had a consistent tendency to reduce metastasis
formation. The average number of metastatic foci in the ticlopidine
group was smaller than that of controls. Table 3 shows the number
of metastatic foci of Lewis lung carcinoma. Neither drug had any
significant influence upon metastasis formation.

TABLE 2

Effect of ticlopidine and acetylsalicylic acid on blood-borne
pulmonary metastasis of B16 melanoma*

Treatments**	No. of metastatic foci in the lung 7 days after inoculation			
	(Trials)	1st	2nd	3rd
Ticlopidine		$29 \pm 6^{\#}$ (9)	41 ± 31 (10)	$24 \pm 11^{\#}$ (10)
Acetylsalicylic acid		54 ± 5 (9)	96 ± 50 (7)	56 ± 21 (9)
Water		54 ± 8 (9)	115 ± 35 (9)	59 ± 20 (12)

*Tumor cells, 5×10^5, 1×10^6 and 2×10^5/0.1 ml were inoculated i.v.
in the 1st,2nd and 3rd trials respectively. **Same treatments as
that in TABLE 1. Number in parentheses shows the number of mice
used. $\#$P<0.001.

TABLE 3

Effect of ticlopidine and acetylsalicylic acid on blood-borne
pulmonary metastasis of Lewis lung carcinoma

Treatments*	No. of metastatic foci in the lung 7 days after i.v. inoculation of tumor cells ($1 \times 10^6/0.1$ ml)	
	1st trial	2nd trial
Ticlopidine	$35.9 \pm 13.5(10)$	43.0 ± 16.1 (10)
Acetylsalicylic acid	$40.9 \pm 16.7(10)$	
Water	37.8 ± 10.1 (9)	69.0 ± 26.8 (10)

*Same treatments as those in TABLES 1 and 2. Number in paren-
theses shows the number of mice used.

DISCUSSION AND SUMMARY

Ticlopidine, which was first described by Podesta et al.,
prevents platelet aggregation induced by various agents including
ADP, collagen, thrombin, arachidonate and prostaglandin endoperoxides and/or thromboxane A_2-like substance (Ashida and Abiko, 1979).

In the present ex vivo studies, it was found that ticlopidine
inhibited completely platelet aggregation induced by AH130 and B16
melanoma as well as by ADP and thrombin. It inhibited not only
platelet aggregation, but also the release reaction, which may play
an important role as a trigger of thrombus formation. These
inhibitory effects are supposed to correlate with the prevention of
blood-borne pulmonary metastasis. Pretreatment with acetylsalicylic
acid failed to prevent the blood-borne metastasis of tumor cells.
This may be due to the potent inhibitory action of acetylsalicylic
acid on PGI_2 generation overcoming the inhibitory action on platelet
aggregation (Ashida and Abiko, 1978). The action of ticlopidine
is not yet fully understood however and enhancement of adenylate
cyclase activity has been described as its main action (Ashida
and Abiko, 1979).

From these results, ticlopidine may be a preferable agent as an
inhibitor for platelet aggregation and the present experiments
suggest the possibility of using this drug for clinical cancer therapy.

152

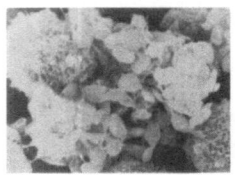

Fig. 5. Platelet adhesion and aggregation by AH130 in PRP of control rat.

Fig. 6. No platelet adhesion and aggregation by AH130 in PRP of rat treated with ticlopidine.

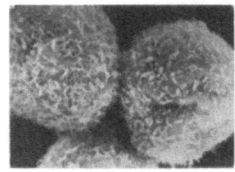

REFERENCES

Ashida, S. and Abiko, Y., 1978. Effect of Ticlopidine and acetylsalicylic acid on generation of prostaglandin I_2-like substance in rat arterial tissue. Thromb. Res., 13: 901-908.
Ashida, S. and Abiko, Y., 1979. Mode of action of Ticlopidine in inhibition of platelet aggregation in the rat. Thrombos. Haemostas., 41: 436-449.

Gasic, G.J., Gasic, T.B., Galanti, N., Johnson, T. and Murphy, S., 1973. Platelet tumor cell interactions in mice. The role of platelets in the spread of malignant disease. Int. J. Cancer, 11: 704-718.
Hilgard, P., Heller, H. and Schmidt, C.G., 1976. The influence of platelet aggregation inhibitors on metastasis formationin mice(3LL). Z. Krebsforsch., 86: 243-250.
Kinjo, M., 1978. Lodgement and extravasation of tumor cells in blood-borne metastasis; an electronmicroscopic study. Br. J. Cancer, 38: 293-301.
Kohga, S., 1978. Thromboplastic and fibrinolytic activities of ascites tumor cells of rats, with reference to their role in metastasis formation. Gann, 69: 461-470.
Kohga, S. and Tanaka, K., 1979. Role of tumor thromboplastin in the mode of distribution of metastatic foci in the lung. Gann, 70: 615-619.
Tanaka, K., Kohga, S., Kinjo, M. and Kodama, Y., 1977. Tumor metastasis and thrombosis, with special reference to thromboplastic and fibrinolytic activities of tumor cells. In: P.G. Stansley and H. Sato (Editors), GANN Monograph on Cancer Research 20: Cancer Metastasis. Jap. Sci. Soc. Press, Tokyo, pp. 97-119.

FAILURE OF RA233 TO AFFECT THE GROWTH OF INTRAVENOUSLY INJECTED MURINE LYMPHOMA CELLS

N. Willmott, A. Baxter, K.C. Calman and A. Malcolm

INTRODUCTION

As regards the welfare of the cancer patient the extravasation of circulating metastatic tumour cells is arguably the most critical event in the development of a tumour. If the extravasated cell is destined to become a focus for further neoplastic growth even the most extensive of surgical exercises is bound to fail (Sugarbaker & Ketcham, 1977). It follows, therefore, that prevention of tumour cells seeding out from the circulation would be highly desirable.

A description of the extravasation of tumour cells that is generally applicable is still awaited. However, it does seem that seeding out of tumour cells is not an inevitable sequel to their being introduced into the circulation since most circulating tumour cells die (Roos & Dingemans, 1979). Nor indeed does the occurrence of a frank metastatic lesion in a certain organ necessarily follow from the detection of tumour cells in that organ by bioassay (Greene & Harvey, 1964; Kim, 1966). Further evidence of the complex relationship between dissemination and seeding comes from the, at first sight, paradoxical observation that the prognosis of cancer patients with tumour cells detected in blood smears is no worse than that of cancer patients where such tumour cells are ostensibly absent (Salsbury, 1975). Although the difficulty of correctly identifying tumour cells in blood smears by morphological criteria should be stressed, it is still perhaps possible to entertain the notion that the detection of circulating tumour cells may be a good prognostic sign since they can do little damage when confined to vascular channels and are probably destined to die anyway.

If a causal relationship is assumed between the frequently observed occurrence of platelet thrombi around embolic tumour cells and the extravasation of the cells (Roos & Dingemans, 1979; Thornes et al, 1968) then one of the ways that tumour cells might be prevented from seeding out of the circulation is by perturbation of haemostasis. Numerous drugs are available that inter alia interfere with the coagulation sequence, the end result being the prevention of thrombus formation. For example: platelet aggregation can be prevented (Gastpar, 1974); the formation of thrombin can be inhibited (Ryan et al, 1968) or lysis of fibrin can be hastened (Chew & Wallace, 1976). In our studies we have chosen to use an inhibitor of platelet function, RA233, to try to prevent tumour cells seeding out of the circulation. The reasons for this were: a) platelets occupy a central position in haemostasis, so if coagulation does facilitate the seeding of circulating tumour

cells inhibition of platelet function should be most likely to prevent it: b) ther
is evidence that in animals depleted of circulating blood platelets the metastatic
capacity of tumours is diminished (Gasic et al, 1973)

The general plan of the experiments was to see if the seeding and subsequent
growth of intravenously(I.V.) injected tumour cells could be influenced when
platelet function of recipient mice was inhibited at the time of tumour cell
injection. RA233 was used to inhibit platelet function and its effect on
haemostasis was assessed as described in the next section.

EFFECT OF RA233 ON EXPRESSION OF PLATELET FUNCTION

RA233 is one of a family of drugs derived from dipyridamole (2,6- bis (dietha
olamino) - 4,8 - dipiperidino-pyrimido (5,4 - d) pyrimidine) by omission of a pipe
idine group from the 8 - position. It has various effects on cell membranes; for
example, it modulates uptake of DNA precursors (De Bono et al, 1976) and it elevate
cyclic AMP levels by inhibiting the action of phosphodiesterases (Rozenberg &
Walker, 1973). In addition, or perhaps because of this, it is an inhibitor of
platelet function and comparative studies have shown that RA233 is more effective
than the parent compound dipyridamole (Mustard & Packham, 1975).

Before investigating whether RA233 had any effect on the seeding and
subsequent growth of circulating tumour cells we first performed experiments to
see under what conditions the drug inhibited the expression of platelet function.
It has been reported that twenty minutes after an I.V. injection of Corynebacteriu
parvum (Wellcome Reagents, Beckenham, Kent) into mice, the circulating platelet
count is reduced (Lampert, et al, 1977). We have confirmed this result and further
more have shown histologically that twenty minutes after C.Parvum I.V. fibrin is
deposited in the capillaries (data not shown). On the basis of this we conclude
that the drop in circulating platelet count following injection of C.parvum I.V.
is due to the expression of platelet function (i.e., aggregation and release) that
triggers the blood coagulation sequence. Thus, if RA233 were capable of preventing
the drop in circulating platelet count following C.parvum injection I.V. then its
capacity to inhibit platelet function would have been demonstrated.

To show under what conditions RA233 was capable of inhibiting platelet functi
the following experiments were performed. CBA female mice, 2-3 months of age were
randomised into three groups and injected I.V. at the times shown in Table I
with medium, C.parvum (16mg/Kg) and RA233 (30mg/Kg). RA233 was prepared for
injection by dissolving in isotonic $\frac{N}{40}$ HCl then neutralised with NaOH. (Under the
conditions the maximum tolerated dose was 100mg/Kg IP or IV). Thus, we have three
experimental groups: a control group injected twice with medium; a group injected
with medium three minutes prior to C.parvum; and a group injected with RA233 three
minutes prior to C.parvum.

TABLE 1

Inhibition of C.parvum-induced platelet aggregation by RA233

TREATMENT (I.V.)		Platelet Count x10^{-9}/L + 20 Min (No. of Mice)		Significance of drop in platelet count compared to control (Wilcoxon Rank Sum test)
-3 Min	0 Min			
Medium	Medium	461	(8)	-
Medium	C.parvum-16mg/kg	371	(7)	P = 0.02
RA233-30mg/kg	C.parvum-16mg/kg	498	(8)	NS

In all cases twenty minutes after the second injection mice were exsanguinated blood samples anticoagulated with EDTA (ethylenediamimetetraacetic acid) and platelet counts performed using a Coulter counter. It can be seen that C.parvum injected IV did indeed elicit a drop in circulating platelet count which was significantly different to controls as assessed by the Wilcoxon Rank-Sum test (P > 0.05 not significant(NS)). Furthermore, this expression of platelet function could be totally inhibited by treatemnt with RA233 administered three minutes prior to C.parvum injection.

An experiment exactly similar in all respects to the above, except that the interval between the two IV injections was extended to twenty minutes, was then performed to see how long-lasting was the effect of RA233 on platelet function. It can be seen from Table 2 that when RA233 was administered twenty minutes prior to C.parvum it had absolutely no effect on platelet function since C.parvum was able to elicit a significant drop in platelet count whether mice were pretreated either with medium or RA233.

TABLE 2

Lack of inhibition of C.parvum-induced platelet aggregation by RA233

TREATMENT (I.V.)		Platelet count x10^{-9}/L + 20 Min (No. of Mice)		Significance of drop in platelet count compared to control (Wilcoxon Rank Sum test)
-20 Min	0 Min			
Medium	Medium	620	(6)	
Medium	C.parvum-16mg/kg	429	(8)	P < 0.005
RA233-30mg/kg	C.parvum-16mg/kg	423	(8)	P < 0.005

From these studies we conclude that following IV administration of RA233 (30mg/Kg) to mice platelet function is inhibited three minutes after treatment but the effect declines rapidly and is not apparent after 20 mins.

EFFECT OF RA233 ON SEEDING AND GROWTH OF CIRCULATING TUMOUR CELLS

The tumour used in these studies was a lymphoma induced in the thymus of a CBA mouse by X-irradiation. It was passaged in the ascites form and tumour cell suspensions contaminated with >20% erythrocytes were purified with Ficol/Hypaque. As can be seen from Fig. 1 it was a highly invasive (note the invasion of striated muscle - light areas in Fig. 1), unencapsulated, rapidly growing (note the abnormal mitotic figures), undifferentiated lymphoma. Its pattern of spread following IV injection or after excision of a small (< 5mm mean diam) subcutaneously growing primary tumour plus regional inguano-femoral lymph node was the same i.e., widespread dissemination to lungs, liver, spleen and kidneys (Data not shown).

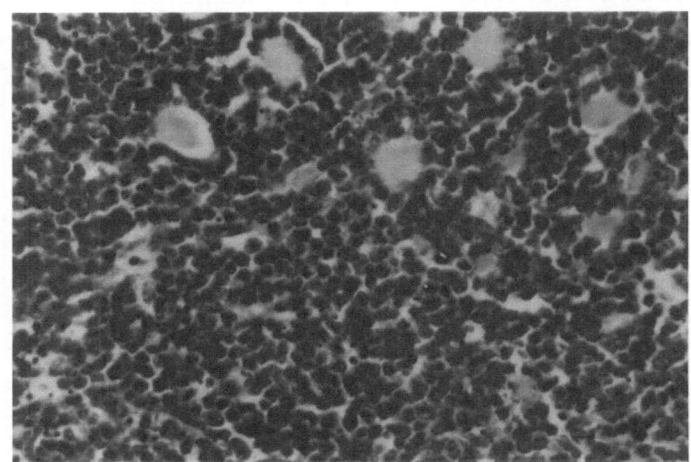

Fig. 1   TLX5 murine lymphoma - see text for description.

The experiment shown in Table 3 was designed so that a low number of tumour cells, 5×10^2, were introduced into the circulation of mice via the IV route at a time when circulating platelet function was inhibited (see Table 1) i.e., 3 mins. after an IV injection of RA233 (30mg/Kg).

TABLE 3

Survival time of TLX-5 lymphoma bearing mice treated with RA233

TREATMENT (I.V.)		Mean survival time in days (No. of Mice)
-3 Min	O Min	
-	5×10^2 TLX-5 Cells	11.5 (6)
Medium	5×10^2 TLX-5 Cells	12.1 (8)
RA233-30mg/kg	5×10^2 TLX-5 Cells	11.2 (9)

However, despite the inhibition of platelet function by RA233 at the time of tumour cell injection the seeding and subsequent growth of the IV injected TLX-5 tumour cells was identical as measured by survival time of mice.

DISCUSSION AND FUTURE DIRECTIONS

There are at least two reasons why inhibition of platelet function by RA233 d: not lead to an increased survival time in this system: 1) inhibition of platelet

function may have been of insufficient duration to prevent tumour cell extravasation, which can take up to eight hours (Poste & Nicholson, 1980: 2) it may be
only tumours that elicit platelet aggregation in vivo or in vitro will be prevented
from seeding out of the circulation by inhibitors of platelet function.

It can be seen from Tables 1 and 2 that the first possibility will have to be
ruled out before any definitive statement can be made regarding the role of RA233
in preventing the extravasation of circulating tumour cells. Thus, from Table 1
we can see that RA233 is an effective inhibitor of platelet function since it
prevents platelet aggregation caused by C.parvum. However, this effect is only
apparent when RA233 is administered IV three minutes before an injection of C.parvum
by the same route and is absent when the interval is extended to twenty minutes.
Since it is known that RA233 levels drop precipitously following IV administration
to rodents and are virtually undetectable after 50 mins. (Boehringer-Ingelheim,
personal communication) it is reasonable to conclude that inhibition of platelet
function by RA233 is strongly dependent on blood levels of the drug. This also seems
to be the case in humans where there is an inverse correlation between blood levels
of dipyridamole, an analogue of RA233, and the capacity of circulating blood
platelets to aggregate (Rajah et al, 1977).

Therefore, since the extravasation of tumour cells can take up to 8 hrs.
(Poste & Nicholson 1980) we are in a situation where to answer the question, does
inhibition of platelet function affect the seeding and extravasation of tumour cells,
we must develop methods to keep the blood levels of RA233 adequate for long-term
anticoagulation. We are currently looking at administering RA233 in drinking water
and also by slow intravenous infusion over a number of hours, with concomitant
monitoring of drug action.

The second possibility is also being explored in order to find a tumour/host
system in which tumour-induced platelet aggregation occurs. Thus, we are screening
a range of transplantable animal sarcomas, carcinomas and lymphomas to see which, if
any, exhibit tumour-induced platelet aggregation either in vivo or in vitro.

In conclusion, under the conditions described above RA233 did not affect the
seeding and growth of IV injected murine lymphoma cells. Accordingly, we have
considered experimental conditions which might account for the lack of effect
of RA233 and have suggested changes in the design of further experiments to determine
whether expression of platelet function is involved in the metastatic process.

REFERENCES

CHEW, E.C. & WALLACE, A.C., 1976. Demonstration of fibrin in early stages of exper-
    imental metastases. Cancer Research, 36, 1904-9.
DEBONO, D.P., GORDON, J.L.,MCINTYRE, D.E.& PEARSON, J.D., 1976. Active transport of
    adenine and adenosine by blood platelets and cultured endothelial cells.
    British Journal of Pharmacology, 58, 466 (abstract).
GASIC, G.J., GASIC, T.B., GALANTI, N. et al, 1973. Platelet - tumour cell inter-
    actions in mice. The role of platelets in the spread of malignant disease.
    Int.J.Cancer, 11, 704-718.

GASTPAR,H., 1974. The inhibition of cancer cell stickiness by the methylxanthine derivative pentoxitylline (BL 191). Thrombosis Research, 5, 277-289.

GREENE, H.S.N. & HARVEY, E.K., 1964. The relationship between the dissemination of tumour cells and tne distribution of metastases. Cancer Research, 24, 799-811.

KIM, U., 1966. Factors controlling metastasis of experimental breast cancer, Cancer Research, 26, 461-4.

LAMPERT, I.A., JONES, P.D.E., SADLER, T.E. & CASTRO, J.E., 1977. Intravascular coagulation resulting from intravenous injection of C.parvum in mice. Br.J. Cancer, 36, 15-22.

MUSTARD, J.F. & PACKHAM, M.A., 1975. Platelets, thrombosis and drugs. Drugs, 9, 19-76.

POSTE, G., NICHOLSON,G.L.,1980. Arrest and metastasis of blood-borne tumour cells are modified by fusion of plasma membrane vesicles from highly metastatic cells. Proc.Natl.Acad.Sci., 77, 399-403.

RAJAH, S.M., CROW, M.J., PENNY, A.F. et al, 1977. The effect of dipyridamole on platelet function : correlation with blood levels in man. Br.J.Clin.Pharmac, 4, 129-133.

ROOS, E. & DINGEMANS, K.P.,1979. Mechanisms of metastasis. Biochemica et Biophysica Acta, 560, 135-166.

ROZENBERG, M.C., & WALKER, C.M., 1973. The effect of pyrimidine compounds on the potentiation of adenosine inhibition of aggregation, on adenosine phosphory-lation and phosphodiesterase activity of platelets. Brit.J.Haematol., 24, 409-415.

RYAN, J.J., KETCHAM, A.S., & WEXLER, H, 1968. Warfarin treatment of mice bearing autochthonous tumours : effect on spontaneous metastases. Science, 162, 1493-1494.

THORNES, R.D., EDLOW, D.W., WOOD, S., 1968. Inhibition of locomotion of cancer cells in vivo by anticoagulant therapy. Johns Hopkins Med.J., 123, 305-316.

SALSBURY, A.J., 1975. The significance of the circulating cancer cell. Cancer Treatment Reviews, 2, 55-72.

SUGARBAKER, E.V. & KETCHAM, A.S., 1977. Mechanisms and prevention of cancer dissemination : an overview. Seminars in Oncology, 4, 19-32.

The authors wish to thank Boehringer-Ingelheim who sponsored this research and Mrs J Willmott and Mrs M McLeod who typed the manuscript.

FAILURE OF FLURBIPROFEN TO AFFECT THE METASTASIS OF RODENT SARCOMAS

S.E. Heckford

INTRODUCTION

An abnormally high production of prostaglandins by some experimental tumours has been noted by several authors (Sykes, 1972; Lynch, 1978) and it has been suggested that this may aid their growth and dissemination by suppressing the immune system of the host (Plescia, 1975). There are many reports that the application of non-steroidal anti-inflammatory drugs (NSAIDs) in various systems will retard tumour growth (Plescia, 1975; Hial, 1976) and this may also be correlated with increased survival of the animals (Lynch, 1978; Strausser, 1975; Trevisani, 1980). However, there is also data suggesting that such treatment has no effect on tumour growth (Sykes, 1972) and may even stimulate cell division (Tutton, 1980). In this study the effect of daily subcutaneous administration of the potent NSAID, Flurbiprofen, on the growth of a variety of rodent fibrosarcomas was investigated. The animals were also observed for the development of metastases following excision of the primary tumour implant and the percentage of phagocytic host mononuclear cells within treated or control tumours was assessed.

MATERIALS AND METHODS

Animals. Male Lister Hooded/Cbi rats and male or female C57Bl/CBi mice over 10 weeks of age were used in this study.
Tumours. MC24 and MC28 are methylcholanthrene induced fibrosarcomas of male rats. FS6 and FS6MI (Mantovani, 1978) are benzo(a)pyrne induced fibrosarcomas maintained in male mice and FS9 was similarly induced in female mice.

Tumour growth, excision and metastasis

Measurements of subcutaneous (s.c.) tumour growth were made on alternate days using vernier calipers following injection of a

single cell suspension (1.10^6 cells) prepared with 0.1% trypsin
and 0.05% DNAse.   These animals were killed at the completion of
the growth study.

Groups of animals received an intramuscular injection of a
mechanically prepared tumour brei and these tumours were excised
after 10-14 days of growth by amputation of the whole limbs;   the
animals were then observed over 300 days for the development of
metastases.

Quantitation of intratumour host mononuclear cells

Using methods which follow those of Evans (Evans, 1972) the
percentages of Fc receptor positive (Fc+ve) phagocytic, mononuclear
host cells within treated or control tumours were assessed.

Drugs

Flurbiprofen (Fp) (Froben, The Boots Company Ltd.) a
prostaglandin synthetase inhibitor, was administered daily s.c.
at a dose of 7mg/kg throughout tumour growth.

RESULTS

Tumour growth

Flurbiprofen had no detectable effect on the s.c. growth of
mouse sarcoma FS6MI (Fig. I) or rat sarcoma MC28 (Fig. II).

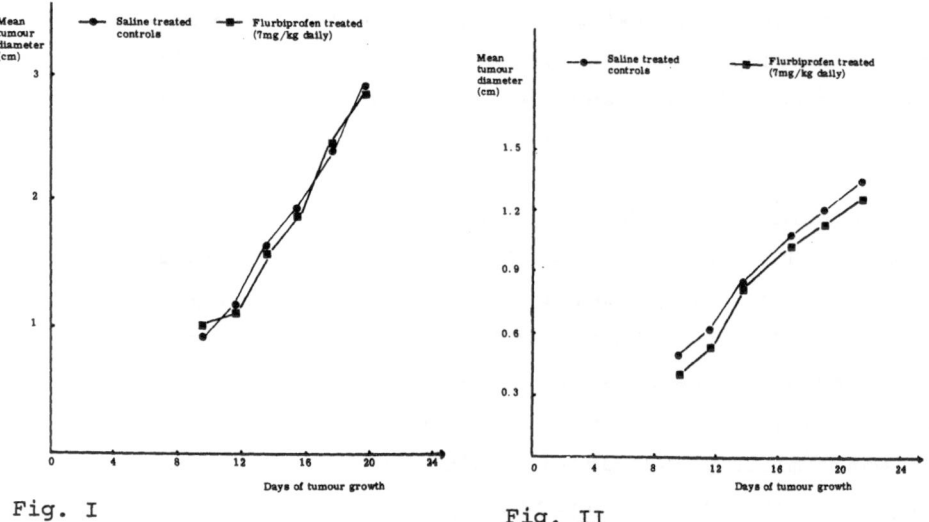

Fig. I   Fig. II

Host cell content

The percentages of Fc+ve, phagocytic host cells within treated and untreated tumours were comparable (Table I).

	Fibrosarcoma	Mean % Fc +ve phagocytic host cells	
		Controls	+ Flurbiprofen
Mice	FS6	28	30
	FS29	24	23
	FS6MI	10	10
Rats	MC24	27	21 N.S.
	MC28	5	4

Table I.

Incidence of Metastases

The incidence of metastases following excision of an intramuscular tumour implant was determined for the mouse fibrosarcomas and was similar in both control and experimental groups (Fig. III).

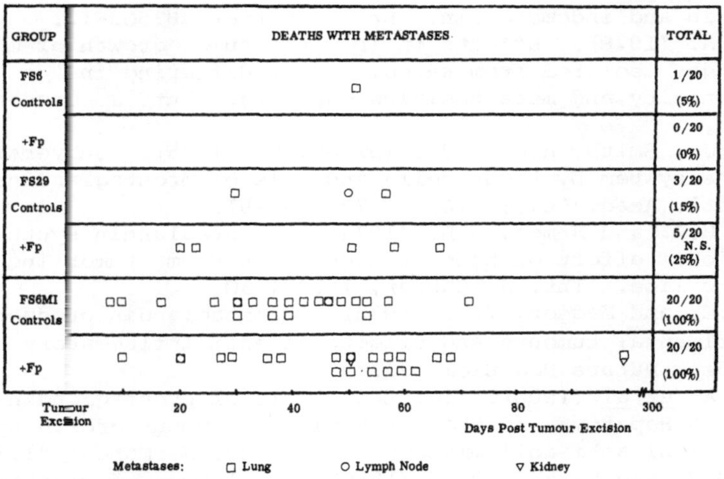

Fig. III. Effect of Fp on the metastasis of murine fibrosarcomas

DISCUSSION

The failure of this potent NSAID to affect the growth and metastasis of these fibrosarcomas argues against an important role for prostaglandins in the success of their progression and dissemination. The data also demonstrate that the infiltration of these tumours by host cells is not simply a response to non-specific inflammatory stimuli produced by the growing neoplasm.

In contrast, immunosuppressive regimens applied to animals bearing these tumours have been shown to decrease the host cell infiltrate and increase the incidence of metastases (Eccles, 1980).

ACKNOWLEDGEMENTS

The supply of Flurbiprofen from The Boots Company Ltd., U.K., is gratefully acknowledged.

REFERENCES

Eccles, S.A., Heckford, S.E. and Alexander, P. (1980). Effect of Cyclosporin A on the growth and spontaneous metastasis of syngeneic animal tumours. Br. J. Cancer. In press.

Evans, R. (1972). Macrophages in syngeneic animal tumours. Transplantation 14:468-73.

Hial, V. et al (1976). Alteration of tumor growth by aspirin and indomethacin: studies with two transplantable tumors in mouse. Eur. J. Pharmacol. 37:367-76.

Lynch, N.R. et al (1978). Mechanism of inhibition of tumour growth by aspirin and indomethacin. Br. J. Cancer 38:503-12.

Mantovani, A. (1978). Effects on in vitro tumor growth of murine macrophages isolated from sarcoma lines differing in immunogenicity and metastasizing capacity. Int. J. Cancer 22:741-6.

Plescia, O.J., Smith, A.H. and Grinwich, K. (1975). Subversion of immune system by tumor cells and role of prostaglandins. Proc. Natl. Acad. Sci., U.S.A. 72:1848-51.

Strausser, H.R. and Humes, J.L. (1975). Prostaglandin synthesis inhibition: effect on bone changes and sarcoma tumor induction in BALB/c mice. Int. J. Cancer, 15:724-30.

Sykes, J.A.C. and Maddox, I.S. (1972). Prostaglandin production by experimental tumours and effects of anti-inflammatory compounds. Nature New Biol. 237:59-61.

Trevisani, A. et al (1980). Elevated levels of prostaglandin E2 in Yoshida Hepatoma and the inhibition of tumour growth by non-steroidal anti-inflammatory drugs. Br. J. Cancer 41:341-7.

Tutton, P.M.J. and Barkla, D.H. (1980). Influence of prostaglandin analogues on epithelial cell proliferation and xenograft growth. Br. J. Cancer, 41:47-51.

IN VIVO AND IN VITRO SELECTION OF EXPERIMENTAL METASTATIC VARIANTS OF RODENT MELANOMA, MAMMARY CARCINOMA AND LYMPHOSARCOMA

G.L. Nicolson, A. Neri, C.L. Reading and K.M. Miner

1. INTRODUCTION

Metastasis via lymphatics and blood does not always result in tumor colonization of tissues and organs based strictly on anatomical considerations (Salsbury, 1975; Sugarbaker, 1952). Many blood-borne experimental metastatic tumor systems show non-random colonization patterns that do not correlate with the initial capillary beds encountered (Dunn et al., 1954; Parks, 1974; Fidler and Nicolson, 1976, 1977; Brunson and Nicolson, 1978, 1979; Conley, 1979). After their initial arrest, malignant cells may die, invade and grow or detach and recirculate to other sites (Zeidman, 1961; Fisher and Fisher, 1967; Fidler and Nicolson, 1976, 1977; Brunson and Nicolson, 1978, 1979) suggesting that factors other than non-specific trapping in the microcirculation determine secondary site location (Nicolson, 1978). In order to determine the host and tumor cell properties important in metastatic tumor spread and survival at distant sites, we have developed animal tumor models in syngeneic hosts that show distinct metastatic behaviors. Several of these models have been based on sequential selection of murine B16 melanoma lines for enhanced blood-borne implantation, survival and growth to obtain sublines capable of preferentially colonizing lungs (Fidler, 1973), brain (Brunson et al., 1978) or ovary (Brunson and Nicolson, 1979). Similarly we have selected _in vivo_ murine RAW117 lymphosarcoma sublines that show enhanced liver colonization after intravenous (i.v.) administration (Brunson and Nicolson, 1978) and rat 13762 mammary adenocarcinoma sublines that show colonization of regional lymph nodes and/or lungs after implantation subcutaneously (s.c.) (Neri et al., 1979). In addition, it has been possible to select tumor cell variant sublines _in vitro_ for loss of sensitivity to cell-mediated toxicity (Fidler et al., 1976), decreased binding to immobilized-lectins (Reading et al., 1980) and increased invasion of tissues (Hart, 1980) or veins (Poste et al., 1980).

2. MATERIALS AND METHODS

2.1. Cells

The murine melanoma line B16-F1 which shows some specificity for lung, but also colonizes a variety of extrapulmonary sites (Fidler and Nicolson, 1976, 1977; Brunson and Nicolson, 1979), was used to select sublines that preferentially colonize brain or ovary (for details see Brunson and Nicolson, 1979). Murine RAW117 lymphosarcoma was selected sequentially for liver colonization by Brunson and Nicolson (1978). Rat 13762 adenocarcinoma cell lines were established from primary tumor, lymph node and lung metastases. Selection for spontaneous lung metastasis was accomplished as described (Neri et al., 1979).

2.2. Biologic assays

B16 melanoma cells were detached with 2 mM EDTA in Ca^{2+}-, Mg^{2+}-free PBS and suspended in serum-free media. Viable, single cells (2.5×10^4) were injected (0.2 ml) i.v. into C57BL/6 mice, and metastases located after 3-4 weeks (Brunson and Nicolson, 1979). RAW117 lymphosarcoma cells grown in suspension were washed three times in serum-free media and injected i.v. (5×10^3 cells in 0.2 ml) into BALB/c, a after 10-15 days the locations of metastases determined (Brunson and Nicolson, 1978). 13762 adenocarcinoma cells were detached with 0.25% trypsin in Ca^{2+}-, Mg^{2}-free PBS and suspended in serum-free media. Viable cells (1×10^6) were injected s into the mammary fat pads of Fisher 344 female rats. After 23 days the sizes of primary tumors, presence of regional lymph node metastases and number of lung meta tases determined (Neri et al., 1979).

2.3. In vitro selections

RAW117 lines were subjected to sequential selection for nonadherence to polyst rene-immobilized concanavalin A (Con A), Ricinus communis I agglutinin (RCA_I), peanut agglutinin (PNA) or wheat germ agglutinin (WGA) according to Reading et al (1980).

2.4. Binding of lectins

RAW117 sublines were examined for lectin-binding sites by quantitating the spe cific amounts of ^{125}I-lectins bound under saturating conditions (Novogrodsky et a 1975).

3. RESULTS

Lung- and ovary-preferring B16 melanoma have been obtained by sequential selec tion for blood-borne implantation, survival and growth. After ten selections for organ preference of colonization, lines B16-F10 or B16-O10 were obtained that sho enhanced experimental metastasis to lung or ovary, respectively (Table 1). Althou some of these lines are not absolutely specific for a given site, strong preferen for the target organ of selection was found (Table 1).

In another system based on rat 13762 mammary carcinoma, selection for spontane lung metastasis yield cell lines that are capable of colonizing lungs from mammar fat pad implants (Neri et al., 1979). Biologic assays on cell clones suggest tha the ability to colonize lungs from s.c. sites exist in subpopulations present in original tumor (Table 2, clone MTF_7). In vivo assays using clones obtained from lung metastases indicate that while most clones are metastatic by 23 days after s implantation, some clones are of low malignancy (Table 2, clone MTLn2) suggesting that the secondary tumors did not arise from individual clones but were formed

TABLE 1. BIOLOGICAL ANALYSIS OF B16 MELANOMA VARIANT LINES SELECTED IN VIVO FOR
LUNG OR OVARY COLONIZATION[a]

B16 Line	Selection Site (Selection No.)	Median No. Lung Metastases (range)	Animals with Ovary Metastases	Metastases at Other Sites
B16-F1	Lung (1X)	25 (2-47)	0/15	4/15 thoracic, 2/15 liver, 3/15 adrenal, 5/15 skin, 3/15 brain
B16-F10	Lung (10X)	89 (44-250+)	1/15	2/15 thoracic, 2/15 skin
B16-O1	Ovary (1X)	22 (0-46)	1/15	5/15 thoracic, 3/15 liver, 2/15 adrenal, 4/15 skin, 1/15 brain
B16-O10	Ovary (10X)	6 (0-19)	13/15	1/15 thoracic, 2/15 adrenal

[a]Animals were injected with 2.5×10^4 viable tumor cells i.v. and experimental metastases were determined after 4 weeks.

perhaps from arrest of multicell aggregates in the lung microcirculation. Alternatively, phenotypic variability of clones obtained from lung metastases could have resulted from biologic drift. Indeed, long-term tissue culture of some of these clones appears to result in phenotypic drift and alterations in metastatic properties (Neri and Nicolson, in preparation).

Variants of malignant cell lines could also be obtained by in vitro selection. Lymphosarcoma cell line RAW117 was selected for sequential nonadherence to immobilized lectins such as PNA, RCA_I or Con A. Selection of low malignant parental lymphosarcoma six times for nonadherence on immobilized-PNA, -RCA_I or -WGA did not affect the biological properties, and few liver experimental metastases form from these cell lines; however, several sequential selections on immobilized-Con A yield cell lines that are highly malignant compared to the parental RAW117-P line (Table 3). After ten selections on immobilized-Con A, a cell line was obtained (RAW117-P Con A^{a10}) that forms >200 visible liver tumor experimental metastases in syngeneic hosts (Table 3). The RAW117-P Con A^{a10} variant line shows a loss in Con A-binding sites per cell. to approximately one-half the number expressed on the parental line, but there is no loss in WGA-binding sites on RAW117-P Con A^{a10} variant (Table 3). When these variant lines are examined by SDS-polyacrylamide gel electrophoresis after cell surface protein labeling by lactoperoxidase-catalyzed iodination, the Con A-selected lines have lost a 70,000 mol. wt. Con A-binding component (Reading et al., 1980).

4. DISCUSSION

Sequential selection of malignant cell populations have yielded variant cell lines with enhanced abilities to form experimental metastases at preferred organ sites. This was accomplished by either i.v. or s.c. administration of tumor cells in syngeneic rodent hosts, and recovery of experimental metastases at various sites. Either the highly metastatic variant cells preexisted in the original tumor cell

TABLE 2. BIOLOGICAL ANALYSIS OF CLONED 13762 ADENOCARCINOMA CELL LINES AND IN VIVC
SELECTED METASTATIC VARIANTS[a]

13762 Clone[b]	Pass. No.	Prim. Tumor Dia. (mm±SD)	Animals with RLN Metastases	Animals with Lung Metastases	Median No. Metastases per Lung (range)
MTC	11	5.67±1.06	0/10	0/10	0
MTF$_7$	12	18.69±2.25	0/21	13/21	16 (1-250+)
MTA	18	2.48±0.95	0/19	19/19	65 (1-250+)
MTLn2	35	13.94±4.05	0/20	1/20	15 (15)
MTLn3	15	10.18±3.05	6/20	16/20	22 (1-250+)

[a]Animals were injected with 1x10^6 viable tumor cells s.c. in the mammary fat pad, a
were sacrificed and examined for metastases at 23 days post-injection.
[b]Clones MTC, MTA and MTF$_7$ were subcloned from different clones obtained from the pr
mary tumor cells. Clones MTLn2 and MTLn3 were subcloned from clones obtained from
secondary tumor cell lines selected twice for lung metastasis.

TABLE 3. BIOLOGICAL ANALYSIS OF RAW117 LYMPHOSARCOMA VARIANT LINES SELECTED IN VI7
FOR REDUCED BINDING TO IMMOBILIZED LECTINS[a]

Cell Line	Selective Lectin (Selection No.)	Median No. Liver Metastases (range)	Binding of ^{125}I-Con A (±SD)[c]	Binding ^{125}I-W((±SD)(
RAW117-P	-	0 (0-20)	3.42±0.46	3.88±0.2
RAW117-P PNA^{a6}	PNA (6X)	0 (0-1)	ND[d]	ND
RAW117-P RCA^{a6}	RCA$_I$ (6X)	0 (0-20)	ND	ND
RAW117-P WGA^{a6}	WGA^I(6X)	0 (0-1)	ND	ND
RAW117-P Con A^{a7}	Con A (7X)	11 (0-50)	2.37±0.49	3.38±0.5
RAW117-P Con A^{a10}	Con A (10X)	200+ (46-200+)	1.72±0.22	4.30±0.4

[a]Animals were injected with 5x10^3 viable tumor cells i.v., and experimental metastases were determined after 14 days.
[b]Lectins were peanut agglutinin (PNA), Ricinus communis I agglutinin (RCA$_I$) and
concanavalin A (Con A).
[c]Specific binding expressed as µg bound per 10^6 cells during saturation labeling
experiments.
[d]Not determined.

population, or the phenotypic variants could have arisen by a process of adaptation
during the selection process. That the cell lines so obtained represent distinct
subpopulations initially present in the original tumor lines has been demonstrated
in cloning experiments using parental, unselected tumor cell populations (Table 2
and Fidler and Kripke, 1977; Kripke et al., 1978; Nicolson, 1978; Reading et al.,
1980). Additionally, attempts to adapt cells to grow at a specific organ location k
direct inoculation was performed. B16-F1 melanoma cells were sequentially adapted
to grow in brain for a series of ten cycles of the same duration in vivo and in
vitro to similar sequential selections performed by i.v. inoculation and recovery c
experimental brain metastases. After ten sequential adaptations for brain survival
and growth, the 10-times-adapted melanoma line was tested for its ability to form
experimental metastases in syngeneic mice. In contrast to B16 lines selected for
blood-borne implantation, survival and growth in brain, the sequentially brain-
adapted melanoma cell lines were no more effective in forming experimental metastas

than the initial B16-F1 line (Brunson and Nicolson, 1980). These data suggest that adaptation _per se_ is not responsible for generating variants with increased meta-static potential. Consistent with these observations are the results here (Table 3) indicating that an entirely _in vitro_ selection for altered cell surface properties of a lymphosarcoma line such as decreased adherence to specific immobilized lectins can lead to variant lines with specific cell surface changes, as well as modifica-tions in metastatic properties. Similar to what we and others have found in many animal tumor systems, cloning of RAW117-P lymphosarcoma yields clones of widely different properties and malignancies (Reading et al., 1980). We are currently examining the stabilities of tumor cell clones _in vitro_ and _in vivo_ with respect to unique characteristics including their malignant properties. Unstable phenotypes that lead to variabilities in malignant properties may be important in allowing survival and growth _in vivo_.

Supported by USPHS NCI grants RO1-CA15122, RO1-CA22950, contract NO1-CB74153 from the Division of Cancer Biology and Diagnosis, NCI and American Cancer Society grant CD71-C to G.L. Nicolson

REFERENCES

Brunson, K.W. and Nicolson, G.L., 1978. Selection and biologic properties of malig-nant variants of a murine lymphosarcoma. J. Natl. Cancer Inst., 61: 1499-1503.
Brunson, K.W. and Nicolson, G.L., 1979. Selection of malignant melanoma variant cell lines for ovary colonization. J. Supramol. Struct., 11: 517-528.
Brunson, K.W. and Nicolson, G.L., 1980. Experimental brain metastasis. In: L. Weiss, H. Gilbert and J.B. Posner (Editors), Brain Metastasis, G.K. Hall & Co., Boston, pp. 50-65.
Brunson, K.W., Beattie, G. and Nicolson, G.L., 1978. Selection and altered tumour cell properties of brain-colonising metastatic melanoma. Nature, 272: 543-545.
Conley, F.K., 1979. Development of a metastatic brain tumor model in mice. Cancer Res., 39: 1001-1007.
Dunn, T.B., 1954. Normal and pathologic anatomy of the reticular tissue in labora-tory mice, with a classification and discussion of neoplasms. J. Natl. Cancer Inst., 14: 1281-1433.
Fidler, I.J., 1973. Selection of successive tumor lines for metastasis. Nature New Biol., 242: 148-149.
Fidler, I.J. and Kripke, M.L., 1977. Metastasis results from pre-existing variant cells within a malignant tumor. Science, 197: 893-895.
Fidler, I.J. and Nicolson, G.L., 1976. Organ selectivity for implantation, survival and growth of B16 melanoma variant tumor lines. J. Natl. Cancer Inst., 57: 1199-1202.
Fidler, I.J. and Nicolson, G.L., 1977. Fate of recirculating B16 melanoma metastatic variant cells in parabiotic syngeneic recipients. J. Natl. Cancer Inst., 58: 1867-1872.
Fidler, I.J., Gersten, D.M. and Budmen, M.B., 1976. Characterization _in vivo_ and _in vitro_ of tumor cells selected for resistance to syngeneic lymphocyte-mediated cytotoxicity. Cancer Res., 36: 3160-3165.
Fisher, B. and Fisher, E.R., 1967. The organ distribution of disseminated ^{51}Cr-labeled tumor cells. Cancer Res., 27: 412-420.
Hart, I.R., 1979. The selection and characterization of an invasive variant of B16 melanoma. Am. J. Pathol., 97: 587-600.

168

Kripke, M.L., Gruys, E. and Fidler, I.J., 1978. Metastatic heterogeneity of cells from an ultraviolet light-induced murine fibrosarcoma of recent origin. Cancer Res., 38: 2962-2967.

Neri, A., Ruoslahti, E. and Nicolson, G.L., 1979. Relationship of fibronectin to th metastatic behavior of rat mammary adenocarcinoma cell lines and clones. J. Supr mol. Struct (suppl. 3), p. 181.

Nicolson, G.L., 1978. Experimental tumor metastasis: Characteristics and organ specificity. BioScience, 28: 441-447.

Novogrodsky, A., Lotan, R., Ravid, A. and Sharon, N., 1975. Peanut agglutinin, a ne mitogen that binds to galactosyl sites exposed after neuraminidase treatment. J. Immunol., 115: 1243-1248.

Parks, R.C., 1974. Organ-specific metastasis of a transplantable reticulum cell sarcoma. J. Natl. Cancer Inst., 52: 971-973.

Poste, G., Doll, J., Hart, I.R. and Fidler, I.J., 1980. In vitro selection of murin B16 melanoma variants with enhanced tissue invasive properties. Cancer Res., in press, May, 1980 issue.

Reading, C.L., Brunson, K.W., Torrianni, M. and Nicolson, G.L., 1980. Malignancies of murine lymphosarcoma correlate with decreased cell surface display of RNA-tumor virus envelope glycoprotein gp70. Proc. Natl. Acad. Sci. U.S.A., in press.

Salsbury, A.J., 1975. The significance of the circulating cancer cell. Cancer Treatment Rev., 2: 55-72.

Sugarbaker, E.V., 1952. The organ selectivity of experimentally induced metastasis in rats. Cancer, 5: 606-612.

Zeidman, I., 1961. The fate of circulating tumor cells. I. Passage of cells through capillaries. Cancer Res., 21: 38-39.

THE ROLE OF TUMOR CELL-BASEMENT MEMBRANE INTERACTIONS IN THE METASTATIC PROCESS

J.C. Murray, S. Garbisa and L. Liotta

INTRODUCTION

Malignant tumor cells must penetrate basement membranes at least once if the metastatic process is to be successful. It has been suggested (Raeminch 1972, Babai 1976) that the penetration of basement membranes occurs in three steps: 1) attachment of tumor cell to BM, 2) local dissolution of BM at point of contact, 3) migration of the tumor cell through the BM. In the experiments described here we have studied the first two steps using an in vitro model. An important constituent of the BM is type IV collagen. Recently much interest has developed in the cell-collagen interaction (Liotta 1978) and we have extended the type of studies initiated by Klebe (Klebe 1974) and others to examine the interaction of metastasizing and non-metastasizing tumor cells with collagen.

Here we show that not only do metastatic cells preferentially adhere to BM collagen but that they also elaborate a specific enzyme which will degrade this substrate. These characteristics are both correlated with the known malignancy of the various cell lines tested in vivo.

MATERIALS AND METHODS

Tumor cell lines

F_1 and F_{10}: variants of B16 melanoma were selected by Dr. Fidler by injecting tumor cells intravenously and culturing cells from lung metastases after one and ten passages respectively: These lines exhibit approximately a ten fold differences in metastatic efficiency (number of lung colonies per cell following tail vein injection).

BL6: this variant with increased invasive capacity in vitro was selected from F_{10} by Dr. I. Hart by culturing the cells in a mouse bladder in vitro as described previously (Poste 1980).

PMT, highly metastatic cell line selected from pulmonary metastases of the T241 mouse sarcoma (Liotta 1980a, Liotta 1980b).

ACT and TACT, normal and spontaneously transformed (but non-metastatic) mouse connective tissue cells (Liotta 1978).

Cell attachment assays

35 mm bacteriological culture dishes were coated with 1 ml of 10 ug/ml collagen solution in 0.5 M acetic acid, and air dried at room temperature. The dishes were preincubated at the same temperature for various times. To remove unattached cells the dishes were rinsed with PBS and the attached cells, removed with 0.1% trypsin - 0.1% EDTA in PBS, were counted by a Coulter Counter ZB1.

Degradation of type IV collagen by tumor cells

Costar cluster of tissue culture wells were first coated by applying 200 μl of (^{14}C)-proline-labeled type IV collagen solution (2.5 x 10^3 cpm) in 10 mM acetic acid, let evaporate and sterilized under U.V. for 10 min. Before using, they were rinsed with serum-free medium (RPMI 1640). Log phase cells were harvested by 0.1% EDTA obtaining 80% viability, washed with complete medium (RPMI 1640 + 10% FCS) and then with serum-free medium. From 1 x 10^3 to 3 x 10^6 viable cells were inoculated into coated wells in 2 ml of serum-free medium and incubated at 37°C. Ten hours later 1 ml of medium was removed, centrifuged at 2000 rpm for 10 min at 4°C and soluble radioactive digestion products checked on a beta counter. Incubation with culture medium alone released approximately 2% of applied counts and with bacterial collagenase (10 units) more than 90%.

Enzyme purification and anti-serum preparation.

The type IV collagenolytic activity was extracted and partially purified from serum-free culture media of the highly metastatic murine sarcoma as described by Liotta et al (Liotta 1980b).

Purified enzyme preparations were run on SDS-Urea-polyacrylamide gel electrophoresis, the gel was stained with Comassie Blue and the enzyme band, at the region of 65,000-70,000 M.W., was removed and minced. The minced gel was injected s.c. in a New Zealand white rabbit, with booster at 3 weeks and 3 months. The serum was stored frozen at -20°C.

RESULTS AND DISCUSSION

Collagen attachment assays

Normal mouse connective tissue cells (ACT), a non metastatic fibrosarcoma derived from ACT (TACT) and a highly metastatic fibrosarcoma (PMT) were compared for their ability to adhere to type IV, type I (stromal) collagen, on bacteriological plastic, in the absence of serum (Table 1). Normal cells attached rapidly to both types of collagen and plastic. The tumorigenic, non-metastatic TACT cells attached to type I and type IV collagen at equal rate but were slower than normal cells in this regard. In contrast the highly metastatic PMT cells attached rapidly and preferentially to type IV collagen. Biochemical studies (data not shown here) showed that PMT cells produced extremely low levels of collagen and undetectable levels of fibronectin. TACT cells produced one fifth as much of these two matrix components as normal ACT cells. Therefore correlated with increased malignancy was a decreased ability to produce extracellular matrix. In addition the metastatic cells appeared to retain a mechanism whereby they could adhere to type IV but not to type I collagen.

Attachment assays with the F_1 and F_{10} variants of the B16 melanoma, supplied by Dr. I. J. Fidler, were also studied for their adhesion to collagen substrates and showed preferential attachment to type IV substrates (Table 2). The degree of preference for type IV being reflected in the "metastatic index", which is generated by successive attachment assays on type I collagen, followed by testing of non-adherent cells on type I or IV collagen. Table 2 shows that the preferential attachment to type IV in the case of the cells so far tested is correlated with spontaneous metastases produced by these cell lines after i.m. implantation in syngeneic mice.

Degradation of type IV collagen by tumor cells

Living metastatic tumor cells, inoculated into labeled type IV collagen coated wells, release soluble degradation products into the media. The degradation takes place after cell attachment to the labeled substrate and is proportional to the cell number and the length of incubation. Only 5% of radioactivity released into the media is detectable on the cells removed from the substrate by EDTA either at short (2 hrs) or long (40 hrs) time period, indicating the degradation is not due to cell phagocytosis.

Several different tumor cell lines were used and compared for type IV collagen degrading activity: Fibroblasts, normal and endothelial cells and TACT cells failed to significantly degrade the substrate. Metastatic tumor cells actively degraded the substrate and the rate was highest in those cells with the greatest incidence of spontaneous metastases.

In addition an in vitro assay to check the presence in the culture media of the latent type IV collagenolytic activity secreted by cells in log phase of growth was used (Liotta 1980a). This second type of assay showed that the tumors with the highest metastatic propensity also had the most enzymatic activity on a per-cell basis.

These findings suggest the existence of specific enzymatic mechanisms by which tumor cells penetrate the basement membrane. Tumor cells can degrade type IV collagen once they are attached to the substrate. On the other hand the enzyme recovered from the culture media required trypsin or plasmin activation. We therefore postulate the enzyme may be present in vivo at the tumor cell surface in latent form and locally activated at the point of contact with the basement membrane. Air dried cover slip cultures of different transformed and normal cell lines were treated for the immunoperoxidase staining of type IV collagenase, using the method described by Liotta et al(Liotta 1979). The results summarized in Table 3 show positive staining for the metastatic cell lines and the absence of a reaction for normal mouse fibroblasts. Additional studies with a large variety of cell and tissue types are in progress using this antisera. In Table I metastatic index, enzyme levels and spontaneous metastases in vivo are compared and appear to show a correlation.

TABLE 1. Attachment to different substrates (% of applied cells) of normal
fibroblasts (ACT), transformed non-metastatic fibroblasts (TACT),
and highly metastatic sarcoma cells (PMT), using serum free media.

	Hours	ACT	TACT	PMT
Plastic	1	19	8	12
	2	62	13	15
	3	69	21	19
Type I collagen	1	35	31	9
	2	74	51	15
	3	95	61	13
Type IV collagen	1	56	24	21
	2	88	46	59
	3	90	50	62

TABLE 2. Attachment assays, Type IV collagenolytic activity and metastases
appearance for different cell lines.

Cell type	Metastatic index*	Type IV degrading activity ($cpm/2.10^5$ cells)	% mice bearing pulm. metastases 18 days after i.m. injection
Normal fibroblasts	0.00	none detected	0
PMT (fibrosarcoma)	0.30	8230 ± 214	100
B16 - F_1	0.05	398 ± 36	0
B16 - F_{10}	0.23	714 ± 62	30

*I.M. $= \dfrac{\text{No cells adherent to Type IV in 2nd assay} - \text{No cells adherent to Type I}}{\text{Total no cells plated on Type I in 1st assay}}$

TABLE 3. Type IV protease positive staining (peroxidase/antiperoxidase method)

Cells studied	Anti-type IV collagen*	Anti-type IV collagen protease	Anti-ovalbumin*
PMT tumor cells	0 / 4+	3+ / 4+	0 / 4+
B16-F_{10} tumor cells	0 / 4+	2+ / 4+	0 / 4+
Human breast (MCF-7) carcinoma cells	1 / 4+	1+ / 4+	0 / 4+
Murine fibroblasts	0 / 4+	0 / 4+	0 / 4+

Positive immunoperoxidase reactions in metastatic tumor cells treated with
antibodies to type IV collagenolytic activity.
* Liotta 1979

REFERENCES

Babai, F., 1976. Etude ultrastructurale sur la patogenie de l'invasion du muscle strie par destumeurs transplantables. J. Ultrastr. Res. 56: 287-303.

Klebe, H. K., 1974. Isolation of a collagen-dependent cell attachment factor Nature 250: 248-251.

Liotta, L. A., Vembu, D., Saini, R. and Boone, C., 1978. Collagen required for proliferation of cultured connective tissue cells but not their transformed counterparts. Nature 272: 622-624.

Liotta, L. A., Foidart, J. M., Gehron-Robey, P., Martin, G.R. and Gullino, P. M., 1979. Identification of micrometastasis of breast carcinomas by presence of basement membrane collagen. The Lancet, July 21: 146-147.

Liotta, L. A., Tryggvason, K., Garbisa, S., Hart, I., Foltz, C. M. and Shafie, S., 1980. Metastatic potential correlates with enzymatic degradation of basement membrane collagen. Nature 284: 67-68.

Liotta, L. A., Tryggvason, K., Garbisa, S., Gehron-Robey, P. and Abe, S., 1980. Partial purification and characterization of a neutral protease which cleaves type IV collagen. Submitted to Biochemistry.

Poste, G., Doll, J., Hart, I. R. and Fidler, I. J., 1980. ·In vitro selection of murine B16 melanoma variants with enhanced tissue-invasive properties. Cancer Res. 40: 1636-1644.

Vlaeminch, M. N., Adenis, L., Houton, Y. and Demaille, 1972. Etude experimentale de la diffusion metastatique chez l'oeuf de poule embryonne. Repartition, microscopic et ultrastructure des foyers tumoraux. Intern. J. Cancer 10: 619-631.

MORPHOLOGICAL AND BIOCHEMICAL DIFFERENCES OF PRIMARY AND METASTATIC HUMAN MELANOMA CELLS

G.D. Birkmayer

INTRODUCTION

One of the crucial events in the multistep process of metastasis formation is the release of transformed cells from the primary tumor and their spread to distant places (Nicolson, 1979). The reason for this phenomenon might be altered intercellular connections and reduced adhesive forces of the tumor cells, which could be due to a change either in the cell membrane structure or in the cytoskeletor These considerations prompted us to investigate human melanoma cells in order to see whether or not this assumption can be substantiated morphologically and biochemically.

MATERIALS AND METHODS

Specimens of primary tumors and lymph node metastases of human melanomas were obtained by surgery and processed for electron micro-scopy, tissue culture experiments and electrophoretic analysis as described previously (Birkmayer et al.,1974; Birkmayer and Stass,198c

RESULTS AND DISCUSSION

Primary human melanomas and their metastases to the regional lymph nodes exhibit a very similar ultrastructure with respect to the cell membrane and the frequent subcellular components such as mitochondria and endoplasmic reticulum (Fig.1: A and B). The most characteristic particles are vesicles of a certain form and size filled with electron dense material which represents the pigment melanin. These pigment-producing melanosomes and their precursor, the premelanosomes (Fig.1: PM), identify these cells as melanoma cells. The number of these vesicles appears considerably higher in cells of the primary tumor than in those of the metastasis. The latter, on the other hand, show an increased content of free and membrane-bound ribosomes as well as of rough endoplasmic reticulum. This finding may provide some indications of an elevated nucleic acid and protein synthesis. A remarkable observation concerns the nucleus of some of the meta-static cells. It exhibits a polymorphic structure with various in-vaginations and extrusions. In addition, a variety of structures can be detected within the nucleus (Fig.1:B,arrows) which are most un-usual. These particles are of different form and size, some of which

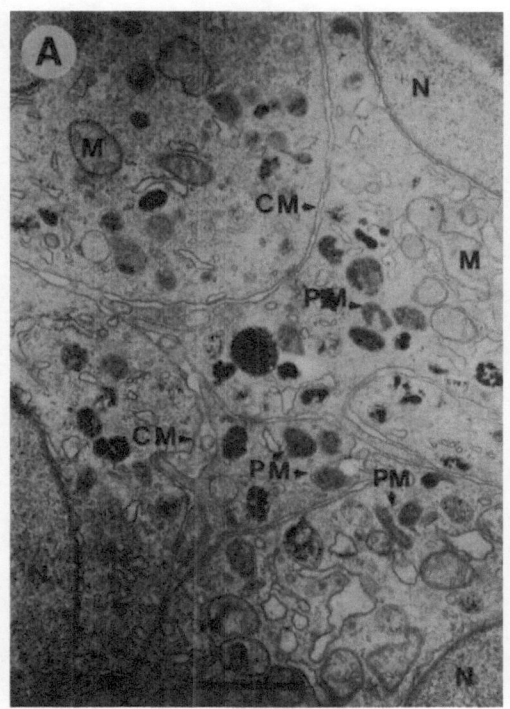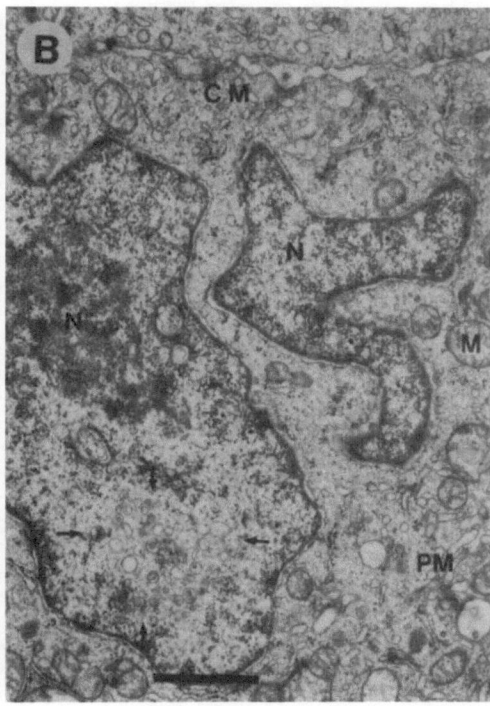

Fig.1: Ultrastructure of cells from a primary human melanoma (A)
        and a metastasis to a regional lymph node (B). The cell
membrane (CM) and the various mitochondria (M) exhibit their usual
structures. The premelanosomes (PM) identify these cells as melanoma
cells. The metastatic cell appears to have two nuclei (N), one of
which shows a polymorphic structure with extrusions and invaginations.
The other contains material (arrows) which is usually observed in the
cytoplasm.   Bar indicates 1 μm.

appear empty and some of which contain electron dense material,thus
resembling virus-like structures. The true intranuclear location of
these particles can be recognized clearly in figure 2 (INI). This is
indicated by the lack of a membrane between these cytoplasmic structure and the nuclear plasma. Thus, they can be distinguished from the
so-called pseudonuclear inclusions (PNI), which occur simultaneously
in these cells. The membrane enveloping the pseudonuclear inclusions
is the nuclear membrane, and they arise very probably from deep in-
vaginations of cytoplasm into the nucleus, which, after thin section-
ing, appear to be within the nuclear area. Morphologically, the particles of the true intranuclear inclusions resemble those of the
pseudonuclear with respect to their appearance and their diversity
(Fig.2:A). The most common of these are vesicles,about 150nm in

176

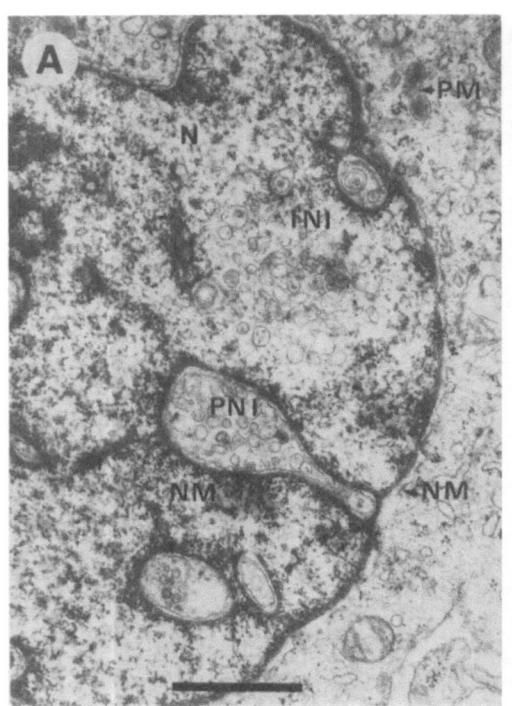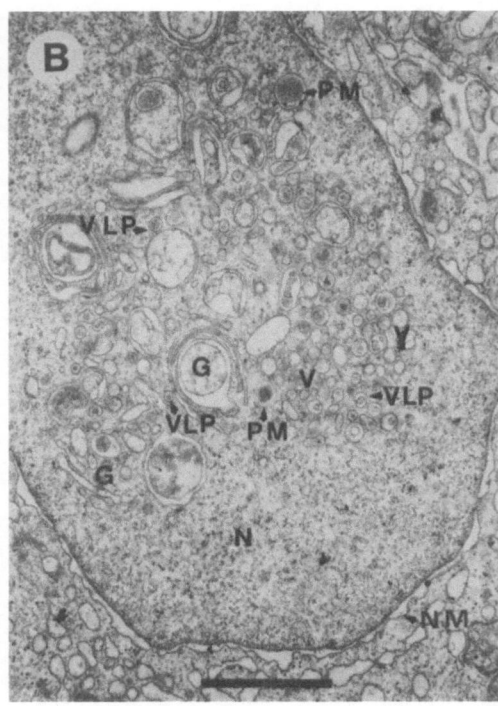

Fig.2: Thin sections of two melanoma cells (A and B) from lymph node
       metastases   of two patients. Both cells show premelanosomes
(PM) and can thus be characterized as melanoma cells. In the nucleus
of cell (A) true intranuclear inclusions (INI) occur simultaneously
with pseudonuclear inclusions (PNI). They can be distinguished from
each other by the absence of a surrounding membrane in the former,
which separates the latter from the nucleoplasm. The amount and the
variety of the true intranuclear inclusion can be recognized in the
nucleus of cell (B). Vesicles (V) of certain size dominate. In addition, Golgi-like cisternae (G) and virus-like particles (VLP) can
be detected. The border between the nucleus (N) and the cytoplasm is
recognizable at the nuclear membrane (NM). Bar indicates 1 um.

diameter, partly empty and partly containing electron dense material.
In addition to these, a variety of other structures can be recognized
(Fig.2:B) which usually occur only in the cytoplasm, for example,
Golgi-like cisternae (G), premelanosomes (PM), and virus-like particle
(VLP). The biological significance of these intranuclear inclusions
is unclear. It might well be that a DNA virus infection is the cause
of this phenomenon, as it is known that these viruses replicate
within the nucleus, leading finally to its destruction and with it to
that of the cell itself. No signs of cell lysis can be observed, howev

and the diversity of the intranuclear inclusions also argues against
a viral infection as the cause of this observation. Another possibility might be that these cells represent macrophages which have
incorporated cytoplasmic material of phagocytosed cells into their
nucleus. Although it has been observed that macrophages are capable
of ingesting a variety of cellular material including melanosomes,
the presence of premelanosomes in the cytoplasm of the intranuclear-
inclusion-carrying cells argues against macrophages. The most reasonable explanation seems to be that these particular cells represent
highly proliferating tumor cells. The very few pictures of true intranuclear inclusions,which have been described in rapidly dividing
animal tumor cells, have been interpreted in a similar way. The
increased proliferation rate leads to a preferential selection of
these cells over the slower growing melanoma cells.

Primary and metastatic melanoma cells also exhibit a somewhat
different biological behaviour. In our hands, cultures from metastatic tumor cells are more easily established and grow faster than
those of primary tumors. Cells from primary melanoma, on the other
hand, show a fibroblast-like morphology and adhere tightly to each
other as well as to the growth matrix. Cells from metastases tend
to dissociate from their neighbour cells and from the plastic surface
of the culture flask. This tendency of disaggregation is accompanied
by a change of their spindle shape to a spherical configuration.

On the basis of these findings we were interested to see whether
these morphological and biological alterations can be correlated to
biochemical changes in the cell and in particular in its membrane.
Primarily the protein and glycoprotein composition of the cell has
been investigated. To gain information on the protein components,
plasma membrane from cells grown in vitro from primary melanoma and
a lymph node metastasis from the same patient have been isolated and
analysed electrophoretically under the disaggregating conditions of
sodiumdodecylsulfate and mercaptoethanol. On the basis of protein
staining with Coomassie-blue a separation into at least 22 polypeptides can be achieved and the pattern of primary and metastatic tumor
cells is remarkably similar. Significant differences can only be
detected in the top area of the gel, which corresponds to the high
molecular weight region. One or two bands can be found only in the
pattern of primary tumor cells. Staining of the gels for carbo-
hydrates with periodic acid-Schiff's reagent reveals two glycoproteins, one in the high molecular weight and one in the low mole-

cular weight region. The one in the high molecular weight region seems to be diminished in the pattern of metastatic cells. As the carbohydrate staining with Schiff's reagent is far less sensitive than the staining for protein with Coomassie-blue, it can not be excluded that further glycopeptides are present in our membrane preparation, some of which might be altered. In order to substantiate this assumption, the glycoprotein synthesis has been investigated by incorporating ^{3}H-fucose and ^{14}C-leucine into melanoma cells grown in vitro. The leucine incorporation of primary and metastatic melanoma cells is comparable, the fucose labelling on the other hand is considerably higher in the metastatic cells. Electrophoretic analysi of the double-labelled melanoma cells reveals only minor differences with respect to the protein synthesis, as measured on the basis of the leucine incorporation. Only one leucine peak in the high molecular weight region of the gel is missing in the pattern of the metastatic cells. A high fucose to leucine ratio can be interpreted as preferential glycoprotein synthesis; in the profile of the primary tumor cells two peaks with a particularly high fucose:leucine ratio occur, one in the high and one in the low molecular weight region. In the pattern of metastatic cells such high fucose to leucine ratios are found only at one peak in the low molecular weight region. However, four or five fucose peaks can be observed in that profile, their counterparts of which are missing or present only in minor amounts in the pattern of primary tumor cells. These differences are found constantly in all cultures from primary and metastatic human melanoma cells. Thus it seems that in the metastatic cells more proteins of the membrane become glycosylated. Whether this observation is directly attributable to the potential of metastasis formation or whether this is merely due to an altered synthetic capacit$\}$ of different melanoma cell lines remains to be elucidated.

REFERENCES

Birkmayer,G.D.,Balda,B.R. and Miller,F.,1974. Oncorna-Viral Informat: in Human Melanoma. Europ.J.Cancer, 10:419-424.
Birkmayer,G.D. and Stass,H.P.,1980. Humoral immune response in glioma patients:A solubilized glioma-associated membrane antigen as a to< for detecting circulating antibodies. Int.J.Cancer, 25:445-452.
Nicolson,G.L., 1979. Cancer Metastasis. Scient.American, 240: 50-60.

LEWIS LUNG CARCINOMA: SELECTING METASTATIC VARIANTS

M. Magudia, P. Whur, Julia Lockwood, Julie Boston and D.C. Williams

Metastasis is a multistep phenomenon, beginning with the invasion of normal tissues, blood vessels and/or lymphatics by malignant cells from the primary tumour. Since only a minute proportion of these cells subsequently form metastatic growths at distant sites, the question has arisen as to whether or not their survival is a random process. If selection operates during metastasis one would expect that variants with differing metastatic potential could be isolated fairly easily. Fidler (1973) reported obtaining "metastatic" variants of B16 melanomas by growing cells from lung colonies in tissue culture and subsequently injecting them intravenously into mice. Repetition of this process over several generations resulted in cell lines with enhanced lung colony forming ability. This technique, however, omits the early stages which probably play a role in selection during spontaneous metastasis. For instance, the processes of detachment and release from the primary tumour may themselves be selective. In addition, the host's immune response to intravenously injected cells is unlikely to resemble that against a progressively growing primary tumour and the cells escaping from it. We have therefore attempted to obtain metastatic variants in a spontaneously metastasising model.

Using a set of fixed conditions to ensure reproducibility of the data, a standard line of Lewis lung carcinoma was established. 10 C57 BL/10 ScSn male mice (8 weeks old) were injected intramuscularly in the hind leg with 20,000 primary tumour cells. The inoculum was prepared as a single cell suspension using the technique described by Stephens et al (1977) and the viability was above 95% as determined by trypan blue exclusion. The mice were sacrificed when the mean primary tumour diameter reached 10mm. The procedure was repeated over twelve generations (Table 1), and the growth rate of the primary tumour and the number of overt lung metastases remained statistically unchanged during this period.

Differential cell counts of primary tumour and metastases were carried out on smears of untreated tumour fragments stained by the May-Grunwald-Giemsa technique. Host cells accounted for 20% of the population of the primary tumours and about 25% in the metastases; the difference being mainly due to the higher macrophage content in metastases (Table 2).

TABLE 1. In vivo characteristics of Lewis lung carcinoma variants compared to a standard line.

Tumour line	Latent period (days)	Growth period (days)	Day sacrificed	No. of overt lung metastases
Standard line	9.9+0.5	8.4+0.4	24.9+0.6	54.6+1.1
Variant F1	11.0+0.3	11.0+0.5	29	75.2+9.9
Variant F2	11.1+0.3	11.1+0.3	28	92.3+14.7
Variant F3	12.4+0.4	10.8+0.6	29	70.0+8.3*
Variant F4	8.1+0.3	11.8+0.6	26	98.2+5.1
Variant F5	10.4+0.4	9.0+0.4	25	124.7+14.2
Cultured primary	14.2+0.6	11.0+0.6	33	8.6+3.9
Cultured metastatic	28.9+2.2	27.1+2.0	66	22.1+4.5

The latent period is the time taken for the tumour to reach 0.5mm diameter, and the growth period is the time taken to grow from 2 to 8mm. The number of lung metastases was counted when the mean primary tumour diameter was 10mm. The data from the standard line is pooled from 12 generations (120 mice). Results are expressed as means ± standard errors.

* Concurrent lung infection obliterated some metastases.

TABLE 2. Differential cell counts of standard and high metastasis Lewis lung carcinomas.

Tumour type	Tumour cells	Macrophages	PMN's ╱	Lymphocytes	Unidentified
Standard primary	80.7+1.9	4.6+0.5*	3.5+1.1	2.9+1.0	8.5
Standard metastases	72.6+1.5	11.7+0.4**	3.9+0.7	3.9+0.7	6.2
High primary	88.0+1.0	1.2+0.5*	1.8+0.2	1.1+0.2	7.6
High metastases	73.0+2.0	8.1+0.6**	8.6+1.7	4.4+0.5	6.1

Unidentified cells were mainly damaged, but fibroblasts and striated muscle cells were subsequently isolated from this fraction.

* and ** indicate the only significant differences between the two lines (P < 0.001).

╱ Polymorphonuclear leucocytes.

If selection occurs during metastasis, the secondary tumours would form a preselected source of cells with higher metastatic potential. The above procedure was therefore repeated, but substituting cells from lung metastases for reinjection at the primary site. The number of lung metastases showed a significant increase (P < 0.01 in the first generation, and further increases with each succeeding passage (Table 1). By the fifth generation the number of metastases had more than doubled. There was no alteration in the growth rate of the primary tumour.

In order to examine some aspects of the process of metastasis in the standard line and high metastasis variant F5, five mice with each tumour were sacrificed sequentially every two days and the metastases were examined. Analysis of this material provided no evidence for earlier seeding or a faster rate of growth in the high metastasis variant; the difference between the two being attributable to a doubling in the rate of seeding.

Differential cell counts on the high metastasis variant showed a significant reduction (P < 0.001) in the number of macrophages (Table 2). Eccles and Alexander (1974) have demonstrated an inverse correlation between the macrophage content of a tumour and its tendency to metastasise. Our findings thus suggest a lowered host immune response to the high metastasis variant.

Attempts to develop a low metastasis variant by in vivo passage were unsuccessful. However, we had previously observed that Lewis lung carcinomas lose much of their metastatic potential when established in monolayer cultures (Whur et al, 1980). Neither cultured primary nor metastatic cells produced as many metastases as the standard line from which they originated (P < 0.001, Table 1), but metastatic cells did produce significantly more than primary cells (P < 0.05). However, the growth rates of the primary tumours differed (Table 1), making rigorous comparison of their relative metastatic potentials uncertain.

These findings suggest that cells with varying metastatic potential exist within the primary tumour cell population of the Lewis lung carcinoma, and that these variants can be selected by appropriate procedures. Our data also suggest that cells of high metastatic potential are selected during spontaneous metastasis.

REFERENCES

Eccles, S.A. and Alexander, P., 1974. Macrophage content of tumours in relation
   to metastatic spread and host immune reaction. Nature, 250, 667-669.
Fidler, I.J., 1973. Selection of successive tumour lines for metastasis. Nature
   New Biology, 242, 148-149.
Stephens, T.C., Peacock, J.H. and Steel, G.G., 1977. Cell survival in B16
   melanoma after treatment with combinations of cytotoxic agents: lack of
   potentiation. Brit. J. Cancer, 36, 84-93.
Whur, P., Magudia, M., Boston, J., Lockwood, J. and Williams, D.C., 1980.
   Plasminogen activator activity of cultured Lewis lung carcinoma cells measured
   by chromogenic substrate assay. Brit. J. Cancer, (in press).

MALIGNANT PROPERTIES OF CLONES ISOLATED FROM A MOUSE FIBROSARCOMA

N. Suzuki, M. Williams and H.R. Withers

INTRODUCTION

One of the features of malignant tumors or tumor cells is their heterogeneity from tumor to tumor and, indeed, within a single tumor. Most tumor cells are aneuploid, and higher in DNA content than normal cells (Atkin, 1966; Stich, 1960). These facts indicate that tumor cells vary in chromosome or DNA content. Chromosome analysis has provided supportive evidence for the concept that tumor cells vary and evolve (Foulds, 1969; Hauschka, 1961; Makino, 1951). In order to investigate the role of variability and heterogeneity of tumor cells in the process of neoplastic development, we have established an experimental system based on freshly isolating clones from a mouse fibrosarcoma. Some of the purposes of the present study were:

(1) to enquire why DNA content of most tumor cells is increased and to determine whether there is a positive correlation between alteration of DNA content and the development of malignant properties.

(2) to determine whether malignancy or malignant characteristics are unifactorial or multifactorial.

(3) to analyze the metastatic process.

MATERIALS AND METHODS

A 3-methylcholanthrene induced fibrosarcoma and syngeneic C_3H host mice were used.

Cloning and plating efficiency (PE) experiments were carried out in 0.14% soft agar containing McCoy's 5A medium supplemented with 20% fetal calf serum (Grand Island Biological Company, Grand Island, N.Y.) (Suzuki and Okada, 1976; Suzuki and Withers, 1978a). A model ZBI Coulter counter and a channelyzer II multichannel analyzer and plotter (Coulter Electronics, Hialeah, Fl.) were used for cell counting and cell volume analyses (Suzuki et al. 1977a). Cell volume was determined from the modal peak channel number of volume distribution profiles of Coulter counter analyses. Late log phase cultures of clones were used as the standard condition for these experiments, although confluent cultures of various clones were chosen for biochemical determination of cellular DNA content (Burton, 1956) or of cellular protein (Lowry et al., 1951).

Lung colony formation, tumor take, host survival and spontaneous metastasis experiments were carried out using C_3Hf/Bu male mice obtained from our specific

pathogen-free breeding colony. Single cell suspensions were obtained by trypsinization of late log phase cultures of various clones. For lung colony formation, single cell suspensions of 10^5 cells in 0.5 ml medium were injected into
tail veins of unirradiated mice without addition of heavily irradiated cells or
microspheres. Lungs were placed in Bouin's fixative overnight before colony
counting.

RESULTS AND DISCUSSION

The clones were isolated by repeated clonings in soft agar containing medium and were designated as FSA1231 through FSA12318. PE of these clones ranged
from 1 to 35% while for the original fibrosarcoma it was 10^{-7} to 10^{-6}. All the
clones were kept in liquid nitrogen when not in experimental use in order to maintain their nascent status for interclonal comparison. PE in vitro, cell size,
cellular DNA content, gross protein content and malignant properties varied from
clone to clone (Suzuki et al., 1977a,b; 1978a,b).

DNA content distribution profiles of these clones determined by flow micro-
fluorometry (FMF) after mithramycin staining are shown in Fig. 1. Heterogeneity
of DNA content of these clones is obvious from the apparently different position
of the G_1 peaks.

The results of biochemical determination of cellular DNA content and protein content of some of these clones agreed with those from FMF DNA analysis and
Coulter counter volume analysis. DNA content, cell volume and protein content
were heterogeneous but correlated with one another.

In the following experiments, malignant properties were compared. Lung
colony forming efficiency of FSA1233 was about ten times higher than FSA1231 as
shown in Figures 2a and 2b. Figure 2a shows the result of an experiment, in which
various doses of cells were injected, and the mice were killed 19 days later,
while Figure 2b shows the number of lung colonies scored at various times after
intravenous injection of the same number of FSA1231 or 1233 cells. Based on
these data, further comparisons of LCFE of various clones were performed using a
constant inoculum of 10^5 cells per mouse and 19 days incubation time to allow for
possible differences of growth rate among clones. There was a positive correlation between LCFE and cell volume; the larger the cell size i.e. the higher the
DNA content, the higher the LCFE.

Host survival was compared after inoculation of 10^6 cells into each of 4
loci on the back using clones 1231 and 1233. The time until death of 50% of the
injected mice was 35 days for the large-cell clone 1233 and 60 days for the small-
cell clone 1231. The tumor take after inoculation of 10^5 cells into each subcutaneous locus was 70% for clone 1233 and 30% for clone 1231. Therefore the
large-cell clone 1233 was more malignant than small-cell clone 1231 in terms of

186

LCFE, subcutaneous tumor take and host survival. PE _in vitro_ of the two clones
was about 20% in McCoy's 5A medium and did not correlate with these differences
in malignant properties.

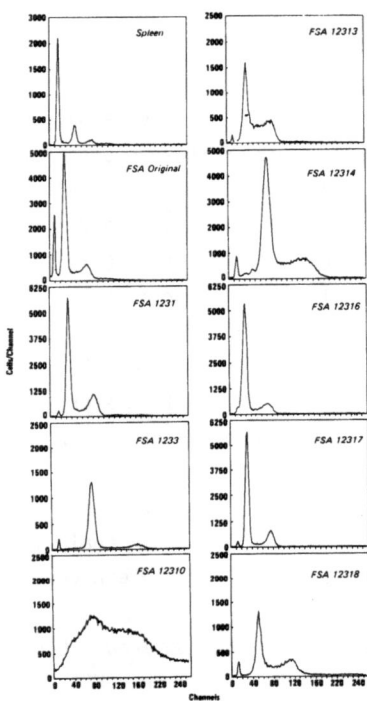

Fig. 1. Histogram of DNA content distribution obtained using FMF. a. Normal
spleen cells, singlet, doublet, triplet; b. the original fibrosarcoma tumor
cell suspension; c. FSA1231; d. 1233; e. 12310; ·f. 12313; g. 12314;
h. 12316; i. 12317 j. 12318. Normal spleen cells were added to the tumor
cell clones as a standard to quantitate DNA content (Courtesy of Nature).

In the next experiment, spontaneous metastasis to the lung from leg tumors
were examined. Mice were killed 49 days after intramuscular inoculation of 10^6
cells into the thigh. The 1233 cell tumors grew to at least 870 mm^2 (the multiplication product of two diameters), while 1231 cell tumors reached only an
average of 600 mm^2. However, the small-cell clone, 1231, produced many more
spontaneous lung metastasis than did the large-cell clone, 1233: only 15% of
the mice bearing the 1233 cell tumor developed lung metastases, compared with
70% of those bearing the 1231 tumor. These results contrast with those for
LCFE, after i.v. inoculation and with tumor take, growth rate and host survival

after subcutaneous inoculation.

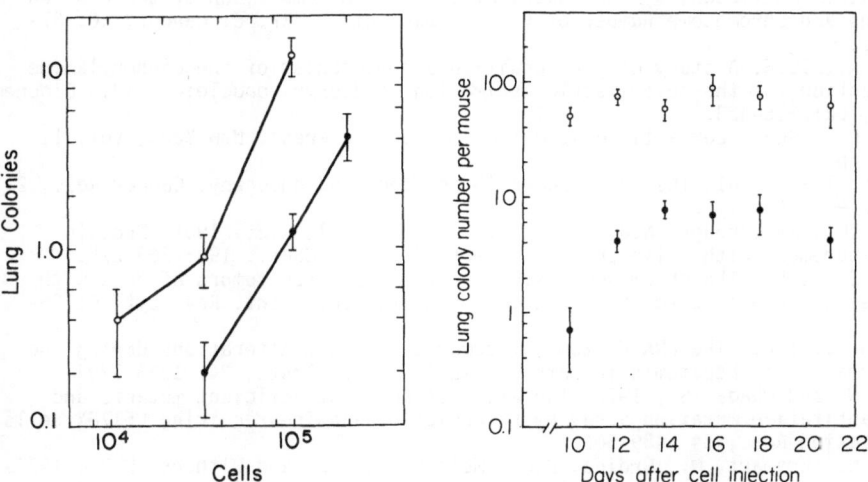

Fig. 2.   Lung colony forming efficiency of FSA1231 (●) and 1233 (o).
a. (left) Lung colony number 19 days after injection of various numbers of cells.
b. (right) Lung colony number at various times after injection of 1.5 x 10⁵ cells
(Courtesy of Cancer Research).

As a summary of the analyses of nascent daughter clones from a single mouse fibrosarcoma;

(1) gross DNA content, protein content and cell volume were heterogeneous among clones but correlated with one another.

(2) variation in DNA content could be the prime reason for the alteration of protein content, cell volume and resulting increase of degree of malignancy in terms of local growth.

(3) the malignant properties of these clones were also heterogeneous and variable: the larger the cell volume, or the higher the DNA content, the more malignant the cell in terms of lung colony formation after intravenous injection of tumor cells, and in subcutaneous tumor "take" and growth rate and host survival. However, the incidence of spontaneous lung metastasis from leg tumors was different, the small-cell clone 1231 being more malignant in this respect than the large-cell clone 1233.

(4) The diverse and discrepant characteristics of subclones from a single tumor suggest that multiple factors are involved in determining malignant characteristics.

REFERENCES

Atkin, N.B., Mattinson, G. and Baker, M.C., 1966. A comparison of the DNA content and chromosome number of fifty human tumors. Br. J. Cancer, 20: 87-101.

Burton, K., 1956. A study of the condition and mechanism of the diphenylamine reaction for the colorimetric estimation of deoxyribonucleic acid. Biochem. J., 62: 315-323.

Foulds, L., 1969. Neoplastic development. Academic Press, New York, Vol. 1, 41 pp.

Hauschka, T.S., 1961. The chromosomes in ontogeny and oncogeny. Cancer Res., 21: 957-974.

Lowry, O.H., Rosebrough, N.J., Farr, A.L. and Randall, R.J., 1951. Protein measurement with folin phenol reagent. J. Biol. Chem., 193: 265-275.

Makino, S., 1957. The chromosome cytology of the ascites tumors of rats with special reference to the concept of the stem cell. Int. Rev. Cyt. 6: 26-84.

Stich, H.F., 1960. The DNA content of tumor cells, II. Alterations during the formation of hepatomas in rats, J. Natl. Cancer Inst., 24: 1283-1297.

Suzuki, N. and Okada, S., 1976. Isolation of nutrient deficient mutants and quantitative mutation assay by reversion of alanine-requiring L5178Y cells. Mutation Res., 34: 489-506.

Suzuki, N., Frapart, M., Grdina, D.J., Meistrich, M.L. and Withers, H.R., 1977a. Cell cycle dependency of metastatic lung colony formation. Cancer Res., 37: 3690-3693.

Suzuki, N., Withers, H.R. and Lee, L.Y., 1977b. Variability of DNA content of murine fibrosarcoma cells, Nature, 269: 531-532.

Suzuki, N. and Withers, H.R., 1978a. Isolation from a murine fibrosarcoma of cell lines with enhanced plating efficiency in vitro. J. Natl. Cancer Inst. 60: 179-183.

Suzuki, N., Withers, H.R. and Williams, M., 1978b. Heterogeneity and variability of artificial lung colony forming ability among clones from mouse fibrosarcoma. Cancer Res., 38: 3349-3351.

CHARACTERISTICS OF TUMOR CELL CLONES WITH VARYING MALIGNANT POTENTIAL

J. Varani, E.J. Lovett, S. Elgebaly and J. Lundy

It has been shown in a number of model systems that uncloned populations of tumor cells maintained in culture contain distinct subpopulations of cells (Fidler, 1973; Kripke, Gruys and Fidler, 1978; Dexter, et al., 1978). The fact that biologically distinct populations can be isolated provides a useful tool for analyzing the relationship between particular characteristics and malignant potential. Working with a 3-methylcholanthrene-induced tumor in C57 bl/6 mice, we have recently isolated subpopulations of cells with differing malignant potential (Varani, Orr and Ward, 1979a, 1979b). Several subpopulations have been characterized. Among all the populations examined so far, high adhesiveness and high motility have been found to characterize cells of high malignant potential while cells of lower malignant potential are less adherent and migrate less actively.

METHODS

Tumor cell populations. A syngeneic 3-methylcholanthrene-induced fibrosarcoma established in a C57 bl/6 mouse served as the parent for all of the cell populations used in this study. It was maintained in vivo by serial transplantation in syngeneic mice (in vivo parent) and in vitro by serial monolayer culture (in vitro parent) over a 4 year period. Nine separate subpopulations were obtained from these parent lines and cloned. Four of the subpopulations were obtained from primary or metastatic tumors induced in syngeneic mice by the in vitro parent. One was obtained from a metastatic tumor induced by the in vivo parent. One was selected from the in vitro parent by serial passage (for 3 months) in medium to which human serum had been added in place of fetal calf serum. Finally, three subpopulations were obtained from primary tumors induced in C57 bl/6 mice by the human serum-adapted cells. All cell lines were maintained on medium 199 with 10% fetal calf serum. All were sub-cultured on a 3-day schedule.

<u>Biological characterization</u>. The malignant potential of each clone was determined. This included establishing the tumorgenicity (percentage of animals developing primary tumors after injection of 1×10^5 cells), the growth rates of the primary tumors and the rate of spontaneous metastasis to the lungs from the primary tumors. Each population was examined <u>in vitro</u> with regard to a number of characteristics including the growth rate and saturation density in monolayer culture, rate of colony formation in soft agar, ability to attach to the surface of plastic culture dishes, sensitivity to trypsin-mediated detachment from plastic culture dishes and motility in the agarose assay. Standard procedures were used for all assays and are described and referenced in our recent reports (Varani, Orr and Ward, 1978; Varani, Orr and Ward, 1979b and 1979c). In addition, two of the subpopulations were examined for ability to adhere in the lungs of animals after intravenous injection and to form tumors in the lungs after intravenous injection.

RESULTS AND DISCUSSION

<u>In vivo behavior</u>. All populations were examined for tumorgenicity and metastasis formation (Table 1).

TABLE 1. TUMORGENICITY AND METASTASIS FORMATION

Population[1]	% of injected animals that develop primary tumors[2]	% of injected animals with pulmonary metastases[2]	Average number of metastases/animal[3]
Parent (in vivo)	75	45	3 ± 2
Parent (in vitro)	100	37	3 ± 1
Clone 1	100	40	2 ± 1
2	100	63	3 ± 1
3	100	45	5 ± 1
4	100	75	7 ± 2
5	100	not done	not done
Clone 6	25	0	-
7	45	5	1
8	14	0	-
9	24	0	-

1. See text for the origin of each clone.
2. A minimum of 20 animals per group were used with each population.
3. Mean ± standard error of mean.

It can be seen that with regard to tumor formation and spontaneous metastases, the clones fall into two distinct groups. Clones 1-5 represent populations which were established from primary or metastatic tumors induced by the in vitro or in vivo parents. All show a high degree of malignancy as do both of the parent populations. Clone 6 refers to the population isolated in vitro from the parent line by selection in medium with human serum. This population has a much lower malignant potential as do clones 7-9, which were established from primary tumors induced in mice by the human serum-adapted cells. Although not shown in this table, there also was a correlation between in vivo growth rates and the other parameters of malignant potential. Clones 1-5 and the parent populations grew much faster in vivo than did clones 6-9.

In vitro characterization. The two parent populations and each cloned sub-population were compared in vitro with regard to a number of biological proper-ties which may contribute to malignancy. These included growth, adhesiveness and motility. With regard to in vitro growth there was no significant difference between any of the populations. All had doubling times of 20-26 hours, grew to a density of 1200-1500 cells per square mm. and formed colonies in soft agar at a high rate.

All of the cell lines were examined for ability to attach to the surfaces of plastic culture dishes and for sensitivity to protease-mediated release from plastic dishes. Working with prototype high and low malignant populations we have previously shown no difference between these variants with regard to rate of attachment to a variety of substrates but did show differences in the rate of trypsin-mediated release. The high malignant variant cells were much more resistant to trypsin mediated release than were the low malignant cells (Varani, Orr and Ward, 1979c). In the present study, all eleven populations were examined and, as shown in Table 2, a 100% correlation between trypsin-sensitivity and malignant potential was obtained. All of the high malignant populations were much more trypsin resistant than were the low malignant populations. Under controlled conditions 15-33% of the high malignant cells were released by trypsin while 48-79% of the low malignant cells were. As was also found in our previous study with a limited number of variants we found in this study no difference between any of the cell types in rates of attachment.

Table 2 also shows motility data obtained with the eleven populations in the agrarose assay. As with trypsin-sensitivity, there is a correlation between increased motility and a high malignant potential.

TABLE 2.   CHARACTERISTICS OF FIBROSARCOMA SUBPOPULATIONS WITH HIGH OR LOW
MALIGNANT POTENTIAL

Population	Characteristic	
	Adhesiveness (% of cells released by trypsin)[1]	Motility (Distance migrated by cells in agarose assay)[2]
Parent (in vivo)	15 ± 8	230 ± 20
Parent (in vitro)	28 ± 4	220 ± 10
Clone 1	18 ± 11	240 ± 10
2	15 ± 7	210 ± 20
3	33 ± 11	240 ± 10
4	28 ± 5	260 ± 10
5	17 ± 6	320 ± 10
Clone 6	55 ± 12	140 ± 10
7	48 ± 8	180 ± 20
8	68 ± 9	160 ± 20
9	79 ± 14	120 ± 10

1. The release of cells from plastic flasks was measured as
    described previously (Varani, Orr and Ward, 1979c). The values
    shown represent the percentage of released cells after treatment
    for 5 minutes under standard conditions.
2. Cell motility was measured using the agarose assay as described
    previously (Varani, Orr and Ward, 1978). The values shown
    represent the distance (± s.e.m.) from the edge of the agarose
    drop to the leading edge of cell migration.

Working with a small number of cloned populations (one high malignant and
one low malignant) we examined both populations for ability to adhere in the
lungs of syngeneic mice after intavenous injection. Cells of each type were
labeled with [I-125]-iododeoxyuridine as described by Fidler (1975) and
injection by the intravenous route. Five minutes after injection, 55-59% of both
the high and low malignant cells were found in the lungs. However, by 4 hours
only 4% of the low malignant cells were still in the lungs while 13% of the
high malignant cells were.   In addition, animals injected by the intravenous
route with unlabeled, high malignant cells developed many more pulmonary tumors
than did animals injected with an equal number of low malignant cells (54 vs. 3).
If these data can be reproduced with a large number of additional tumor cell
populations, it will lend strong support for the concept that high adhesiveness
contributes to malignant potential.

It is interesting that other investigators working with other model systems have also found a correlation between high adhesiveness and malignant or metastatic capability (Fidler, 1975; Nicolson and Winklehake, 19765; Briles and Kornfeld, 1978). It is not known how high adhesiveness contributes to malignancy. It may be that in vivo these cells need to be substrate-attached in order to divide or in order to avoid host defense mechanisms.

This study was supported in part by NIH Grant CA 26263.

REFERENCES

1. Briles, E.B. and Kornfeld, S. 1978. Isolation and metastatic properties of detachment variants of B16 melanoma cells. J. Nat. Cancer Inst. 60:1217-1222.
2. Dexter, D.L., Kowalski, H.M., Blazar, B.A., Fligiel, Z., Vogel, R. and Heppner, G.H. 1978. Heterogeneity of tumor cells from a sirgle mouse mammary tumor. Cancer Res. 38:3174-3181.
3. Fidler, I.J. 1970. Metastases: A quantitative analysis of distribution and fate of tumor cell emboli labeled with I-125-idodeoxyuridine. J. Nat. Cancer Inst. 45:773-782.
4. Fidler, I.J. 1973. Selection of successive tumor lines for metastasis. Nature New Biol. (London) 242:148-194.
5. Fidler, I.J. 1975. Biological behavior of malignant melanoma cells correlated to their survival in vivo. Cancer Res. 35:218-224.
6. Kripke, M.L., Gruys, E. and Fidler, I.J. 1978. Metastatic hetercgeneity of cells from an ultraviolet light-induced murine fibrosarcoma of recent origin. Cancer Res. 38:2962-2967.
7. Nicolson, G.L. and Winkelhake, J.L. 1975. Organ specificity of blood-borne metastases as determined by cell adhesion. Nature (London) 225:230-232.
8. Varani, J., Orr, W. and Ward, P.A. 1978. Comparison of the migration patterns of normal and malignant cells in two assay systems. Am. J. Path. 90:159-172.
9. Varani, J., Orr, W. and Ward, P.A. 1979a. Comparison of subpopulations of tumor cells with altered migratory activity, attachment characteristics, enzyme levels and in vivo behavior. Euro. J. Cancer 15:585-592.
10. Varani, J., Orr, W. and Ward, P.A. 1979b. Hydrolytic enzyme activities, migratory activity and in vivo growth and metastatic potential of recent tumor isolates. Cancer Res. 39:2376-2380.
11. Varani, J., Orr, W. and Ward, P.A. 1979c. Adhesive characteristics of tumor cell variants of high and low malignant potential. J. Nat. Cancer Inst. (in press).

INVASION OF LUNG AND LIVER TISSUE BY DIFFERENT TYPES OF TUMOUR CELLS

K.P. Dingemans and M.A. Van den Bergh Weerman

The pattern of invasion of mouse lung and liver tissue by different types of tumours was compared. To this end, cell suspensions from the following tumours were ·
jected either into a tail vein or into the portal system of syngeneic mice: MB 6A
lymphosarcoma; B16/F1 and B16/F10 melanomas, and M 8013, Ta3/Ha, and TA3/St mammary
carcinomas. In contrast to previous studies, in which we concentrated on the initia
events (for references, see Roos and Dingemans, 1979), the tumour colonies were al·
lowed to invade the target organs for periods ranging from a few days to several
weeks. After this time, the livers and lungs were fixed by vascular perfusion or in
tracheal instillation, respectively, and tissue was prepared for ultrastrucutral ex
amination.

Lymphosarcoma cells injected into a tail vein were trapped almost instantaneous·
in capillaries all over the lungs. Within a few days, the cells had proliferated t(
fill many capillaries (Fig. 1), but evidence of penetration of the endothelium was
never detected (Fig. 2). Melanoma cells were also trapped in the lung capillaries
after tail vein injection, but only those cells that escaped from the vascular lume
survived. From a few days after the injection, areas diffusely invaded by tumour
cells were present and within 2 weeks developed into irregular tumour foci with sle
der extensions in many directions. Such foci usually spread along the lung surface
(Fig. 3) or were located in the lung parenchyma at a very short distance from the
surface. Ultrastructural examination revealed that the great majority of the cells
were located in the interstitial spaces (either immediately under the mesothelial
cells (Fig. 3), between pulmonary epithelial and endothelial cells (Fig. 4), or
around small vessels) where they were in direct contact with basal laminae, collage
fibres, etc. (Fig. 4); in addition, a number of tumour cells were found in the alve
lar air spaces in which case macrophages containing large melanin-laden phagosomes
were invariably present near the tumour cells (Fig. 5). Despite their rapid spread
through both tissue compartments, tumour cells migrating through the basal laminae
the cell layers separating these compartments were not observed. This indicates tha
such migration, although apparently occurring, is a very rare event. Mammary carcin
ma cells growing in the lungs exhibited a growth pattern similar to that of the mela
noma cells but for the fact that they did not form prominent collars around blood
vessels.

Lymphosarcoma cells reaching the liver (either directly, after injection into th
portal system, or indirectly via the lungs) penetrated the endothelium almost immedi
ately after their trapping in the sinusoids. At the same time they started to invag

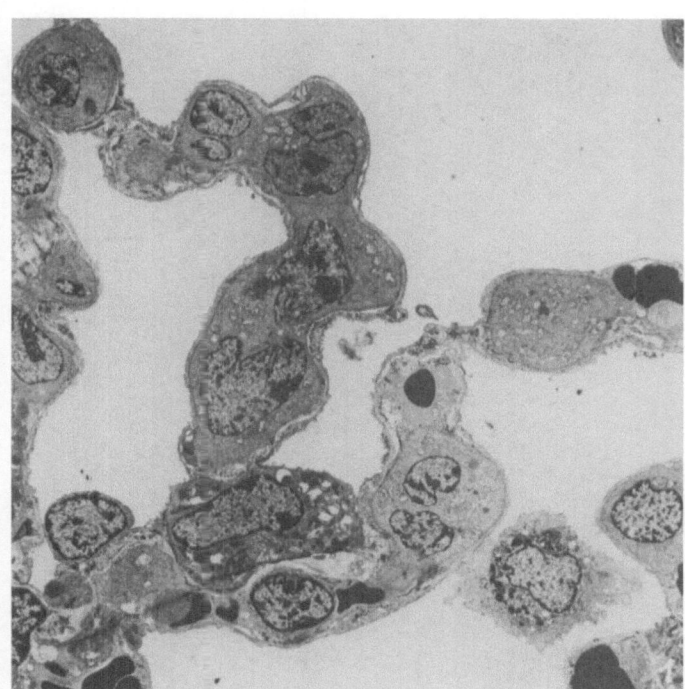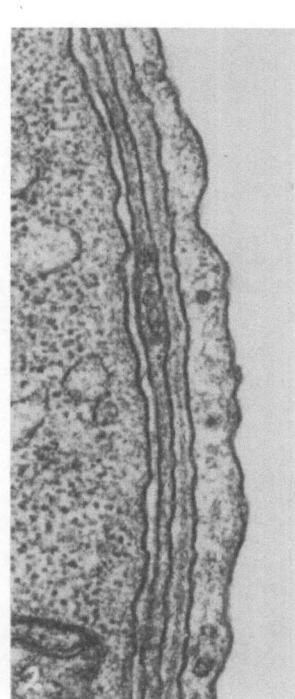

Fig. 1. Lymphosarcoma cells filling many lung capillaries. X 2100.
 Fig. 2. Detail of lymphosarcoma cell in lung capillary, showing that tumour cell (left) is separated from alveolar air space (right) by intact endothelium, basal lamina, and pulmonary epithelial cell. X 47.500.

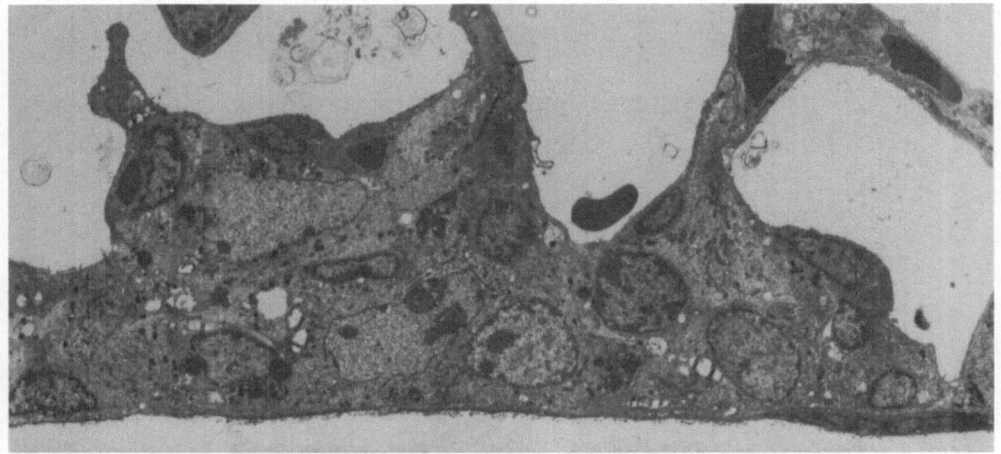

Fig. 3

Fig. 3. Melanoma colony, spreading along lung surface and situated between alveolar spaces (top) and mesothelium (bottom). X 2100.

196

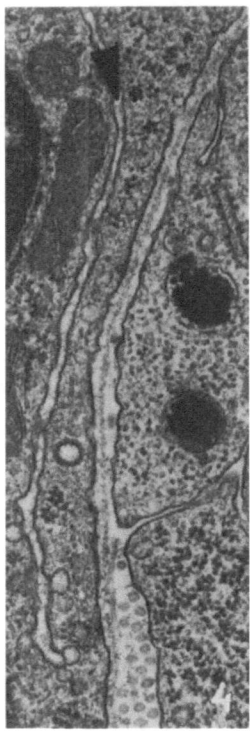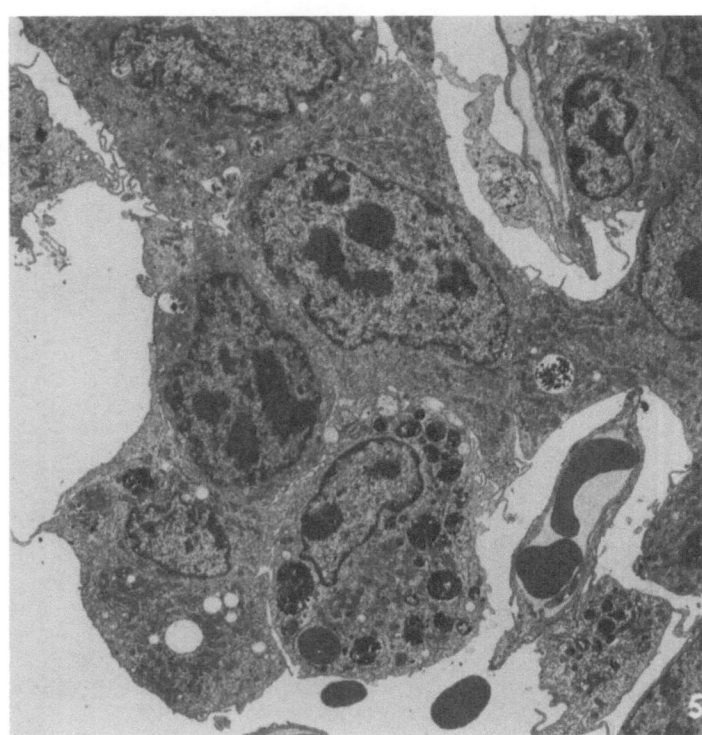

Fig. 4. Melanoma cell, recognizable by melanosomes, growing in lung. Cell is in direct contact with basal lamina and collagen fibres, and compresses capillary lume (arrow head). X 34.500.

Fig. 5. Melanoma cells in alveolar space. Note presence of macrophage with mela-nin-containing phagosomes. X 2600.

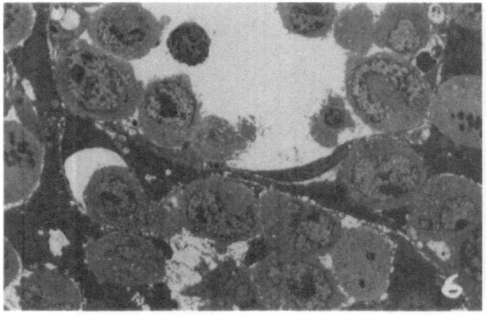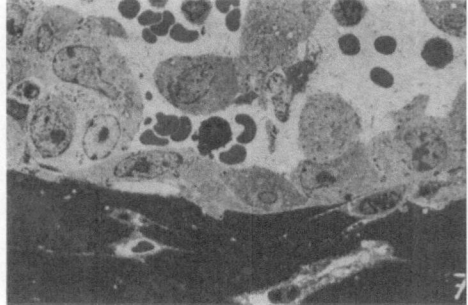

Fig. 6. Lymphosarcoma cells in liver tissue, situated both inside and outside ve sels, and compressing hepatocytes. X 715.

Fig. 7. Melanoma nodule in liver. Note smooth edge of nodule, compression of su rounding liver tissue, and large spaces within nodule that contain fluid, erythro-cytes, and leucocytes. X 715.

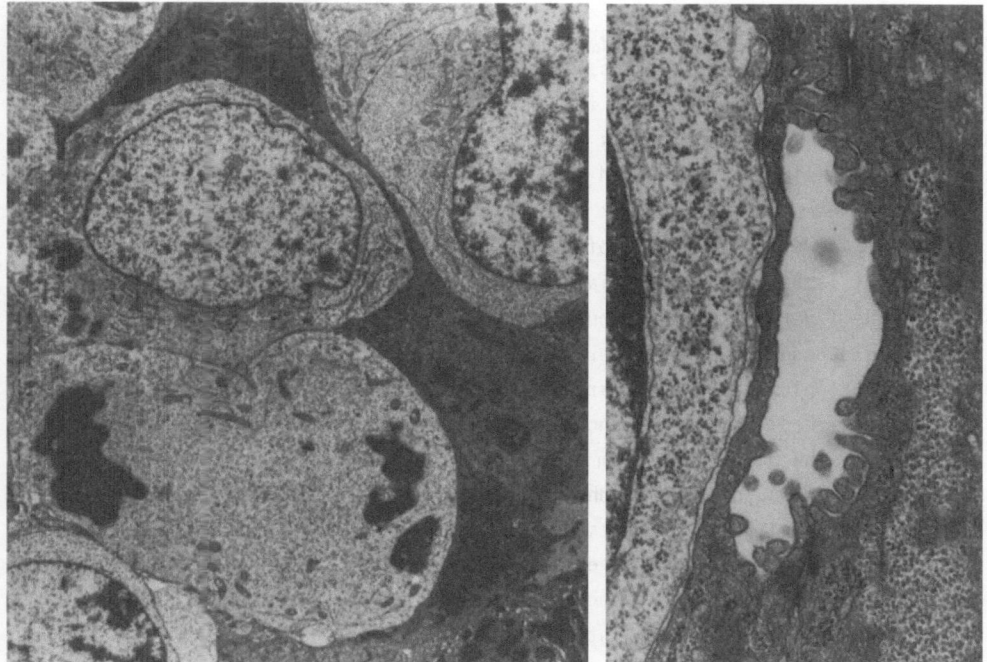

Fig. 8   Fig. 10

Fig. 8. Edge of mammary carcinoma nodule in liver. Note deep invagination of tumour cells into hepatocytes. X 3500.

Fig. 10. TA3/Ha mammary carcinoma cell, separated from intact bile canaliculus by
exceedingly deformed hepatocyte. X 25.000.

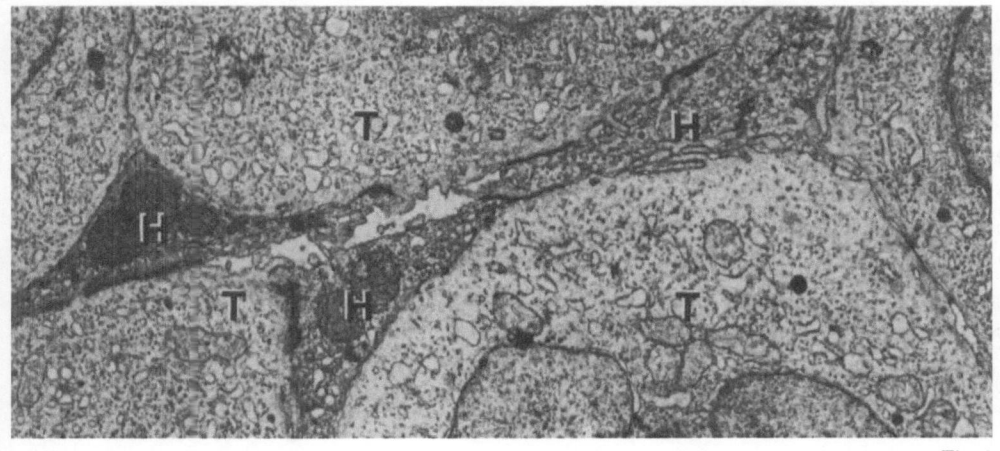

Fig. 9

Fig. 9. M 80_3 mammary carcinoma cells (M) and hepatocytes (H) forming bile canaliculus that is sealed by a junction at every cell interface. Note distorted shape of
hepatocytes. X 8100.

inate the adjacent hepatocytes, resulting in tumour cells nearly completely buried in exceedingly deformed hepatocytes. Ultimately, large areas of the liver were crow ed with tumour cells, located both inside and outside vessels (Fig. 6). Unlike the lymphosarcoma cells, melanoma cells growing in the liver barely invaginated the he- patocytes, and ultimately developed into smooth-edged nodules pushing aside rather than invading the surrounding liver tissue (Fig. 7). Another characteristic of the melanoma nodules was the presence of large, cystic spaces containing various blood components but lacking an endothelial covering (Fig. 7). Connections between these spaces and the liver vasculature could not be detected. Mammary carcinoma cells als formed discrete nodules in the liver. When the edges of such nodules were studied electron microscopically, the mammary carcinoma cells appeared to invade the hepatc cytes almost as deeply as the lymphosarcoma cells (Fig. 8). This suggests that the main reason for the difference from the diffuse growth pattern of the lymphosarcoma cells might be a stronger mutual adhesion of the mammary carcinoma cells. On the other hand, the in vitro experiments by Roos, described in this book, demonstrate that considerable differences between the interaction of individual lymphosarcoma a mammary carcinoma cells with hepatocytes also exist.

Next to the deep invagination into hepatocytes, which was similar for the three different types of mammary carcinoma cells studied, there was another type of inter action with hepatocytes, in which the three cell types differed considerably: M 801 cells frequently broke the junctions between hepatocytes and inserted themselves be ween the hepatocytes around bile canaliculi, which resulted in well-organized lumin lined by both hepatocytes and tumour cells and sealed by junctions at every cell in terface (Fig. 9); TA3/Ha cells also formed many junctions with adjacent hepatocytes but these were localized haphazardly, and the cells never reached the lumen of a bi canaliculus (Fig. 10); finally, TA3/St cells only occasionally formed junctions wit hepatocytes, located at fully arbitrary places. In all probability, this differenti behaviour reflects the degree of differentiation of the types of mammary carcinoma tested. However, the in vitro experiments by Roos do not suggest that the presence absence of junctions is an important factor in the invagination of hepatocytes by t tumour cells.

The above observations demonstrate considerable variations in the interaction be ween growing tumour nodules and surrounding host tissues, depending on both the typ of the tumour and the type of the invaded tissue. Such variations may have importan consequences for the mode and speed of tumour spread.

REFERENCE

Roos, E. and Dingemans, K.P., 1979. Mechanisms of metastasis. Biochim. Biophys. Act
    560: 135-166.

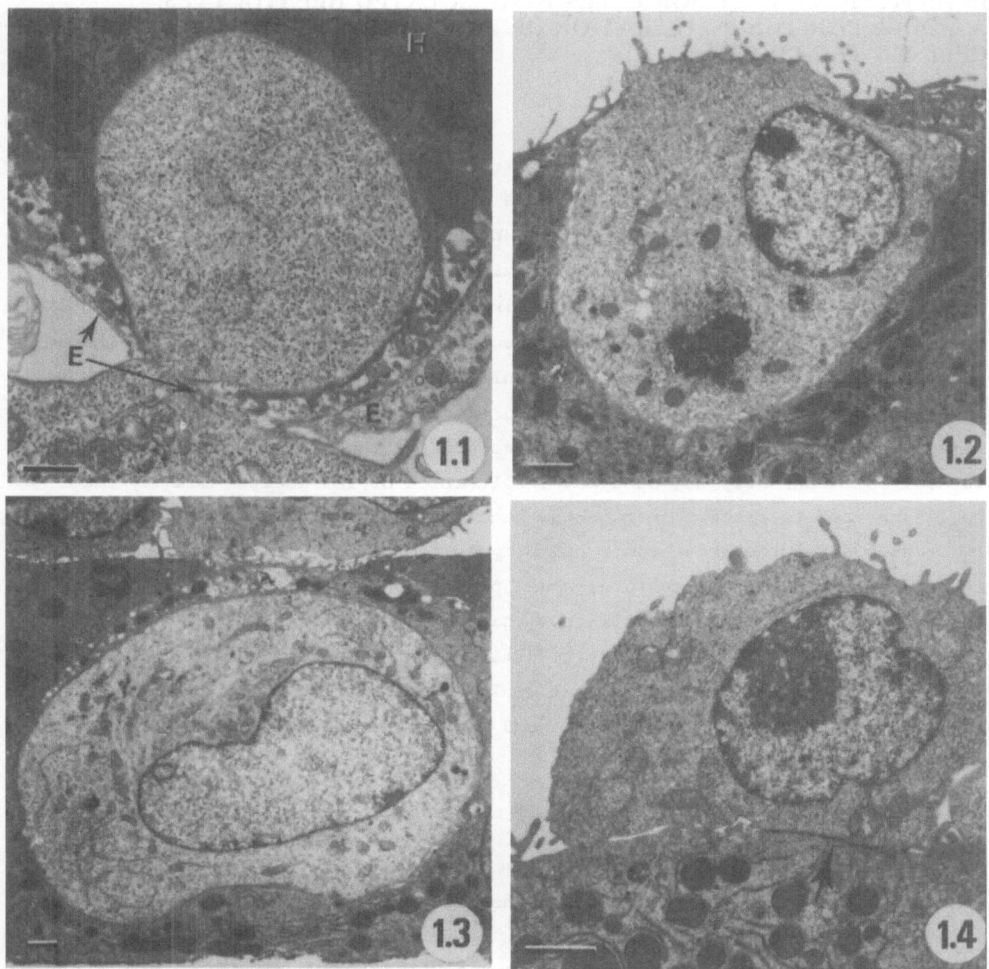

Fig. 1. Interactions of TA3 mammary carcinoma cells with hepatocytes.
1.1 A TA3 cell pseudopod extending through a small opening in liver endothelium
(E) and invaginating a hepatocyte (H). (Perfused mouse liver, 4 hours after addition of tumor cells to the perfusion medium)
1.2. A TA3 cell invaginating a hepatocyte, 4 h after addition to a 24 h hepatocyte culture.
1.3. A TA3 cell completely encircled by hepatocytes (within the plane of the
section), 24 h after addition to a hepatocyte culture. Substrate side of hepatocyte (bottom) slightly damaged by scraping it off the dish. Non-invaginating
TA3 cells are present on top of the hepatocytes.
1.4. Non-invaginating TA3 cell on a hepatocyte in culture. Note tight junction
(arrow). Also invaginating cells form tight junctions. Bar = 1 um

INTERACTIONS OF TUMOR CELLS WITH ISOLATED HEPATOCYTES. A MODEL FOR THE INFILTRATION OF BLOOD-BORNE TUMOR CELLS IN THE LIVER

E. Roos

1. INTRODUCTION

We have studied infiltration into the liver, both *in vivo* and in the perfused mouse liver, using electron microscopy. We found (Roos et al., 1977) that MB 6A lymphosarcoma cells penetrated through sinusoidal endothelium by extension of small protrusions through multiple openings in, rather than between, endothelial cells. These protrusions enlarged to pseudopods that deeply invaginated the hepatocytes underlying the endothelium. Enlargement of pseudopods continued until finally the whole tumor cell was located extravascularly (fig. 2.1). The invaginated hepatocytes, that fitted tightly around the tumor cells, were strongly deformed, but apparently not damaged. Infiltration of TA3 ascites mammary tumor cells appeared to proceed in much the same way (Roos et al., 1978; see fig. 1.1).

We have added the above tumor cells types to cultures of isolated rat hepatocytes, hoping that these cultures would prove to be a suitable model to study the described phenomena. We will show that the interaction between tumor cells and hepatocytes in these cultures is similar to that observed in the intact liver. The more detailed morphological analysis, that these cultures allowed for, seems to indicate that lymphosarcoma and mammary carcinoma cells do differ in their infiltration mechanism.

2. MATERIALS AND METHODS

2.1 Tumor cells

MB 6A ascites lymphosarcoma and TA3 ascites mammary carcinoma cells were maintained as described previously (Roos et al., 1977,1978). B16-F10 melanoma and PA3 prostate adenocarcinoma cells were grown in DMEM + 10% FCS and harvested with trypsin-EDTA.

2.2 Hepatocyte cultures

Rat hepatocytes were isolated by collagenase perfusion. They were cultured on gas-permeable membranes (Petriperm) in DMEM + 10% FCS, 20 mM HEPES and 1% adult rat serum.

Hepatocytes were washed 24 hours after isolation, and incubated in DMEM + 20 mM HEPES. Tumor cells were added and the cultures were fixed after different intervals and embedded *in situ*. Sections were cut perpendicular or parallel to the substrate. Alternatively, cells were gently scraped off the dish and embedded as a pellet.

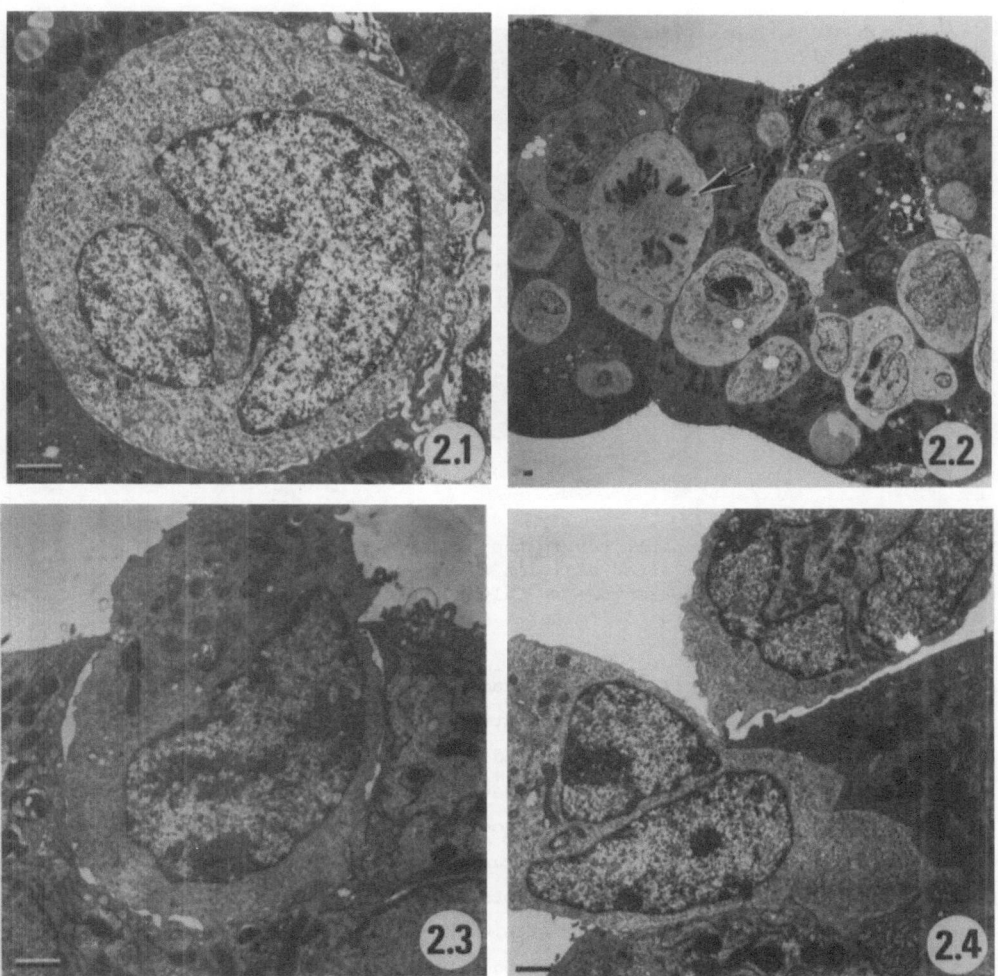

Fig. 2. Interactions of MB 6A lymphosarcoma cells with hepatocytes.
2.1. MB 6A cell in an extravascular location in the perfused liver, 3 h after
addition to the perfusion medium. The cell deeply invaginates one of the hepatocytes, between which it is located.
2.2. MB 6A cells, accumulated within a hepatocyte aggregate, 24 h after their
addition to a hepatocyte culture. Note cell in mitosis (arrow).
2.3. Invagination of a hepatocyte by a MB 6A cell, 3 h after addition to the
culture.
2.4. Intrusion of a MB 6A cell between two hepatocytes. Bar = 1 μm.

3. RESULTS

3.1 TA3 mammary carcinoma cells

TA3 cells adhered to the hepatocytes. Part of the TA3 cells invaginated the
hepatocytes (fig. 1.2), much like in the intact liver (fig. 1.1). Some TA3 cells
were completely encircled by hepatocytes in the plane of the section (fig. 1.3).

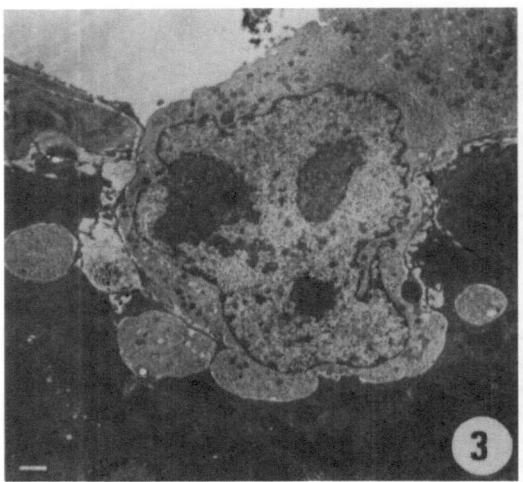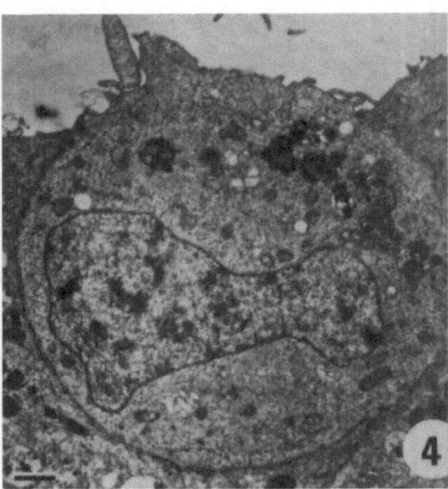

Fig. 3. Invagination of hepatocytes in the perfused liver, by pseudopods of a B16-F10 melanoma cell, 2 h after addition to the perfusion medium.
Fig. 4. Invagination of hepatocytes in culture by a PA3 prostate adenocarcinoma cell, 24 h after addition to the culture. Bar = 1 μm.

Another part of the TA3 cells did not invaginate (fig. 1.4). Several of these cells spread on the hepatocyte surface, attaining a flattened shape. Both non-invaginating and invaginating cells formed tight junctions with the hepatocytes (fig. 1.4). Studying serial sections, we established that TA3 cells invaginated all over the exposed surface of the hepatocytes. In order to quickly assess the extent of invagination, subconfluent cultures were scraped off the dish and pelleted. In sections through these pellets, the percentage of adherent TA3 cells that was completely encircled, within the plane of the section, by hepatocytes or contained between hepatocytes and substrate, was taken as an index for extent and average depth of invagination. This percentage was approx. 3% after 3 hours and approx. 12% after 24 hours.

3.2 MB 6A lymphosarcoma cells

MB 6A cells also adhered to the hepatocytes. They rapidly infiltrated (fig. 2.4) between and under the hepatocytes, and after 24 h most of the cells were located within the hepatocyte aggregates (fig. 2.2). Infiltrating cells deeply invaginated hepatocytes (fig. 2.3), as in the intact liver (fig. 2.1). Observation of serial sections indicated that, in contrast to TA3 cells, invagination did not occur all over the exposed surface, but only at interhepatocyte boundaries and between hepatocytes and substrate. Using the same quantification method, as described for TA3 cells, we found approx. 60% completely encircled cells after only 3 h, and approx. 90% after 24 hours.

3.3 B16 melanoma

Invagination of hepatocytes by B16 melanoma cells was sometimes seen in the perfused liver (fig. 3), but it was a rather rare phenomenon. In the cultures, invagination was observed, but most B16 cells spread over and under the hepatocytes, and became extremely flattened.

3.4 PA3 prostate adenocarcinoma

In preliminary experiments we have observed that interaction of the metastasizing rat prostate carcinoma PA3 (see contribution of M. Pollard) with hepatocytes was comparable to that of TA3 cells (fig. 4).

4. DISCUSSION

An *in vitro* model is presented for the interaction between tumor cells and hepatocytes during infiltration of tumor cells into liver parenchyma. Both in liver and in the cultures, hepatocytes were deeply invaginated by both MB 6A lymphosarcoma and TA3 mammary carcinoma cells. The MB 6A cells rapidly accumulated within the hepatocyte cultures, in keeping with their massive infiltration in the intact liver (Dingemans, 1973). In contrast, a minor proportion of the TA3 cells infiltrated, and much more slowly than MB 6A cells, as in the intact liver. The slowness of infiltration might be one of the reasons why few TA3 cells survive to form a limited number of liver nodules (Roos et al., 1978).

In contrast to what had appeared to be the case in the intact liver, the observations in the cultures seem to indicate that TA3 and MB 6A cells differ in their infiltration mechanism. Whereas MB 6A cells rapidly invaginated at interhepatocyte boundaries, the TA3 cells invaginated slowly all over the exposed surface, even when fixed to the hepatocytes by tight junctions. We propose that this invagination is due to a phagocytosis-like activity of the hepatocytes, leading to encirclement of TA3 cells. Encirclement does not occur when TA3 cells spread on the hepatocytes. Thus, invagination may be due to part of the TA3 cells being less able to spread on the hepatocytes.

Invagination by B16 cells was rare, both in the intact liver and in the cultures. Most B16 cells spread extensively over the hepatocytes. This might indicate that B16 cells in the liver might move under the endothelium, but over the hepatocytes, as is also suggested by the smooth boundaries between B16 liver nodules and the surrounding hepatocytes as described by Dingemans in this book.

REFERENCES

Dingemans, K.P., 1973. Behavior of intravenously injected malignant lymphoma cells. A morphologic study. J. Natl. Cancer Inst. 51: 1883-1895.
Roos, E., Dingemans, K.P., et al., 1977. Invasion of lymphosarcoma cells into the perfused mouse liver. J. Natl. Cancer Inst. 58: 399-407.
Roos, E., Dingemans, K.P., et al., 1978. Mammary-carcinoma cells in mouse liver: infiltration of liver tissue and interaction with Kupffer cells. Br. J. Cancer 38: 88-99.

ULTRASTRUCTURAL FEATURES OF INTRAVASCULAR AND EXTRAVASCULAR MIGRATION OF CANCER CELLS

T. Kawaguchi, S. Tobai, M. Endo and K. Nakamura

We have attempted to characterize the events in metastasis formation by electron microscopy through the examination of either embolic tumor cells or invading tumor cells into the vascular wall (Kawaguchi and Nakamura, 1976, Nakamura et al., 1977, Sakurai et al., 1977, Kawaguchi et al., 1978, Kawaguchi et al., 1979, Tobai et al., 1980). Female Donryu strain rats were used. The tumors used were Yoshida sarcoma (YS) and five strains of rat ascites hepatoma, AH-7974F, AH13, AH130, AH601 and AH 974.

The Mode of Intravasation

Soon after i.p. injection YS cells were found in circulating blood. The target site for early invasion of these cells were the milky spots in the omentum. In these sites the tumor cells were in close contact with the newly proliferating blood vessels or lymphatic vessels and were packed with elongated cytoplasmic processes of the endothelial cells resulting in their transport into the vascular lumen (Figs. 1-3).

The Mode of Extravasation

Examinations were undertaken of the brain, lungs, liver, kidneys, and adrenal glands, from 1 to 7 days after i.a. and i.v. injection of tumor cells. The tumor cells were arrested and lodged in the blood vessels without being enclosed by fibrin thrombi and platelet aggregates. They were in close contact with the endothelial cells by two particular junctional structures: one type being characterized by a parallel gap of about 100 A between the cells (Fig.4), and the other type having a coupling between adjacent cells with the insertion of a cytoplasmic protrusion of one into the depression of the other. The following three ways of extravasation were demonstrated. 1) Locomotion type (Fig.5). The tumor cells migrated actively through the endothelial linings and basement membranes. From the shape of the pseudopodia formed, they could be divided into three types:

filopod type (AH7974-brain, AH7974-glomerulus), lobopod type
(YS-liver, AH13-adrenal gland), and rhizopod type (AH13-liver).
2) Explosion type. The wall of the blood vessels was swollen
by the intravascular growth of a number of tumor emboli resulting
in explosive extravasation. This type of extravasation was
observed in the combination of AH7974-glomerulus (Figs. 6 and 7)
and AH601-lungs. 3) Segregation type. Tumor emboli in the blood
vessels were covered by repairing endothelial cells and thus
separated out from the blood stream. This type of extravasation
was observed in the combination of AH7974-brain (Fig.8) and
AH7974F-liver.

Attack of Tumor Cells Against Hepatic Cells

Destruction of hepatic cells by the tumor was found at one
day after i.v. inoculation. Some parts of the hepatic cells
adjacent to the tumor were actually attacked by microvilli or
cytoplasmic protrusions from the tumor cells. The destruction
of hepatic cells by AH7974F and AH13 cells was particularly noted.
The vesicles which were seen to be coated in many cases on the
cell surface of the hepatic cells, were filled by tips of microvilli or cytoplasmic protrusions of the tumor cells. The cytoplasmic protrusions of the tumor cells intruded deeply into the
hepatic cells, and some areas of the hepatic cells, were occupied
by many elongated cytoplasmic protrusions of the tumor cells and
were fragmented (Fig.9). Comments: Some workers have reported
that the intravasation of tumor cells are due to the direct
migration of tumor cells. In the present paper, we have demonstrated a new mode of intravasation of tumor cells. Principal
cellular events of hematogenously disseminated tumor cells in the
processes of metastasis formation have been suggested to be
arrest in organs, extravasation and establishment of growing foci.
Results in the present study seem to correspond with this scheme,
and indicate moreover the importance of the interaction of tumor
cells and normal host cells in every process.

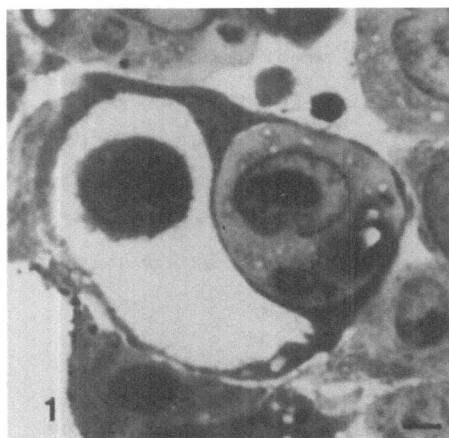 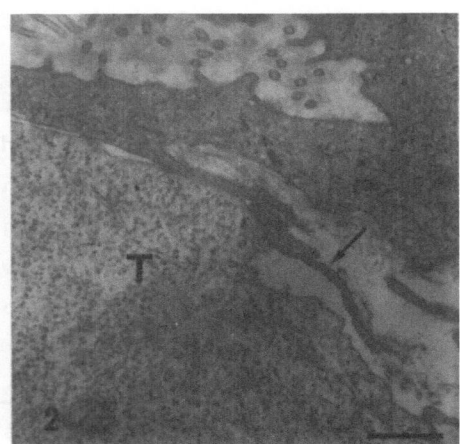

Fig. 1. A YS cell enclosed in endothelial cells. 24 hr. The scale is 2 micron.

Fig. 2. Endothelial cell of lymphatic vessel extending its cytoplasmic processes (arrow) toward the surface of YS cell (T) and in close contact with it. 24 hr. The scale is 1 micron.

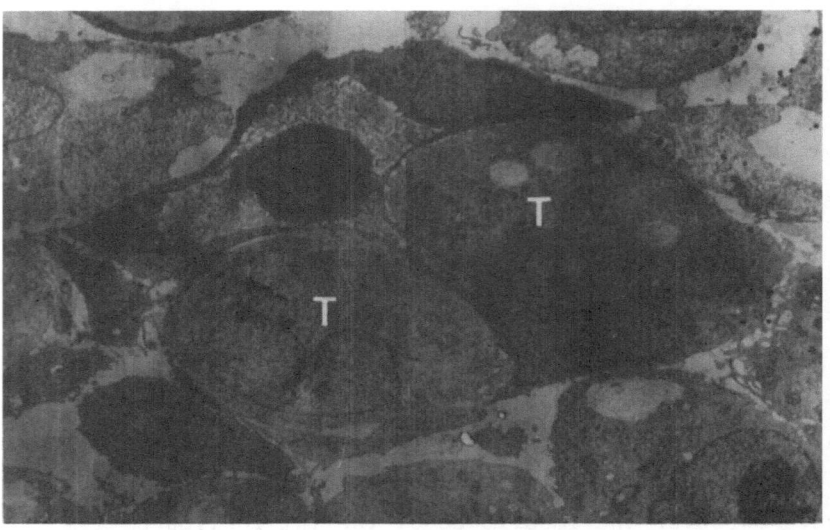

Fig. 3. Two YS cells (T) enclosed in endothelial cells of lymphatic vessel; tumor cells packed completely with cytoplasmic processes of endothelial cells. 24 hr. The scale is 2 micron.

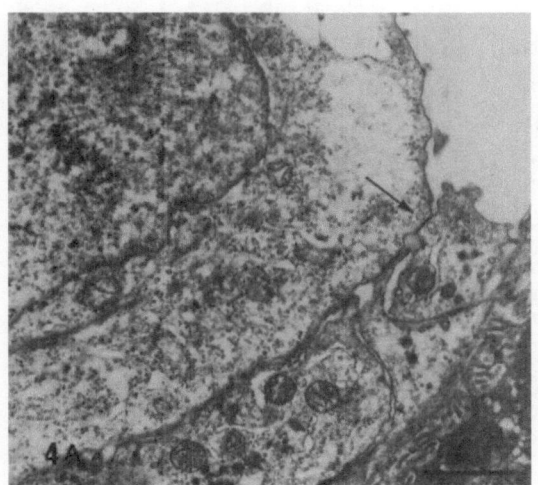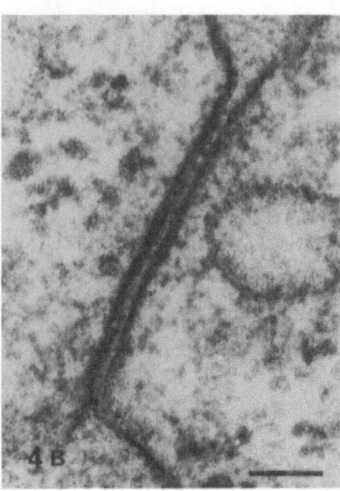

Fig. 4. (A) AH7974F cell in the liver sinusoid. This cell is attached to the endothelial cell at the arrow. The scale is 1 micron.
(B) A higher magnification of the contact region. The opposing cell
membranes show a parallel and straight arrangement across the gap
of about 100 A. The scale is 500 A.

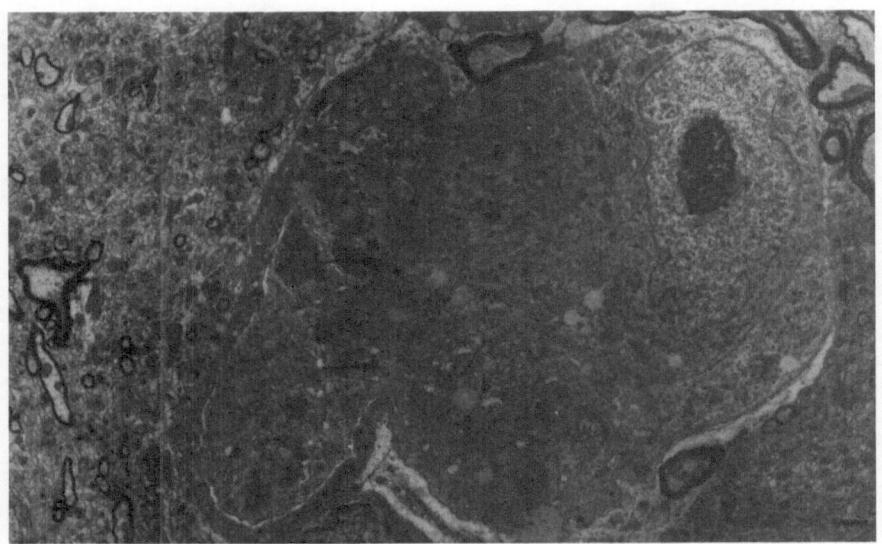

Fig. 5. Through two splits (arrows) of the wall, tumor cells look
as if they are emigrating from the vessel. Continuity of the cyto-
plasms of each of tumor cells is clear. AH7974-brain, 3 days.
The scale is 1 micron.

208

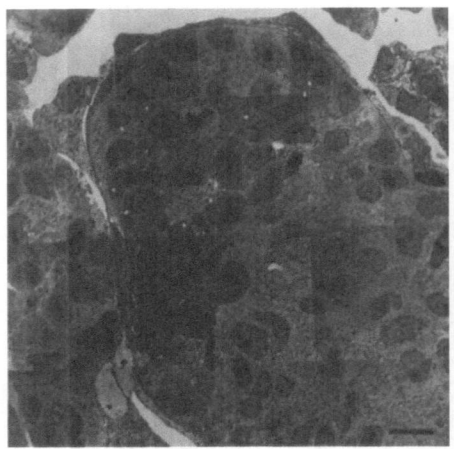

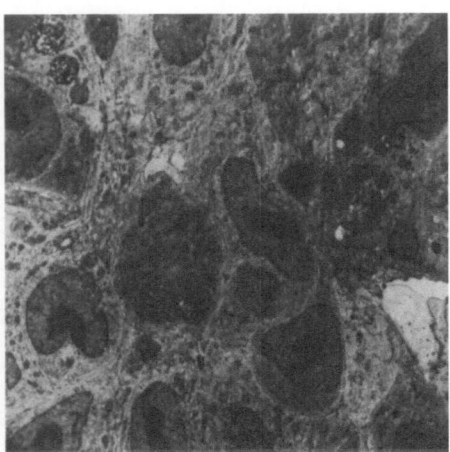

Fig. 6. Proliferated and metastatic AH7974 cells in the renal
corpuscle at 9 days after i.a.
One part of glomerular capillary
is swollen by proliferating tumor
cells (in the center). The scale
is 10 micron.

Fig. 7. Extravasation of the
tumor cells from the glomerular
capillary to the Bowman's space.
This breached portion was obtained from deeper sections of the
specimen shown in Fig. 6. The
scale is 1 micron.

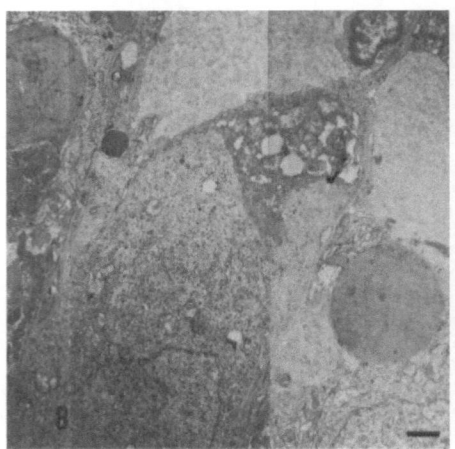

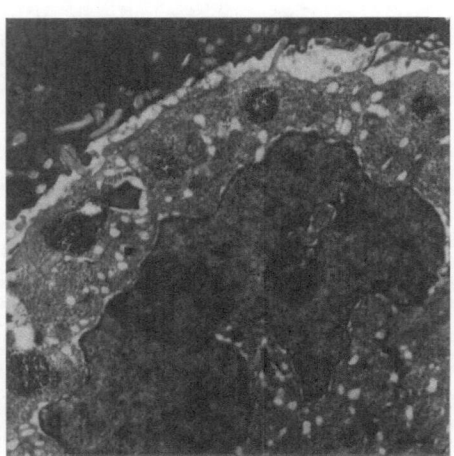

Fig. 8. AH7974 cells are segre-
gated from capillary space by repairing cytoplasm of endothelial
cells. 3 days-brain. The scale
is 1 micron.

Fig. 9. Many elongated cytoplasmic protrusions are seen in the
hepatic cell. AH13, 4 days. The
scale is 1 micron.

REFERENCES

Kawaguchi, T. and Nakamura, K., 1976. Electron microscopic studies on destructive action of tumor cells to normal cells. Saibo, 8: 447-450.
Kawaguchi, T., Tobai, S. and Nakamura, K., 1978. Electron-microscopic studies on stickiness of tumor cells to normal cells. Saibo, 10: 573-579.
Kawaguchi, T., Endo, M., Tobai, S. and Nakamura, K., 1979. Behavior pattern of rat ascites tumor cells arrested in liver sinusoids: An electron microscopic study. Gann, 70: 277-290.
Nakamura, K., Kawaguchi, T., Asahina, S., Sakurai, T., Ebina, Y. and Morita, M., 1977. Electronmicroscopic studies on extravasation of tumor cells and early foci of hamatogenous metastasis. Gann monogr., 20: 57-71.
Sakurai, T., Ebina, Y., Yokoya, S. and Nakamura, K., 1977. Electron microscopic studies on extravasation of ascites hepatomas in the kidney and lungs. Fukushima J. Med. Sci., 24: 1-21.
Tobai, S., Kawaguchi, T., Asahina, S. and Nakamura, K., 1980. Some findings on intravasation of Yoshida sarcoma cells in the onentum. Gann, submitted.

CHARACTERISTICS OF METASTASIZING AND NON-METASTASIZING TUMORS AND THEIR INTERACTION WITH THE HOST IMMUNE SYSTEM IN THE DEVELOPMENT OF METASTASIS

U. Kim

INTRODUCTION

Most animal solid tumors grow expansively at the site of origin without invading the surrounding soft tissue stroma or metastasizing to distant organs, even when they become very large. On the other hand, the single most critical attribute of human cancers is their capacity to invade and metastasize to vital secondary organs resulting in death of the patient. However, the lack of invasion and metastasis in laboratory animal tumors is not because the tumor cells do not enter into the systemic circulation of the host, for a large number of viable tumor cells are readily harvested from the venous as well as the arterial blood of animals bearing a localized tumor (Kim, 1966; Butler and Gullino, 1975), and yet such cells seem incapable of establishing secondary colonies. Thus, there seems to be fundamental difference in the biological property between human and animal tumor cells, and it may lie in the manner by which these tumors are developed. Laboratory investigators in general tend to favor fast growing tumors with a short latent period irrespective of the type of oncogenic agents used. Such tumors are frequently highly immunogenic (Prehn, 1975), due probably to insufficient time for the developing tumor cells to undergo immunological and other host-generated selective processes. Human cancers, on the other hand, particularly carcinomas are usually a late event in our life, and also most of them are non-immunogenic. Such characteristics are likely to have been brought about by more subtle oncogenic exposures and by repeated selective pressures produced by host immune surveillance mechanism during the life of patients. These suppositions were experimentally tested in young adult female rats by exposing them to chemical carcinogen together with the application of non-specific and specific immuno-suppression and stimulation to bring out weakly or non-immunogenic tumor cells slowly over an extended period of time. Such laboratory manipulation yielded many spontaneously meta-stasizing rat mammary carcinomas with many of their characteristics similar to those of breast cancer in women (Kim, 1970, 1977). Table 1 lists 9 representa-tives of such tumors that have been established and are maintained in the highly inbred strain of W/Fu rats in our laboratory to carry out various studies outlined in this paper. In order to learn the nature of metastatic potential of tumor cells, their biological, biochemical and immunological properties were compared with those of conventional, non-metastasizing, chemi-cally-induced, syngeneic rat tumors that had been matched according to the degree of glandular differentiation and growth rate in normal syngeneic rats.

TABLE 1

Established spontaneously metastasizing rat mammary carcinomas and their metastatic pattern.

Tumor strain	Metastasizing capacity[a]	Latency (days)[b]		Metastatic route and site
		Primary	Metastasis	
TMT-50	0-+	8	48	Hematogenous: lung only
STMT-058	+-++	8	30	Hematogenous & lymphatic: lymph node, lung
MT-449	++	10	40	Hematogenous & lymphatic: lymph node, lung
SMT-077	++-+++	60	50-60	Lymphatic: lymph node, lung, liver, bone
DMBA-4	++-+++	14	26	Lymphatic & hematogenous: lymph node, lung
MT-450	+-+	24	60	Hematogenous & lymphatic: lymph node, lung
SMT-2A	++-+	15	27	Lymphatic: lymph node, lung, liver, bone, others[c]
SMT-2B	++-+	60	60-70	Lymphatic: lymph node, lung, liver, bone, others
TMT-081	++-+	18	23	Hematogenous & lymphatic: lymph node, lung, liver, others

[a] After a standardized amount of tumor mince (0.05-0.1 ml) is injected into the right inguinal mammary fat pad, the spontaneously metastasizing capacity is arbitrarily graded as: + = slight; ++ = moderate; +++ = marked; ++++ = extensive, according to the speed and extent of metastasis.

[b] The time required for the primary implant to become palpable: 3-5 mm for the primary and 5-10 mm for the right axillary lymph node involvement. Metastasis to lung, liver, etc. are checked by surgical exposure.

[c] Spleen, kidney, heart, adrenal, soft tissues.
Five non-metastasizing, syngeneic rat mammary tumors (MT-W9A, MT-W9B, MT-66, MT-91, MT-100) are used as controls.

METASTATIC POTENTIAL OF TUMOR CELLS

Biological properties

After studying many spontaneously metastasizing and non-metastasizing rat mammary tumors, and comparing them with other rodent tumors and human breast cancer, the following general statements can be made (Kim, 1979). 1) In the development of metastasizing tumors we have learned that the acquisition of metastasizing property by these tumor cells seemed to have taken place already subclinically, for there was no grossly recognizable karyotypic difference between the primary and metastatic tumors either in the autochthonous host at the beginning or after many syngeneic transplantation generations.

Furthermore, the same metastatic potential seems to be inherent in all cells regardless of which organ they colonize, for an identical metastatic pattern can be maintained by transplanting either the primary tumor itself or any affected organ. Therefore, at least in this tumor system, one may conclude that there are no factors inherent in tumor cells that may be identified as having special affinity for a particular organ or tissue. 2) The structural or functional differentiation in connection with gland formation in mammary carcinomas, is independent of metastasizing capacity, for non-metastasizing tumors do not become metastasizing ones even when they have progressed from well differentiated to undifferentiated tumors during many generations of syngeneic transplantation. Among the metastasizing tumors, on the other hand, poorly differentiated tumors tend to be more aggressive by widely infiltrating an already involved organ than well differentiated ones. However, with respect to the distant metastasis, well differentiated ones are capable of disseminating just as far as poorly differentiated ones can. It is the capacity of blood borne tumor cells in traversing the pulmonary vasculature and entering into the greater circulation that will determine the distance of their journey. 3) As to the growth rate, poorly differentiated cells grow faster than well differentiated ones, but it is not necessarily correlated with the metastasizing capacity. Among the metastasizing ones, however, rapidly growing ones may spread faster, but not necessarily more extensively. Conversely, tumors with longer latency may metastasize more slowly, but often involve many more organs. 4) All metastasizing rat mammary tumors tested in our laboratory so far are either weakly or non-immunogenic. However the absence of immunogenicity does not seem to assure conferring the metastatic potential to tumor cells, for Baldwin (1973) observed that 2-aminofluorene-induced rat hepatomas were non-immunogenic, but also non-metastatic. The tumors that metastasize via the blood stream only to the lung seem to be immunogenic to a certain extent, and tend to lose their metastasizing capacity after successive syngeneic transplantations. 5) In vivo, the metastasizing tumor has microscopically distinct invasive periphery, in contrast to the sharply defined, expansive border of a non-metastasizing tumor mass. 6) In vitro, when they are cultivated in suspension with latex beads, the former tends to grow as free-floating single cells, while the latter attaches to the bead forming cohesive clusters (Horng and McLimans, 1975), suggesting that the metastasizing cells have reduced adhesiveness or bonding defect. 7) When the amount of blood flowing through the primary tumor mass was determined by the technique of infusing radiolabeled microspheres (^{125}I, ^{109}Cd, ^{141}Ce) into the left cardiac ventricle of tumor-bearing rats (Jirtle, et al., 1978), it was found that almost twice as much blood flowed through non-metastasizing tumors than metastasizing ones (Jirtle, unpublished data). This finding contradicts the Folkman's postulation of "tumor angiogenesis factor" playing an important role in tumor metastasis.

Immunological and biochemical properties

The metastasizing tumor cells can further be characterized as follows. 1) They share a common, organ (mammary gland)-specific antigen (Ghosh, et al., 1978), as is often the case with onco-fetal and other tumor-associated antigens of human cancers, while the non-metastasizing cells have individual, tumor-specific antigens similar to other chemically-induced rodent tumors (Prehn, 1975). 2) They also shed this antigen rapidly into their microenvironment, and it can be quantitated by the radioimmunoassay technique in their culture fluid as well as in the host sera. The amount of antigen released by these cells in vitro in a 24 hour period can be several hundred to several thousand times that of non-metastasizing cells (Ghosh, et al., 1979). Thus, the lack of immunogenicity in them may not only be due to its loss, but also to its nonspecificity. 3) The degree of shedding can be estimated by the level of plasma membrane marker enzymes in the cells, e.g., 5'-nucleotidase, phosphodiesterase I, which is inversely correlated with the metastasizing capacity (Kim, et al., 1975). The rate of antigen turnover or synthesis is reflected in the glycosyltransferase activity in the cells (Bernacki and Kim, 1977; Chatterjee and Kim, 1977, 1978). The serum enzyme levels also rise with the circulating antigen level in the tumor host, which probably help to prolong the half-life of the antigen by hyperglycosylating it, and contributing to the state of antigen excess in these animals. 4) Such organotypic antigen may also be characterized as "thymus-independent" and the tumor specific ones as "thymus-dependent." When the metastasizing cells were implanted into athymic nude mice, they were either rejected immediately or accepted only temporarily but eventually rejected, without developing metastasis (Kim, et al., 1980). Similarly, human cancers are extremely difficult to grow in these mice without prior cultivation in vitro, and even when some are successfully xenografted, they rarely metastasize (Rygaard, 1973; Sharkey and Fogh, 1979). On the other hand, the non-metastasizing ones were readily accepted by these mice, and grew rapidly to a large size, and produced blood-borne metastasis to the lung and liver of the mice, thus, reversing the metastatic potential.

CONCLUSIONS

The most outstanding characteristic of metastasizing tumor cells seems to be the extreme structural instability of their plasma membranes, causing them to unceasingly shed membrane constituents in the form of organotypic or onco-fetal antigens, with constant renewal of the loss. Such membrane defects may also permit the leakage of various degradative and other enzymes as well as some potent biological mediators, e.g., prostaglandins, plasminogen activator. These substances may not only weaken or break cell-to-cell bonds and clear the path for freed cells

214

to disperse, but also help subverting the host immune mechanism. Thus, cells with such property will be metastatic actively through their own power, and those without it will not, unless the host immune milieu is modified to T-cell deficient state.   In either tumor cell initiated or host mediated event, the phenomenon of tumor metastasis is brought about by their intricate interaction.

REFERENCES

Baldwin, R. W., 1973. Immunological aspects of chemical carcinogenesis. Adv. Cancer Res., 18: 1-75.
Bernacki, R. and Kim, U., 1977. Concomitant elevation in sialyltransferase activity and sialic acid content in rats with metastasizing mammary tumors. Science, 195: 577-580.
Butler, T. P. and Gullino, P. M., 1975. Quantitation of cell shedding into efferent blood of mammary carcinoma. Cancer Res., 35: 512-516.
Chatterjee, S. and Kim, U., 1977. Galactosyltransferase activity in metastasizing and nonmetastasizing rat mammary carcinomas and its possible relationship with tumor cell surface antigen shedding. J.Natl.Cancer Inst., 58: 273-280.
Ibid., 1978. Fucosyltransferase activity in metastasizing and nonmetastasizing rat mammary carcinomas. J.Natl.Cancer Inst., 61: 151-162.
Folkman, J., 1975. Tumor angiogenesis. In: F.F. Becker (editor), Cancer, a Comprehensive Treatise. Plenum Press, New York, pp. 355-388.
Ghosh, S., Grossberg, A., Kim, U. and Pressman, D., 1978. Identification and purification of an organ specific, tumor membrane-associated antigen from a spontaneously metastasizing rat mammary carcinoma. Immunochemistry, 15:345-352.
Ibid., 1979. A tumor-associated organ specific antigen in rat mammary carcinoma, present at high levels in metastatic and at low levels in nonmetastatic tumors. J. Natl. Cancer Inst., 62: 1229-1233.
Horng, C. and McLimans, W., 1975. Primary suspension culture of calf anterior pituitary cells on a microcarrier surface. Biotech. Bioengin., 17: 713-732.
Jirtle, R., Clifton, K.H. and Rankin, J.H.G., 1978. Measurement of mammary tumor blood flow in unanesthetized rat. J.Natl.Cancer Inst., 60: 881-886.
Kim, U., 1966. Factors controlling metastasis of experimental breast cancer. Cancer Res., 26: 462-464.
Ibid., 1970. Metastasizing mammary carcinomas in rats: Induction and study of their immunogenicity. Science, 67: 72-74.
Ibid., 1977. Pathogenesis of spontaneously metastasizing mammary carcinomas in rats. Gann Monogr., 20: 73-81.
Ibid., 1979. Factors influencing metastasis of breast cancer. In: W.L. McGuire (editor), Breast Cancer, vol. 3, Current Topics. Plenum Press, N.Y., pp.1-49.
Kim, U., Baumler, A., Carruthers, C. and Bielat, K., 1975. Immunological escape mechanism in spontaneously metastasizing tumors. Proc. Natl. Acad. Sci. USA, 72: 1012-1016.
Kim, U., Han, T., Ghosh, Freedman, V.H., Shin, S.I. and Pressman, D., 1980. Immunological mechanisms of selective graft resistance to certain malignant tumors and prevention of metastasis by athymic nude mice. In: N. Reed (editor), 3rd Internatl. Workshop on Nude Mice. Gustav-Fisher Verlag, New York, in press.
Prehn, R.T., 1975. The relationship of tumor immunogenicity to the concentration of the inducing oncogen. J. Natl. Cancer Inst., 55: 189-190.
Rygaard, J., 1973. Thymus and Self: Immunology of the Mouse Mutant Nude. Wiley, New York.
Sharkey, F. E. and Fogh, J., 1979. Metastasis of human tumors in athymic nude mice. Int. J. Cancer, 24:733-738.

(This work was supported in part by the grant CA-24215 from the National Cancer Institute, U.S. Public Health Service.)

METASTATIC POTENTIAL OF TUMOR CELLS FROM SPONTANEOUS METASTASIS

A. Mantovani, R. Giavazzi, G. Alessandri, F. Spreafico
and S. Garattini

Metastasis is one of the crucial events in malignancy but the mechanisms involved in the processes of cancer cell dissemination and metastasis still largely remain to be defined (Fidler, 1978; Poste and Fidler, 1980). Tumor cell clones from primary murine neoplasms can be markedly heterogeneous in several biological characteristics including metastasizing capacity (Fidler and Kripke, 1977; Kripke et al., 1978; Suzuki et al., 1978; Dexter et al., 1978; Miller and Heppner, 1979). Tumor lines have been selected which, upon intravenous inoculation, show enhanced metastatic capacity (Fidler, 1973) or which selectively seed at specific anatomical sites (Brunson and Nicolson, 1978; Brunson et al., 1978; Tao et al., 1979). Essentially on the basis of these findings, it has been proposed that metastases originate from variant cells with greater intrinsic metastasizing capacity, pre-existing within the primary neoplasm, and that metastasis formation is the ultimate expression of a strongly selective multistep process (Fidler, 1978; Kripke et al., 1978; Poste and Fidler, 1980).

This hypothesis predicts that cells from spontaneous metastases are better able to undergo the multistep process of metastatic dissemination. This prediction was not verified in the present study, in which we investigated the metastatic potential of cells from spontaneous metastases in transplanted murine tumors.

In a first series of experiments, lung metastases from a transplanted, chemically-induced sarcoma (mFS6, Mantovani, 1978) were studied. Individual lung lesions were transplanted s.c. in syngeneic mice, and the metastatic capacity of the resulting neoplasms was studied (Table 1). Cell lines derived from individual metastatic lung deposits were heterogeneous in their capacity to give spontaneous metastases after i.m. inoculation. Compared to the primary tumor, the M4 and M7 lines showed significantly greater metastatic capacity, whereas the M8 and M9 lines had little metastatic potential. Cell lines from the remaining nodules(M1,M2, M3, M5 and M6) were not significantly different from the primary mFS6 sarcoma in this respect. No consistent difference was detected in the growth rate of the lesions, as judged from the survival time of tumor-bearing mice (Table 1) and from tumor diameters measured twice per week with calipers (results not presented).

TABLE 1

Spontaneous metastases of tumor cell lines derived from lung secondaries of the mFS6 sarcoma.

Tumor line	MST[a]	Mice with metastases/total	Metastases number ($\pm$S.E.)[b]	Metastases weight (mg$\pm$S.E.)[b]
Primary	33 (25-50)	17/32	3.3 $\pm$ 0.3	18.2 $\pm$ 5.4
Cell line from metastasis				
No. M1	38 (25-49)	4/8	5.2 $\pm$ 3.2	50.1 $\pm$ 40.9
M2	33 (28-55)	6/15	3.2 $\pm$ 1.2	7.8 $\pm$ 7.0
M3	36 (25-48)	10/16	8.7 $\pm$ 3.0	48.9 $\pm$ 33.2
M4	36 (30-49)	13/14[c]	16.7 $\pm$ 3.6[c]	122.5 $\pm$ 38.5[c]
M5	33 (25-41)	10/15	8.7 $\pm$ 1.8	45.7 $\pm$ 20.0
M6	31 (27-42)	10/15	7.8 $\pm$ 2.9	11.3 $\pm$ 4.0
M7	44 (33-52)	15/15[c]	13.8 $\pm$ 2.6[c]	170.2 $\pm$ 12.7[c]
M8	35 (26-27)	1/16[c]	1.0	0.5
M9	38 (30-51)	0/15[c]	-	-
Pool of data for metastases	36 (25-52)	69/129	10.5 $\pm$ 1.19	57.1 $\pm$ 21.1

4-5 weeks after inoculation of the spontaneously metastasizing mFS6 sarcoma (Mantovani, 1978), C57B1/6 male mice were killed. The lungs were aseptically removed and examined with a dissecting microscope. Lung secondaries were dissected free of gross lung parenchyma, rinsed with basal medium Eagle (BME) and transplanted s.c. into the back of individual mice with the aid of a trochar. The resulting tumors, each deriving from an individual lung nodule and designated M1 through M9, were aseptically collected when weighing 4-6 g, and stored in liquid nitrogen. To evaluate metastasizing capacity, the tumors were disaggregated with trypsin (0.3%) and 10^4 cells in 0.1 ml BME were injected i.m. in the right hind thigh. At death the number and weight of lung secondaries was measured as previously described (Spreafico et al., 1975). The incidence of mice with metastases was analysed by Fisher's exact test, and Duncan's new multiple range test was used for metastases weight and number.
[a]Median survival time with range shown in parentheses
[b]Number or weight of lung metastases/mouse
[c]$p < 0.01$ compared to primary mFS6 sarcoma.

When cell lines from metastases, kept frozen in liquid nitrogen, were repeatedly tested over a period of 1 year, the same pattern of metastasing capacity was observed.

Metastasizing capacity after i.v. inoculation was also measured (Table 2) and under these conditions too, cell lines from individual metastases were to some extent heterogeneous though on the whole they showed no consistent tendency to increased metastatic potential. It is noteworthy that for some lines (e.g. M7) there was little correlation between their capacity to metastasize by the i.v. and i.m. route, relative to other lines and the primary tumor.

Since s.c. passage of metastases in mice may have altered their properties, in a series of experiments individual lung lesions (≥ 3 mm in diameter) were dissected free of lung parenchyma, disaggregated and injected immediately i.m. (Table 3) or i.v. (results not presented) into test animals. None of the 8 metastatic cell preparations had greater metastatic potential than the primary tumor; metastasis No. 18 gave fewer spontaneous lung metastases than the primary neoplasm.

TABLE 2

Artificial metastases of tumor cell lines derived from lung secondaries of the mFS6 sarcoma

Tumor line	Mice with metastases/total	Metastases number ($\pm$S.E.)[a]	Metastases weight (mg$\pm$S.E.)[a]
Primary mFS6	7/8	34.8 ± 4.8	21.2 ± 5.0
Cell lines from metastasis No. 41	8/8	3.0 ± 0.4[b]	3.4 ± 0.9[b]
42	8/8	123.5 ± 21.9[c]	97.5 ± 0.5[c]
43	8/8	39.5 ± 8.8	20.5 ± 5.1
M4	8/8	83.0 ± 10.4[c]	43.2 ± 5.4
M5	7/8	2.9 ± 0.9[b]	1.5 ± 0.4[b]
M6	8/8	2.5 ± 0.2[b]	1.3 ± 0.1[b]
M7	8/8	49.6 ± 6.3	25.7 ± 3.3
M8	7/8	6.3 ± 1.6[b]	3.3 ± 0.8[b]
M9	7/8	22.8 ± 5.0	13.5 ± 2.3
Pool of data for metastases	69/72	40.7 ± 5.9	24.5 ± 6.18

Tumor lines were the same as in Table 1. To evaluate artificial metastases, 10^5 cells in 0.2 ml basal medium Eagle were injected i.v. in the tail vein and the mice were killed 18 days later.

[a] Number or weight of lung metastases/ mouse
[b] $p < 0.05$ compared to primary mFS6 sarcoma
[c] $p < 0.01$ compared to primary mFS6 sarcoma

TABLE 3

Spontaneous metastases from lung secondaries of the mFS6 sarcoma

Tumor cells	Tumor palpable on day[a]	MST[b]	Metastases number (+S.E.)	Metastases weight (mg+S.E.)
Primary tumor	14	37	13.5 + 6.3	49.0 + 27.3
Metastases No. 11	14	42 (35-48)	8.7 + 2.6	26.4 + 13.1
	12	15	42 (33-48)	7.6 + 3.5	14.1 + 7.7
	13	14	36 (28-50)	16.6 + 5.6	38.2 + 16.3
	14	14	35 (30-37)	8.3 + 2.7	7.8 + 2.6
	15	13	37 (29-39)	9.5 + 2.4	24.8 + 15.2
	16	12	32 (26-39)	4.4 + 1.5	3.8 + 1.1
	17	12	37 (32-40)	18.0 + 7.5	48.2 + 28.8
	18	12	35 (27-37)	2.5 + 0.9[c]	5.4 + 3.2
Pool of data for metastases	14	37 (27-50)	9.43+1.47	20.7 + 5.1

Individual lung metastases were disaggregated immediately after isolation from the lung parenchyma; 10^4 cells were injected i.m. and metastases were evaluated at death.

[a] Day on which 50% of injected mice showed a palpable tumor
[b] Median survival time with range
[c] $p < 0.05$ compared to the primary tumor

In the experiments discussed above, lung metastases from a sarcoma were examined In a further series of experiments the metastasizing capacity of secondaries from the M5076/73A (M5) ovarian carcinoma was investigated (Mantovani et al., 1980). As shown by the typical findings presented in Table 4, this tumor (of spontaneous origin, histologically an anaplastic carcinoma, obtained though the courtesy of Dr. A.E. Bogden, Mason Res. Inst., Worcester, Mass.) after i.m., s.c. or even i.v. inoculation, selectively metastasizes to abdominal organs, lung lesions being rarely observed (Mantovani et al., 1980). After i.p. inoculation the tumor grows as scattered lesions on the abdominal wall and, at late stages, causes ascites (results not presented). Thus this neoplasm selectively metastasizing to various abdominal organs represents a unique experimental model. As illustrated by the representative experiment shown in Table 4, individual metastases from the M5

TABLE 4

Metastasizing capacity of metastases from the M5 ovarian carcinoma

Tumor line from	Metastases at[a]					
	Spleen	Kidney	Liver	Lung	Ovary	Uterus
Primary tumor	9/16	7/16	16/16	0/16	12/16	10/16
[b]Metastasis from spleen No.						
1	0/6	1/6	4/6	0/6	3/6	2/6
2	1/3	0/3	2/3	0/3	2/3	2/3
3	0/4 (5/22)[c]	0/4 (5/22)	0/4 (14/22)	0/4 (0/22)	1/4 (12/22)	0/4 (6/22)
4	4/5	3/5	5/5	0/5	2/5	0/5
5	0/4	1/4	3/4	0/4	4/4	2/4
Liver No.						
1	3/6	2/6	6/6	0/6	3/6	2/6
2	4/5 (8/16)	3/5 (5/16)	3/5 (11/16)	0/5 (0/16)	3/5 (6/16)	3/5 (5/16)
3	1/5	0/5	2/5	0/5	0/5	0/5
Ovary No.						
1	0/6	1/6	3/6	0/6	2/6	1/6
2	2/5 (3/16)	1/5 (6/16)	5/5 (12/16)	0/5 (0/16)	3/5 (9/16)	0/5 (4/16)
3	1/5	4/5	4/5	0/5	4/5	3/5
Kidney No.						
1	2/7	0/7	6/7	0/7	2/7	2/7
2	1/7 (8/22)	1/7 (5/22)	4/7 (16/22)	0/7 (0/22)	2/7 (11/22)	0/7 (5/22)
3	5/8	4/8	6/8	0/8	7/8	3/8

C57Bl/6 female mice were injected s.c. with cells from the primary tumor or individual mestastases. Mice were killed 28 days after tumor inoculation. Presence or absence of metastases in various organs was confirmed histologically. As no differences were detected in the number and weight of the lesions, these data are not presented, for clarity's sake.

[a]Mice with metastases/total 28 days after s.c. inoculation of tumor cells.
[b]Each tumor line was obtained from an individual nodule after one subcutaneous passage
[c]Pool of data for metastases from each anatomical site

ovarian carcinoma were heterogeneous in their metastatic capacity, but also in this model on the whole tumor cells from spontaneous metastases showed no apparent tendency to express increased metastatic potential. In Table 4 results are presented as incidence of mice with metastases, but similar conclusions were drawn from the number and weight of the lesions.

Results similar to those described herein with the mFS6 sarcoma and M5 ovarian carcinoma were obtained in a series of experiments on spontaneous lung metastases from the B16 melanoma, colon 26 carcinoma and MCA1 sarcoma, a tumor recently induced in our laboratory with methylcholanthrene.

Thus, tumor cells from spontaneous metastases at different anatomical sites are, to some extent, heterogeneous in their metastatic potential, both among themselves and compared to the primary tumor. Although individual metastases were heterogeneous in their metastatic potential, overall tumor cells from spontaneous metastases in this series of murine neoplasms showed no tendency to express a better ability than the primary tumor to undergo the multistep process of metastasization.

Cell clones from primary murine tumors can be markedly heterogeneous in their metastatic potential (Fidler and Kripke, 1977; Kripke et al., 1978; Suzuki et al., 1978). In the B16 melanoma, used also in the present study, of 17 clones examined, 2 were similar to the parent tumor cell population, 8 were more metastatic and 7 were less metastatic (Fidler and Kripke, 1977). Similar results were obtained with some of the tumors used in the present study. For instance, in one experiment of 7 clones from the primary MN/MCA1 sarcoma, two were more metastatic than the primary neoplasm, the remaining being comparable to or less metastatic than the parent tumor population (unpublished data). On this basis one would have expected spontaneous metastases to derive mainly from those clones with greater metastatic potential and therefore to express a better capacity to undergo the multistep process of metastasis formation. This prediction was not verified in the present study. Individual metastases were to some extent heterogeneous in their metastatic potential, but overall tumor cells from spontaneous metastases showed no tendency quantitative or qualitative, to express a better ability to undergo the multistep process of metastasis formation. It would therefore appear that in the murine tumors considered in the present study, metastasis is not the ultimate expression of a strong selection of variant cells endowed with greater intrinsic metastasizing capacity. Thus the possibility that metastases are to some extent a random representation of the cell populations present within the primary tumor still merits serious consideration.

Acknowledgement

This work was supported by Grant ROI-CA-12764 from the National Cancer Institute and by Contract 78.02792.96 from Consiglio Nazionale delle Ricerche, Rome, Italy.

We thank Dr. A. Anaclerio for discussions and criticisms and Miss Anna Mancini for typing the manuscript.

References

Brunson, K.W., Beattie, G. and Nicolson, G.L., 1978. Selection and altered properties of brain-colonising metastatic melanoma. Nature, 272: 543-545.

Brunson, K.W. and Nicolson, G.L., 1978, Selection and biologic properties of malignant variants of a murine lymphosarcoma. J. Natl. Cancer Inst., 61: 1499-1503.

Dexter, D.L., Kowalski, H.M., Blazar, B.A., Fligiel, Z., Vogel, R. and Heppner, G.H., 1978, Heterogeneity of tumor cells from a single mouse mammary tumor. Cancer Res., 38: 3174-3181.

Fidler, I.J., 1973, Selection of successive tumour lines for metastasis. Nature New Biol., 242: 148-149.

Fidler, I.J., 1978, Tumor heterogeneity and the biology of cancer invasion and metastasis. Cancer Res., 38: 2651-2660.

Fidler, I.J. and Kripke, M.L., 1977, Metastasis results from preexisting variant cells within a malignant tumor. Science, 197: 893-895.

Kripke, M.L., Gruys, E. and Fidler, I.J., 1978, Metastatic heterogeneity of cells from an ultraviolet light-induced murine fibrosarcoma of recent origin. Cancer Res., 38: 2962-2967.

Mantovani, A., 1978, Effects on in vitro tumor growth of murine macrophages isolated from sarcoma lines differing in immunogenicity and metastasizing capacity. Int. J. Cancer, 22: 741-746.

Mantovani, A., Giavazzi, R., Polentarutti, N., Spreafico, F. and Garattini, S., 1980, Divergent effects of macrophage toxins on growth of primary tumors and lung metastases in mice. Int. J. Cancer, in press.

Miller, F.R. and Heppner, G.H., 1979, Immunologic heterogeneity of tumor cell subpopulations from a single mouse mammary tumor. J. Natl. Cancer Inst., 63: 1457-1463.

Poste, G. and Fidler, I.J., 1980, The pathogenesis of cancer metastasis. Nature 283: 139-146.

Spreafico, F., Vecchi, A., Mantovani, A., Poggi, A., Franchi, G., Anaclerio, A., and Garattini, S., 1975, Characterization of the immunostimulants levamisole and tetramisole. Eur. J. Cancer, 11: 555-563.

Suzuki, N., Withers, H.R. and Koehler, M.W., 1978, Heterogeneity and variability of artificial lung colony-forming ability among clones from mouse fibrosarcoma. Cancer Res., 38: 3349-3351.

Tao, T.-w., Matter, A., Vogel, K. and Burger, M.M., 1979, Liver-colonizing melanoma cells selected from B-16 melanoma. Int. J. Cancer, 23: 854-857.

CELL SURFACE CHANGES ASSOCIATED WITH THE SELECTION OF SPONTANEOUS METASTASES

G.A. Turner, D. Guy, A.L. Latner and G.V. Sherbet

INTRODUCTION

Recent studies (Fidler, 1973; Brunson et al., 1978; Tao et al., 1979) have suggested that tumour cell populations are heterogeneous with respect to their metastatic ability, and that certain subpopulations can be selected with characteristics which specify both the site and/or the degree of metastatic spread. Furthermore, in some cases these differences in biological behaviour have been shown to be accompanied by changes in the composition of the cell surface (Bosmann et al., 1973; Yogeeswaran et al., 1978; Brunson et al., 1978). The significance of these changes, however, to the metastatic process as a whole is still unclear because they have been demonstrated with cells selected after intravenous implantation and not with cells spontaneously released from a primary tumour. The object of the present study was to try to relate any change in cell surface structure with the process of spontaneous metastasis. For this purpose, cells were isolated from the primary and secondary growths of a metastasizing lymphoblastic lymphoma (ML) and the same tumour which had been subjected to a number of alternate passages through the secondary site.

MATERIALS AND METHODS

Unselected tumours were grown in Syrian hamsters by the subcutaneous transplantation of pieces of chopped tumour from a primary (1°) growth. Selected tumours were obtained by the isolation of secondary (2°) tumour cells from the liver of hamsters bearing a subcutaneous 1°. These cells were then transplanted subcutaneously into another hamster, and this whole procedure repeated five times. Single cell suspensions from 1° and 2° growths were prepared using collagenase, and non-viable cells and erythrocytes were removed by centrifugation on Ficoll-Hypaque (Guy et al., 1977, 1979a). Collagenase treatment resulted in the release of approximately the same number of cells from the 1° growths of unselected and selected tumours; however, with the 2° growths more cells were released by the selected tumours.

The adhesion of 1° and 2° cells to monolayer cultures was investigated using the method described by Walther et al. (1973). Tumour cells were labelled with ^{51}Cr and 10^5 labelled cells were added to fully confluent washed monolayers (Chang, BHK, HaK and 3T3) grown in multiwell dishes. These were agitated for fixed times between 5 and 60 min and the number of adherent cells determined by lysing the washed monolayer with ammonium hydroxide and measuring the bound radioactivity. Results were expressed either as maximum adhesion or as the adhesive rate constant (Walther et al., 1973).

Adhesion to immobilized lectins was determined using the method described by Guy et al. (1979b). Lectins were coupled to 60 mm diameter polystyrene Petri dishes (bacteriological grade) using 1 cyclohexyl-3-(2-morpholinoethyl) carbodiimide metho-p-toluene sulfonate. The number of adherent cells was determined microscopically after shaking 2×10^6 cells for 10 min.

Cell surface proteins were labelled with ^{125}I as described previously (Guy et al., 1979a). Extracts of this labelled material were analysed by carrying out electrophoresis in 7.5% (^{w}/v) polyacrylamide gels. After electrophoresis, the distribution of radioactivity was determined by counting 1 mm slices of the gel.

RESULTS

Table 1 compares the adhesion of the unselected and selected cells to various monolayers of cultured cells. For all monolayers investigated both the adhesive rate constant and the maximum adhesion significantly increased ($P < 0.01$) after selection. The same result was obtained whether 1° and 2° cell preparations were compared.

Table 2 compares the adhesion of the unselected and selected cells to immobilized lectins. In this case, selection resulted in a considerable change in the adhesion profile of the ML cells. Significantly less ($P < 0.025$) selected cells were observed to adhere to WGA and ricin II, but significantly more ($P < 0.025$) of the selected cells adhered to Gorse I. Again, similar changes were observed with both the 1° and 2° selected cells. As these lectins have certain sugar specificities, the findings suggest that the surface expression of N-acetylglucosamine and D-galactose on the selected cells is reduced and the expression of L-fucose is increased.

TABLE 1

Adhesion of Unselected and Selected 1^O and 2^O ML Cells to Cell Monolayers

Cell Monolayer	Tumour Cell	mean $\pm$ SD	
		Adhesive Rate Constant (% min^{-1})	Maximum Adhesion (%)
Chang	Unselected 1^O	0.62 ± 0.01	17.1 ± 0.2
	2^O	0.60 ± 0.03	17.8 ± 0.3
	Selected 1^O	0.66	20.0
	2^O	0.68	21.0
BHK	Unselected 1^O	0.52 ± 0.03	17.4 ± 0.4
	2^O	0.50 ± 0.01	17.1 ± 0.2
	Selected 1^O	0.68	20.5
	2^O	0.68	19.5
HaK	Unselected 1^O	0.33 ± 0.04	9.6 ± 0.4
	2^O	0.33 ± 0.02	9.4 ± 0.2
	Selected 1^O	0.42	11.5
	2^O	0.39	10.0
3T3	Unselected 1^O	0.13 ± 0.02	4.9 ± 0.4
	2^O	0.14 ± 0.03	5.8 ± 0.2
	Selected 1^O	0.18	6.5
	2^O	0.19	6.0

Values for unselected and selected cells were calculated from triplicate measurements made on each cell suspension prepared from 3 and 2 different tumours respectively.

TABLE 2

Adhesion of Unselected and Selected 1^O and 2^O ML Cells to Immobilized Lectins

	Number of Adherent Cells/Field (mean $\pm$ SD)			
	Unselected ML		Selected ML	
Lectin	1^O	2^O	1^O	2^O
Con A	103 ± 6	105 ± 5	102 ± 6	103 ± 3
WGA	85 ± 4	84 ± 3	76 ± 3	77 ± 6
Ricin I	113 ± 7	114 ± 5	116 ± 7	118 ± 5
Ricin II	154 ± 10	155 ± 10	141 ± 8	136 ± 10
Gorse I	91 ± 4	90 ± 3	99 ± 4	101 ± 3

Values were calculated from 20 observations made on each cell suspension prepared from 2 different tumours.

Qualitatively, the radiolabelling patterns of the unselected and selected cells were very similar to those previously reported for ML 1° and 2° cells (Guy et al., 1979a). There were, however, indications of possible quantitative differences in the patterns. Therefore, in order to have an objective assessment of these differences the patterns were divided into six sections, each section consisting of a defined range of R_f values. Subsequent comparisons were then made by expressing the total count for each section as a percentage of the overall total count. Such an analysis (Table 3) showed that selection was accompanied by a significant decrease ($P < 0.025$) in the incorporation in section V of the pattern. This section contained molecules with a molecular weight of approximately 20K. The same change was observed for both 1° and 2° cells prepared from selected tumours.

TABLE 3

Distribution of ^{125}I in Surface Proteins of Unselected and Selected 1° and 2° ML Cells

Tumour Cell	Distribution of ^{125}I in Different Sections of Gel (mean % $\pm$ SD)					
	I	II	III	IV	V	VI
Unselected 1°	11.7 $\pm$ 1.1	24.9 $\pm$ 1.5	13.4 $\pm$ 0.8	18.6 $\pm$ 0.6	14.3 $\pm$ 1.2	17.0 $\pm$ 1.3
Unselected 2°	11.6 $\pm$ 0.8	26.1 $\pm$ 2.2	13.0 $\pm$ 0.7	18.7 $\pm$ 0.7	13.3 $\pm$ 0.6	17.1 $\pm$ 1.5
Selected 1°	11.8 $\pm$ 0.9	25.6 $\pm$ 0.7	13.5 $\pm$ 0.8	19.1 $\pm$ 0.8	11.9 $\pm$ 0.4	17.8 $\pm$ 0.9
Selected 2°	11.6 $\pm$ 0.2	25.8 $\pm$ 1.3	13.2 $\pm$ 0.4	19.4 $\pm$ 0.1	12.0 $\pm$ 0.7	17.9 $\pm$ 0.7

Sections I to VI correspond to R_f ranges 0 - 0.13; 0.14 - 0.4; 0.41 - 0.53; 0.54 - 0.73; 0.74 - 0.87; 0.88 - 1.00 respectively. Bromophenol blue band taken as $R_f = 1$. Values for unselected and selected cells were calculated from measurements made on each cell suspension prepared from 5 and 3 different tumours respectively.

DISCUSSION

These results suggest that the passage of ML tumour cells through the process of spontaneous metastasis, rather than experimental metastasis, is also associated with changes in cell surface structure; however, the reasons for some of these changes occurring with selection is still uncertain. Obviously, the increased adhesion of the selected tumour cells to cell monolayers could be linked with an increased ability of circulating tumour cells to form attachments to vascular

endothelium. Furthermore, maximum rates of adhesion of the selected
ML cells did occur with monolayers which consisted of cells originally
isolated from the liver, and this organ is the predominant site for
secondary localisation of the ML cells. Previous results (Brunson et
al., 1978; Tao et al., 1979) have suggested that organ specificity
may be important in determining the site of secondary localisation.

The changes we observed for surface sugars and proteins are more
difficult to interpret. Probably they are associated with the changes
in cell adhesion. It might be expected that altered expression of
surface macromolecules would be accompanied by rearrangement, and
this in itself implies involvement with cell adhesion. In relation
to one of the observed changes, the increased expression of fucose,
it is interesting to note that it has been shown that metastasizing
mammary carcinomas have higher levels of a fucosyl transferase enzyme
than are present in non-metastasizing mammary carcinomas (Chatterjee
and Kim, 1978).

REFERENCES

Bosmann, H.B., Bieber, G.F., Brown, A.E., Case, K.R., Gersten, D.M.,
Kimmerer, T.W. and Lione, A., 1973. Biochemical parameters corre-
lated with tumour cell implantation. Nature, 246: 487-489.
Brunson, K.W., Beattie, G.B., and Nicolson, G.L., 1978. Selection and
altered properties of brain-colonising metastatic melanoma. Nature,
272: 543-544.
Chatterjee, S.K. and Kim, U., 1978. Fucosyltransferase activity in
metastasizing and non-metastasizing rat mammary carcinomas. J.
Natl. Cancer Inst., 61: 151-162.
Fidler, I.J., 1973. Selection of successive tumour lines for metastasis. Nature New Biology, 242: 148-149.
Guy, D., Latner, A.L. and Turner, G.A., 1977. Radioiodination studies
of tumour cell surface proteins after different disaggregation procedures. Br. J. Cancer, 36: 166-172.
Guy, D., Latner, A.L. and Turner, G.A., 1979a. Surface protein distribution in cells isolated from solid tumours and their metastases.
Br. J. Cancer, 40: 634-640.
Guy, D., Latner, A.L. and Turner, G.A., 1979b. A simple lectin-mediat
cell-adhesion method for investigating the cell surface. Exp. Cell
Biol., 47: 312-319.
Tao, T-W., Mather, A., Vogel, K. and Burger, M.M., 1979. Liver-colonizing melanoma cells selected from B-16 melanoma. Int. J. Cancer,
23: 854-857.
Walther, B.T., Ohman, R. and Roseman, S., 1973. A quantitative assay
for intercellular adhesion. Proc. Natl. Acad. Sci. USA, 70: 1569-15
Yogeeswaran, G., Stein, G.S. and Sebastian, H., 1978. Altered cell
surface organisation of gangliosides and sialylglycoproteins of mous
metastatic melanoma variant lines selected in vivo for enhanced lung
implantation. Cancer Res., 38: 1336-1344.

INTRINSIC AND EXTRINSIC FACTORS GOVERNING THE EXPRESSION OF METASTATIC POTENTIAL

S.A. Eccles

INTRODUCTION

Rodent tumours of apparently similar type may exhibit widely differing capacities for spontaneous metastasis when transplanted in syngeneic recipients. Comparisons of the biological properties of these tumours and their spontaneous metastases may yield information regarding intrinsic properties which favour successful metastasis, and manipulation of host immunity will indicate the extent to which this factor modifies the expression of metastatic potential of different tumours.

METHODS

In this study, tumours were grown intramuscularly (i.m.) from mechanically prepared cell suspensions and excised by amputation after 10-14 days of growth. The subsequent development of metastases was determined in immunocompetent and immunodeprived hosts. Individual metastases were selected from various organs and transplanted i.m. to further groups of syngeneic recipients for comparison with the 'parent' tumours. The tumour systems, means of immune deprivation, assessment of tumour host cell infiltration and immunogenicity have been described previously (Eccles and Alexander, 1976; Eccles et al, 1979; Eccles, Heckford and Alexander, 1980).

RESULTS

Figure 1 shows the different patterns of metastasis of 3 chemically-induced rat sarcomas HSBPA, HSN and MC28, and that the degree of dissemination was inversely related to their immunogenicity as indicated by TD_{50} values in immunised animals and levels of intratumour host cells. The first animal in each group succumbing to metastases (✶) was used as a source of metastatic tumour for transplant. The tumours which developed from either lung (LM) or lymph node (LNM) metastases showed no trend towards increased metastatic efficiency, and cells which had disseminated via the lymphatic route were equally able to metastasize via the haematogenous route and vice versa. Also, the spontaneous metastases shown here yielded tumours of host cell infiltration and immunogenicity broadly comparable to the parent tumours.

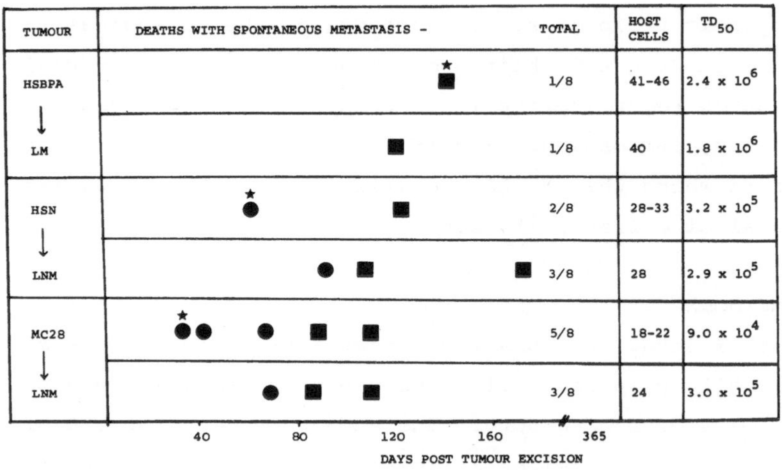

TUMOUR	DEATHS WITH SPONTANEOUS METASTASIS –	TOTAL	HOST CELLS	TD_{50}
HSBPA	★ ■ (≈140)	1/8	41–46	2.4×10^6
↓ LM	■ (≈120)	1/8	40	1.8×10^6
HSN	★ ● (≈70) ■ (≈120)	2/8	28–33	3.2×10^5
↓ LNM	● ■ (≈110) ■ (≈365)	3/8	28	2.9×10^5
MC28	★ ●● (≈45) ● (≈80) ■ (≈100) ■ (≈120)	5/8	18–22	9.0×10^4
↓ LNM	● (≈80) ■ (≈100) ■ (≈120)	3/8	24	3.0×10^5

Days post tumour excision axis: 40   80   120   160   365

DAYS POST TUMOUR EXCISION

Fig. 1. Properties of rat sarcomas and their metastases
lung; ■ lymph node; ●

In a further series of 30 transplanted lymphatic, pulmonary and visceral metastases from 10 different sarcomas, lymphomas and carcinomas, similar results were obtained. There was a slight trend towards decreased immunogenicity in the metastases as a whole, but not greater than the degree that may be seen when primary tumours are transplanted. These data suggest that the metastasis progenitor cells did not possess unique metastasizing potential or specific organ colonising ability.

Figure 2 shows that an immunogenic rat sarcoma which is
generally 'non-metastatic' in normal animals (N-1), when grown
in athymic recipient rats (ATX-1) contained a much reduced host
cell infiltrate and rapidly produced pulmonary, lymphatic and
visceral metastases. A lymph node metastasis derived from the
first athymic animal which died when transplanted back into
normal animals (N-2) yielded tumours with a very low rate of
overt metastases, and transplanted visceral and pulmonary metastases
in a further 24 recipients gave no secondary disease. If the
local tumours from the N-2 rats were transplanted back into
athymic hosts (ATX-2) widespread metastases again ensued.
Similar results were obtained using this and other sarcomas
in animals immunosuppressed with Cyclosporin A (Eccles, Heckford
and Alexander, 1980).

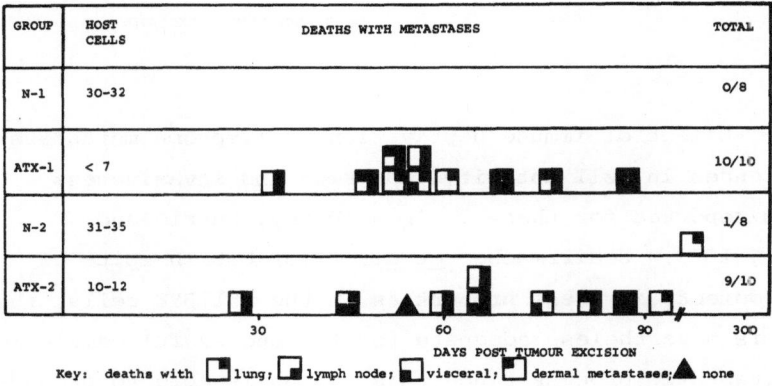

Fig. 2.   Rat sarcoma metastases in normal and athymic hosts.

The effect of immunosuppression on the metastatic pattern of the DBA/2 Lymphoma L5178Y has also been determined. There are 2 lines of this tumour; L5178YES which gives a 100% incidence of metastases and rapidly kills the hosts with widespread disease, and L5178YE which kills only about 10% of mice with metastases as illustrated in Figure 3.

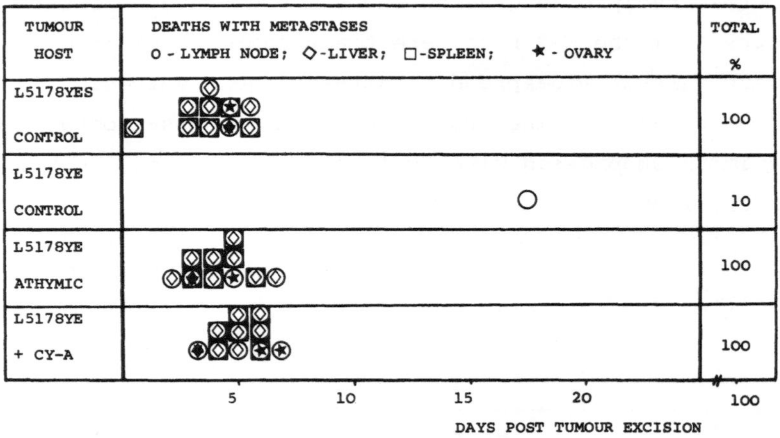

TUMOUR HOST	DEATHS WITH METASTASES O - LYMPH NODE; ◇-LIVER; □-SPLEEN; ★ - OVARY	TOTAL %
L5178YES CONTROL		100
L5178YE CONTROL		10
L5178YE ATHYMIC		100
L5178YE + CY-A		100

DAYS POST TUMOUR EXCISION

Figure 3. Effect of immune deprivation on lymphoma metastases.

Differences in cell motility, adhesion and invasiveness have been reported for these 2 lines (Davey, Currie and Alexander, 1979; Schirrmacher et al, 1979) but in spite of apparent defects in these properties in the L5178YE cells, their activity is nevertheless adequate for the successful completion of the metastatic process since this tumour is able to produce widespread metastases in immunosuppressed hosts. Figure 3 shows that the behaviour of L5178YE is indistinguishable from that of the 'metastatic variant' ES when grown in athymic or Cyclosporin A treated mice.

Transplanted lymphatic, splenic or liver metastases again yielded tumours with metastatic patterns not significantly different from those of the parent tumours, and no specific organ selectivity was apparent.

In the cases illustrated so far, the intrinsic ability of tumour cells to disseminate and colonise 2° sites was no different for 'metastatic' and 'non-metastatic' tumours, or for primary implants and their metastases, rather the host immune environment determined the expression of overt disease; most organs being susceptible to the development of metastases in immune-deprived hosts.

In marked contrast to this, immunosuppression failed to influence the metastatic patterns of weakly immunogenic murine squamous cell carcinomas and mammary adenocarcinomas (Eccles, Heckford and Alexander, 1980). These tumours were originally well-differentiated and had low rates of spontaneous metastases (unlike their sarcoma and lymphoma counterparts), but in later transplant generations many became anaplastic, and their tumorigenicity and metastatic capacity increased. Whether these observations are causally related, and due to tumour-intrinsic or host modifying factors remains to be determined.

REFERENCES

Davey, G.C., Currie, G.A. and Alexander, P. (1979). Immunity as the predominant factor determining metastasis by murine lymphomas. Br. J. Cancer, 40:590-6.
Eccles, S.A. and Alexander, P. (1976). Macrophage content of tumours in relation to metastatic spread and host immune reaction. Nature 250:667-9.
Eccles, S.A. et al (1979). Metastasis in the nude rat associated with lack of immune response. Br. J. Cancer, 40:802-5.
Eccles, S.A., Heckford, S.E. and Alexander, P. (1980). Effect of Cyclosporin A on the growth and spontaneous metastasis of syngeneic animal tumours. Br. J. Cancer. In press.
Schirrmacher, V. et al, (1979). Tumor metastases and cell-mediated immunity in a model system in DBA/2 mice.
    1. Tumor invasiveness in vitro and metastasis formation in vivo. Int. J. Cancer 23:233-44.

METASTATIC POTENTIAL OF SK-Br-3 CELLS TREATED WITH L-CYSTEINE OR ASCORBIC ACID*

L. Ozzello and C. Leuchtenberger

INTRODUCTION

L-cysteine and ascorbic acid, which had previously been shown to inhibit the carcinogenic effects of tobacco and marihuana smoke on hamster and human lung cultures by interfering with the SH-reactive components of the gas vapor phase of the smoke (Leuchtenberger and Leuchtenberger, 1977), were found to modify the morphology and to enhance the growth rate of a human mammary carcinoma cell line (SK-Br-3 (Leuchtenberger and Ozzello, submitted for publication). When these cells were grc in media enriched with L-cysteine they underwent a progressive fibroblast-like transformation indicative of cellular dedifferentiation. This transformation persisted after the modified cells were returned to the original (cysteine-free) medi um. On the other hand, ascorbic acid favored the in vitro differentiation of SK-Br-3 cells which became uniformly smaller and tended to arrange themselves in rosette-like patterns. When ascorbic acid was withdrawn from the medium, the cells gradually became dedifferentiated and resembled those modified by L-cysteine.

Therefore, it appeared important to determine whether the alterations produced by these substances on SK-Br-3 cells in vitro also affected the behavior of the cells in vivo. For this purpose we transplanted SK-Br-3 cells previously modified by L-cysteine and by ascorbic acid into nude thymus-deficient mice and compared their neoplastic potential to that of untreated cells. In this report we shall foc on the metastatic patterns of the tumors produced by the transplanted cells. A mor extensive report will be published elsewhere (Ozzello et al., submitted for publication).

MATERIALS AND METHODS

Cell cultures. SK-Br-3 cell lines were derived from the pleural effusion of a m tastatic mammary carcinoma in a 43-year-old woman (Fogh and Trempe, 1975). Their human mammary nature has been recently confirmed (Engel and Young, 1978). Cultures for transplantation, handled as previously described (Leuchtenberger and Leuchtenberger, 1977), included:

---

*Supported by grant FOR.084.AK.79 from the Swiss League against Cancer, and by grants from A.S.F.C., Switzerland.

1. Control cultures: SK-Br-3 cells grown as monolayers in plastic flasks using Eagle-Dulbecco's medium supplemented with 20% calf serum (ED);

2. Experimental cultures:

a. 1st set: SK-Br-3 cells grown for 73 weeks in ED with 0.3 g L-cysteine per liter, and SK-Br-3 cells grown for 62 weeks in ED followed by 11 weeks in ED with 8 mg ascorbic acid per liter;

b. 2nd set: SK-Br-3 cells grown in ED with L-cysteine (0.3 g/liter) or with ascorbic acid (8 mg/liter) both for 71½ weeks.

Nude mice. BALB/c nu/nu mice were handled under pathogen-limited conditions as described elsewhere (Ozzello and Sordat, 1980). Adult virgin females were used.

Transplantations. For the original transplantations trypsinized cells were injected sc in the lateral thoracic region of the mice. Subsequent passages were carried out by mincing surgically removed tumors and implanting them (2-3 mm^3) sc by means of a trocar.

Tumors. Some of the tumors were surgically excised after variable periods of time and the animals allowed to survive. The other tumors were permitted to grow until the death of the animals. Both operated and nonoperated mice were ultimately subjected to a complete autopsy. All specimens were examined histologically using conventional techniques. In addition, the presence of human α-lactalbumin was checked in selected tumors by Dr. J. Hurlimann (Dept. of Pathology, Lausanne) using the immuno-peroxidase technique (PAP) or indirect immunofluorescence. Antigens and antisera were prepared as described by Hurlimann and Dayal (1978).

RESULTS

The salient features of the tumors and of their metastatic spread are summarized in table 1. Further details are described below.

Tumorigenicity. Successful takes of the original transplants of untreated (control) cultures were obtained with inocula of 30×10^6 cells after latent periods of 95 to 105 days. On the contrary, cells treated with L-cysteine or ascorbic acid produced tumors with original inocula as small as 1.5×10^6 after latency periods of 10-11 and 10-17 days respectively.

Tumors. While the tumors of the control group were moderately differentiated carcinomas (Fig. 1) composed of broad sheets of polygonal cells some of which contained α-lactalbumin and no appreciable mucin, those produced by L-cysteine-treated cells were undifferentiated carcinomas (Fig. 2) made up of spindle cells the epithelial nature of which was confirmed by the demonstration of α-lactalbumin in some of them. In contrast, the tumors of the ascorbic acid-treated cells were well differentiated adenocarcinomas (Fig. 3) whose cells produced mucin and more

TABLE - 1   Tumors produced in BALB/c nu/nu mice by SK-Br-3 cells

Cultures grown in	Transplants/ takes	Passages in nude mice	Tumors			Mice with metastases[c]	Metastatic sites		
			Histology	Volume (cm³)[a]	Growth index[b]		Lymph nodes	Lungs	Others[d]
Eagle-Dulbecco (ED)	31/28	10	mod. diff carcinoma	2.0±0.3	3.4±0.4	0/28	0	0	0
ED + L-cysteine									
1st set (73 wks)	47/47	37	undiffer. carcinoma	4.9±0.5	24.3±1.8	28/47	9	27	19
2nd set (71½ wks)	27/27	11	undiffer. carcinoma	4.5±0.5	20.4±1.6	22/27	1	22	10
ED + ascorbic ac.									
1st set (11 wks)	5/5	2	well diff. adenoca.	1.6±0.4	3.5±0.8	1/5	1	1	0
	31/31	27	undiffer. carcinoma	4.7±0.7	21.5±1.8	17/24	2	17	18
2nd set (71½ wks)	44/44	11	well diff. adenoca.	1.7±0.2	4.1±0.3	23/44	19	14	5

a $V = \frac{\pi}{6} (d_1 \cdot d_2 \cdot d_3)/6$, where $d_{1,2,3}$ represent the 3 largest diameters. Mean ± S.E.

b   Estimation of the daily increase in size. $GI = \dfrac{Volume}{age\ of\ tumor\ in\ days} \times 100$

c   Expressed as number of mice with metastases/number of mice with adequate follow-up (to death with a minimum of 8 postoperative days). Many mice had multiple metastatic foci.

d   Mediastinum, pleura, pericardium, kidneys.

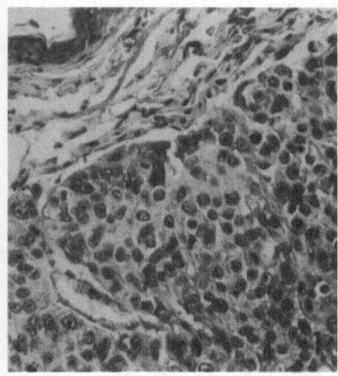 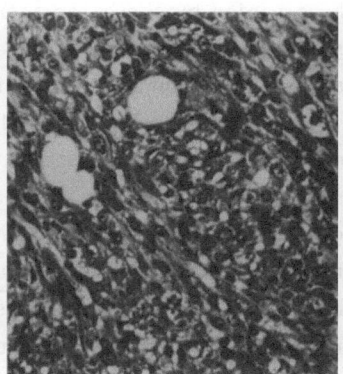 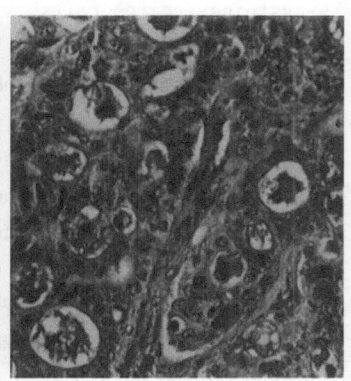

Fig. 1. Tumor of untreated SK-Br-3 cells. X 100
Fig. 2. Tumor of SK-Br-3 cells treated with L-cysteine. X 100
Fig. 3. Tumor produced by ascorbic acid-treated SK-Br-3 cells. X 100

α-lactalbumin than those of the other groups. However, the tumors from the 1st set of cultures grown in ED with ascorbic acid retained the features of well differentiated adenocarcinomas only for 116 days (original transplant and first passage), after which they became undifferentiated. All tumors were invasive, but the undifferentiated carcinomas were much more aggressive than the others.

Metastatic spread. Metastases were accepted as such when the neoplastic cells formed a well defined nodule. Isolated tumor cells in vessels or in lymph node sinuses were not included. Lymphatic metastases were more frequent in the homolateral axillary lymph nodes than in the inguinal and upper mediastinal nodes. They displayed a tendency to break through the capsule of the nodes and to invade the surrounding tissues. Hematogenous metastases were commonly multiple. This was particularly true in the lungs where they were frequently peribronchial and surrounded blood vessels sometimes causing massive pulmonary infarcts.

It is important to stress that the undifferentiated carcinomas metastasized predominantly via the blood stream, whereas the well differentiated adenocarcinomas more frequently gave rise to lymphatic metastases.

DISCUSSION

L-cysteine and ascorbic acid exert important effects on SK-Br-3 cells cultured in vitro. These effects are manifested in vivo by enhanced tumorigenicity and by profound morphological alterations which parallel those observed in the cultures. It would appear that L-cysteine leads to a dedifferentiation of the cells while ascorbic acid enhances their epithelial features and their degree of differentiation. Furthermore, the morphological undifferentiation of the tumors produced by

L-cysteine-treated cells is accompanied by a greater aggressiveness.

Of particular interest is the observation that the metastatic potential of SK-Br-3 cells is greatly enhanced by exposing the cells in vitro to L-cysteine or ascorbic acid, two naturally occurring metabolites. Further, the pathway of metasta tization is predominantly hematogenous in the L-cysteine group and lymphatic in the ascorbic acid group. The difference in metastatic pattern, however, appears to be also related to the degree of differentiation of the neoplastic cells as shown by the ascorbic acid group whose rate of blood-born metastases increased when the carcinomas became undifferentiated and ultimately resembled the tumors of the L-cysteine group in their morphology, aggressiveness, and metastatic behavior. At present we are unable to explain why a loss of differentiation occurred in the 1st set of our transplanted tumors while the carcinomas of the 2nd set did not change over the entire period of experimentation. The cultures of the 1st set were exposed to ascorbic acid for 11 weeks while the treatment of those of the 2nd set lasted 71½ weeks. It is possible that a relatively long (more than 11 weeks) period of exposure to ascorbic acid is necessary to produce long-lasting effects.

A relationship between degree of differentiation of the tumors and the frequency of metastases is less apparent as it is difficult to explain why the well differenti ated ascorbic acid tumors give rise to metastases whereas no metastases are observed in the less well differentiated carcinomas of the control group.

The results reported above suggest that the morphology and the behavior of some human carcinoma cells may be altered by naturally occurring substances. No general conclusion is justified in the present state of our investigations. Additional work has to be done to find out the mechanisms of action of these substances and the types of cells affected by them.

REFERENCES

Engel, L.W. and Young, N.A., 1978. Human breast carcinoma cells in continuous culture: a review. Cancer Res., 38: 4327-4339.

Fogh, J. and Trempe G., 1975. New human tumor cell lines. In: J. Fogh (Editor), Human Tumor Cells in Vitro, Plenum Press, New York, pp. 115-159.

Hurlimann, J. and Dayal, R., 1978. Antigens of a human breast carcinoma cell line (BT 20). I. Synthesis of serum proteins, membrane-associated antigens, and oncofetal-associated antigens. J. Natl. Cancer Inst., 61: 677-686.

Leuchtenberger, C. and Leuchtenberger, R., 1977. Protection of humster lung cultures by L-cysteine or vitamin C against carcinogenic effects of fresh smoke from tobacco or marihuana cigarettes. Br. J. Exp. Path., 58: 625-634.

Ozzello, L. and Sordat, M., 1980. Behavior of tumors produced by transplantation of human mammary cell lines in athymic nude mice. Eur. J. Cancer, in press.

EFFECT OF PRE-TREATMENT WITH ANTISERA AGAINST CHORIOGONADOTROPIN ON THE METASTATIC POTENTIAL OF A RAT ADENOCARCINOMA

J.A. Kellen, A. Kolin, J.A. Teodorczyk-Injeyan and A. Malkin

INTRODUCTION

The synthesis of gonadotropin-like polypeptides (CG) by a variety of nontrophoblastic neoplasms (Braunstein et al., 1973; Muggia et al., 1975) has recently been demonstrated. This finding is of interest because of the similarity of some of the biologic characteristics of malignant cells to those of the trophoblast. Sensitive and relatively specific assay methods together with a systematic screening for the presence of CG have revealed the surprisingly ubiquitous character of CG-like materials in normal as well as in malignant cells (Braunstein et al., 1979; Yoshimoto et al., 1979).

CG-like polypeptides have been found in tissue sections and cell cultures of an experimental rat mammary tumor, the R3230AC adenocarcinoma, using immunohistochemical, radioimmunoassay and bioassay methods respectively (Malkin et al., 1979). CG is known to enhance amino acid incorporation into cells (Golbus and Siiteri, 1976), induces a variety of enzymes (Maudsley and Kobayashi, 1974), suppresses mixed lymphocyte culture reactions and phagocytic activity (Fernitcheve-Rostaing et al., 1979), all of which can be considered to enhance malignant growth.

The R3230AC adenocarcinoma can be propagated in cell culture; the cells retain their morphology and malignant characteristics for at least five passages. Intravenous injection of these cell cultures into isologous Fischer 344 rats gives rise to numerous foci of this tumor in the animals' lungs within 8 to 10 days.

In an effort to determine whether CG plays a role in the process of nidation after i.v. seeding, we subcultured parallel passages of the R3230AC in the presence of anti-human CG (beta subunit) rabbit antiserum. Judging from previous histochemical studies, extensive binding of the antiserum to CG determinants could be expected. We tested the metastatic potential of these pretreated cell cultures, compared to those which were exposed to normal rabbit IgG as control.

MATERIALS

Throughout the experiments, Fischer 344 femals rats, weighing 130-150g were used; the rats were fed Purina Chow and tap water <u>ad libitum</u> and caged in twos.   The R3220 AC rat adenocarcinoma was obtained from the Mason Research Tumor Bank, (courtesy of Dr. A Bogden) and maintained by transplantation of 10 mg Stadie slices).

METHODS

The R3230AC rat mammary adenocarcinoma was cultured from explants of subcutaneous tumors, grown for 20-21 days in Fischer 344 female rats.   Cultures were maintained in RPMI 1640, supplement with 12% fetal calf serum.   Upon reaching confluency, cells were dispersed by 0.1% hyaluronidase and 0.05% collagenase treatment and passaged three times.

To test the effect of rabbit antiserum against the β subunit of BCG, parallel cell cultures were grown in standard medium supplemented with reconstituted anti-HCG β (Ayerst) at a concentration of 1:100 (v/v), with rabbit serum as control in the untreated cultures.   At the early stationary growth phase, the cultures were dispersed for <u>in vivo</u> administration.   The cell density was determined using a hemocytometer and viability was checked by the Trypan blue exclusion method. 1×10^6 cells were then injected into the tail vein of female Fischer 344 rats weighing 130-150g.   The animals were sacrificed by cervical dislocation on the 10th day after the injection and autopsied.   The livers, spleen, kidneys and lungs were carefully examined and processed for paraffin sections and H & E staining in order to detect metastasis.

RESULTS

The qualitative histological appearance of pulmonary tumor deposits in both groups of animals is practically identical, i.e. poorly differentiated adenocarcinoma rarely producing glandular lumina.   The mitotic rates are high; tumor necroses and inflammatory reactions around tumor nodules are absent in both the pretreated and control groups.   However, there is a striking contrast in numbers and sizes of the tumor deposits between these groups.   In

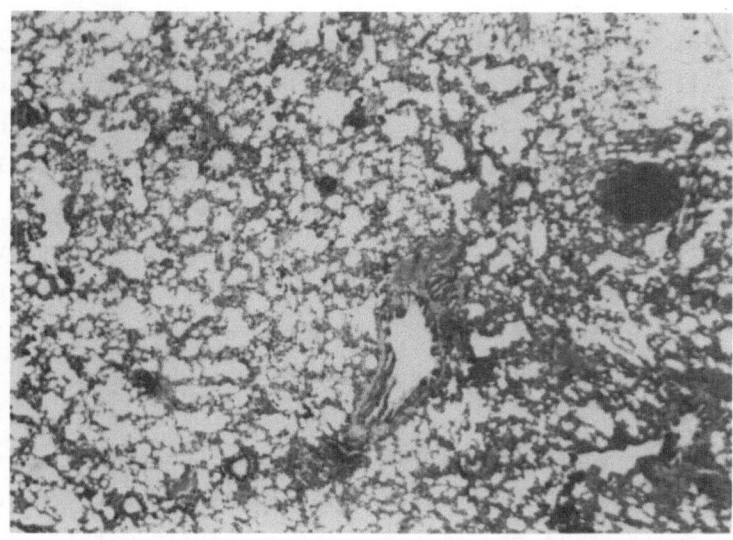

Figure 1. Lung section from rat injected with R3230AC cells exposed
to anti-CG B 10 days ago. A single metastatic nodule is
seen.

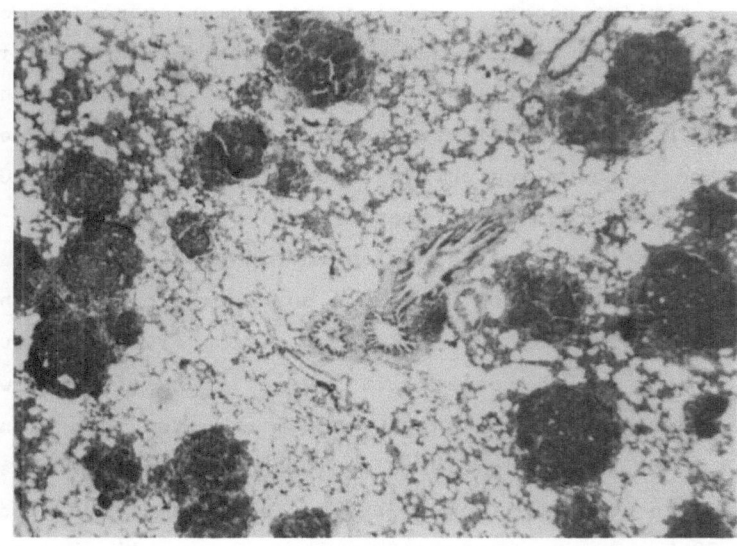

Figure 2. Lung section from rat, injected with R3230AC cells exposed
to normal rabbit serum 10 days ago. Numerous tumor nodules
are present.

Both figures : H & E Stain, 37,5 X

the control group, metastatic tumor nodules ranging in size from
a few cells to 1 mm in diameter were uniformly distributed through
the lung parenchyma. 5-15 tumor nodules could be found in every
low power camera field (obj. 2,5x). In lungs of animals injected
with anti-HCG treated tumor cells, 1-4 metastatic nodules were found
in the entire lung sections, so that only rarely a low power field
could be found containing a metastatic focus. Most lung parenchyma
was completely free of tumor. The sizes of these rare metastatic
nodules did not exceed 0.3 mm in diameter.

CONCLUSIONS

The tumor model chosen for this study, when maintained by
transplantation, does not metastasize spontaneously. However, when
cultured tumor cells are injected intravenously within the time
limits of this study and the number of cells administered, lung foci
are observed in all animals so treated.

While a concentrated effort is being made on studies with antibodies to CG in the field of contraception, there are only sporadic
data on a similar approach testing anti-tumor properties of such
antisera. Knecht (1980) used active immunization against the beta
subunit of CG coupled to the tetanus toxoid and reported negative
results with a transplantable choriocarcinoma. In our design, we
did not try to induce an active immune response against CG in vivo;
we endeavoured rather to develop a model for studying the role of
CG-like peptides on tumor nidation and invasiveness.

The R3230AC cells did not show any morphological changes nor
changes in the rate of multiplication during five subcultures;
injection of 1×10^6 viable cells i.v. after cultivation with an
antiserum against CG-beta in the medium resulted in a significant
decrease in the number and size of tumor foci in the lungs. We
would like to conclude that under the conditions presented, exposure
to anti-CG-β antisera appears to select tumor cell clones which
show decreased metastatic potential.

Supported in part by a grant from the National Cancer Institute
of Canada.

REFERENCES

Braunstein, G.D., Vaitukaitis, J.L., Carbone, P.P. and Ross, G.T., 1973.
  Ectopic production of human chorionic gonadotropin by neoplasms.
  Ann. Int. Med. 78: 39-45.
Braunstein, G.D., Kamdar, V., Rasor, J., Swaminathan, N. and Maclyn, E.W.,
  1979. Widespread Distribution of a Chorionic Gonadotropin-Like Substance
  in Normal Human Tissues. J. Clin. End. & Met. 49: 917-925.
Golbus, M.S. and Siiteri, P.K., 1976. Effects of Human Chorionic Gonadotropin
  in Preparations on Amino Acid Uptake and Incorporation into Protein In Vitro.
  End. Res. Comm. 3: 273-279.
Knecht, M., 1980. The Lack of an Effect of Active Immunization with the
  B-Subunit of Chorionic Gonadotropin Coupled to Tetanus Toxoid on the Growth
  of Human Choriocarcinoma Maintained in the Hamster Cheek Pouch.
  Endocr. 106: 150-154.
Malkin, A., Kellen, J.A., Reviczky, M.I. and Kolin, A., 1979. Immunohistochemical
  detection of ectopic hormones in experimental rat tumors. In: F.J. Lehman, Ed.
  Carcino-Embryonic Proteins, Vol. II, Elsevier/North Holland Biomedical Press,
  751-758.
Maudsley, D.V. and Kobayashi, Y., 1974. Induction of Ornithine Decarboxylase
  in Rat Ovary after Administration of Luteinizing Hormone or Human Chorionic
  Gonadotropin. Biochem. Pharm. 23: 2697-2703.
Muggia, F.M., Rosen, S.W., Weintraub, B.D. and Hansen, H.H., 1975. Ectopic
  Placental Proteins in Nontrophoblastic Tumors. Cancer 36: 1327-1337.
Pernitcheva-Rostaing, E., Fontagne, J., Adolphe, M., Engellman, P., Morin, P.
  and Lechat, P., 1979. Effect of Human Chorionic Gonadotropin on Phagocytic
  Activity and Proliferative Capacity of Rat Peritoneal Macrophages in Culture.
  Acta Endocr. 92: 187-192.
Yoshimoto, Y., Wolfsen, A.R., Hirose, F. and Odell, W.D., 1979. Human Chorionic
  Gonadotropin-Like material: presence in normal human tissues. Am. J. Obst.
  Gyn. 134: 729-733.

METASTASES OF MAMMARY TUMOURS IN BR6 MICE

L.S.C. Pang, A.E. Lee, L.A. Rogers and K.J. Miller

The mammary tumours described in these studies occur in BR6 mice, a strain originally developed by Foulds (1949). The mice carry a mammary tumour virus, and 94% of breeding females and 48% of virgin females develop tumours (Lee, 1970). We wished to find out whether these tumours metastasized; if so, with what frequency, and whether there was any correlation between the morphology of the tumour and its ability to metastasize.

The structure of the primary tumours varied from those with well differentiated acini organized into uniform clusters (Fig. 1) and which showed secretion during pregnancy, through intermediate stages sometimes showing papillary formation with the epithelial elements forming slit-like clefts (Fig. 2), to poorly differentiated irregular masses. For convenience, three main types were designated, though there was continuous transition between them.

The tumours could be readily transplanted by scraping a cut surface of the tumour and diluting the tissue so obtained with a little isotonic saline. Samples of this brei were then injected subcutaneously into the flanks of syngeneic host mice.

In the first survey, 101 mice bearing syngeneic transplants of mammary tumours were examined. Secondaries were found most commonly in the lungs, occurring in 97% of mice with poorly differentiated (Group III) tumours, and in 48% of mice with the intermediate (Group II) tumours. The well differentiated (Group I) tumours rarely produced metastases. Some pulmonary lesions were quite large and easily discernible with the naked eye (Fig. 3), but others were only detected by light microscopy. In some cases they consisted of a small embolus of cells within a blood vessel (Fig. 4) and had not invaded the lung parenchyma. The lung secondaries were usually slow growing and well differentiated, with signs of secretion during pregnancy. When they were transplanted to subcutaneous sites however, they grew rapidly in size, and produced further lung metastases with a frequency similar to that of the parent tumour, viz: 67% when the original tumour was Group II, and 100% when it was Group III.

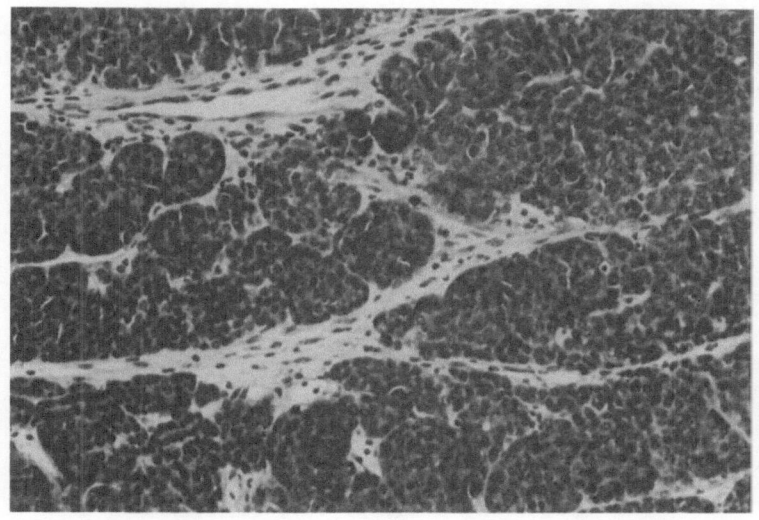

Fig.1. Primary tumour consisting of uniform clusters of acini.   x200

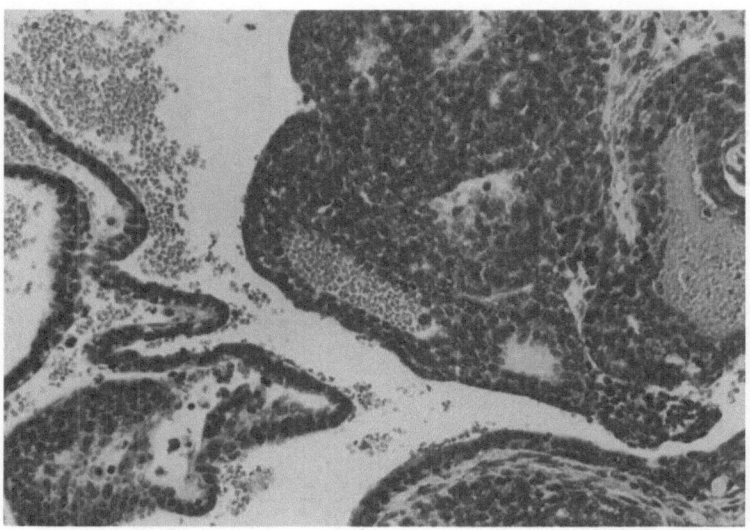

Fig.2. Primary tumour with papillary formation.   x200

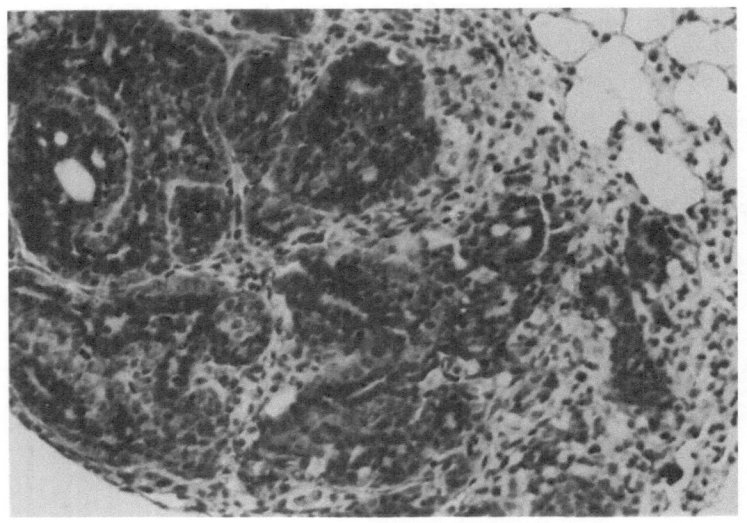

Fig.3. Lung showing metastasis from mammary tumour.   x200

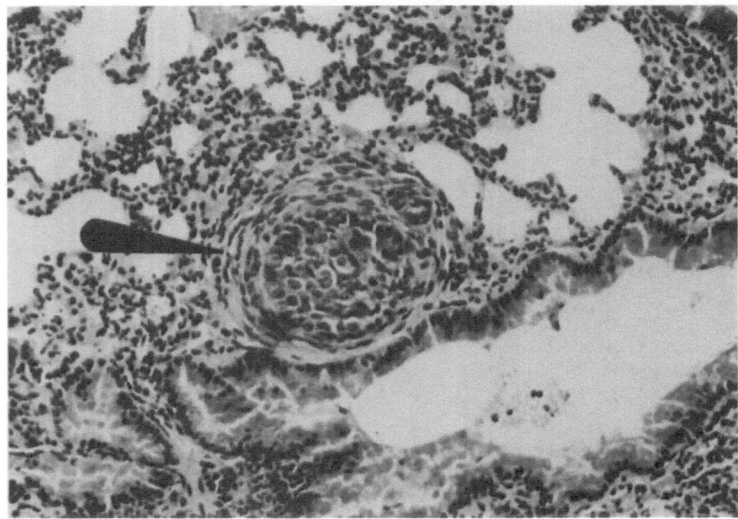

Fig.4. Lung showing embolus of mammary tumour cells (arrowed) within
       pulmonary artery.   x200

The metastatic potential appeared to be a stable characteristic of each type of mammary tumour, and was linked with its morphology. Twenty tumour lines were established by subcutaneous transplantation into syngeneic hosts, and examination of 500 mice showed that the tumours could be separated into those giving rise to consistently low (5/90, 6%) or higher (139/410, 34%) incidences of lung secondaries in the hosts. From these lines, two have been selected showing 3% and 57% incidences of lung metastases, and maintained for 72 and 53 passages respectively. The transplants still morphologically resemble the two parent tumours and are distinguishable by light microscopy and SEM.

BR6 mammary tumours are similar to other tumours described by Poste and Fidler (1980) in that they appear to consist of several subpopulations of cells, some of which are more capable of surviving the hazards of the meta-static process than others. The balance of the subpopulations within a tumour depends on its degree of differentiation, and is maintained through many sub-cutaneous passages. The consistent and high rate of metastasis of some BR6 mammary tumour lines makes them a useful model for investigating the control of tumour spread.

Foulds, L., 1949. Mammary tumours in hybrid mice: the presence and trans-
    mission of the mammary tumour agent. Br.J.Cancer, 3: 230-239.
Lee, A.E., 1970. Mammary tumour development in BR6 mice: ovarian
    influences and 5-hydroxytryptamine. Br.J.Cancer, 24: 561-567.
Poste, G. and Fidler, I.J., 1980. The pathogenesis of cancer metastasis.
    Nature, 283: 139-146.

FIXATION OF α-MELANOCYTE STIMULATING HORMONE (α-MSH) TO HUMAN METASTATIC MELANOMA CELLS IN VITRO AND IN VIVO

F. Legros, A. Verhest, J. Coel, P. Hanson, S. Legros, A. Liteanu,
A. Nuchowicz, N. van Tieghem and F.J. Lejeune

1. INTRODUCTION

α-MSH binds to the plasma membrane of a human metastatic melanoma cell line, increases intracellular cyclic AMP level, stimulates
tyrosinase activity and inhibits cell division and DNA replication
(Legros et al., 1979).

An immunocytochemical method based upon α-MSH immunoreactivity
(Barbea et al., 1977 ; Vaudry et al., 1978) and immunocytochemical
localization in the nervous system (Remy and Dubois, 1974 ; Swaab
and Visser, 1978) has been elaborated in order to visualize hormonal fixation to various human metastatic melanoma cell cultures
and to metastatic tissues. A highly specific antibody against human
α-MSH has been used (Usategui et al., 1976).

2. MATERIALS

After surgical excision, melanoma metastatic tumour fragments
were implanted in 25 cm^2 Falcon tissue culture flasks. HAM F-10
nutrient medium or MEM, supplemented with 10% heat inactivated fetal calf serum, antibiotics and CO_2 was added. The flasks were incubated at 37°C. Usually, the first subculture was obtained after
1 month by gentle trypsinization of the cells. After 4 or 5 subcultures, only fibroblast-like cells were observed, whereas redif-
ferentiation occured at the 10-12th subculture. For histological
studies, melanoma metastatic fragments were fixed in 10% neutral
formaldehyde and embedded in parafin.

3. METHODS

3.1 - Cell harvesting.

Confluent melanoma cells were incubated in the presence and in
the absence of α-MSH (Bioproducts) 10^{-8}M at 37°C. They were rapidly
rinsed in 0.5 ml of versene-tris buffer saline (VTS) pH8.0 and
harvested by a 10 minute treatment with the same buffer. After dilution to a concentration of 10^5 cells/ml in phosphate buffer saline,

cells were layered on microscope slides coated with gelatin by cy-
tocentrifugation (12 minutes at 750 rpm in a **cytofuge**).
of O.5 ml of cell suspension/slide and fixed with methanol 99% for
5 to 10 minutes.

3.2 - Tissue sections.

Metastatic tissues embedded in parafin were cut at 6 u.
Sections were layered on gelatin coated slides. Parafin was removed
in toluene and slides were hydrated by successive rinsings in decreasing alcohols to distilled water.

3.3. - Immunocytochemistry and Immunohistochemistry.

Rinsings and dilutions of antibodies were performed in Coons-
Veronal buffer, pH7.4.

Cells or tissues were treated for 10 minutes by 1% H_2O_2 in order to suppress endogenous peroxidase activity. After three rinsings,
they were immersed for 15 minutes in O.2% bovine serum albumin.

Slides were incubated for 20 minutes in each antibody and rinsed three times for 5 minutes. The successive series of antibodies
was as follows : 1) Rabbit Ig against human ∝-MSH (Bioproducts ;
Titre 1/38.000 ; dilution 1/30 ; cross-reactivity with ACTH and
related hormones inferior to 0.01%) : 2) Goat Ig against rabbit Ig
(GAR Nordik ; dilution 1/50) and 3) Anti-rabbit Peroxidase-antiper-
oxidase complex (R/PAP Nordik ; dilution 1/100).

Two different staining media were alternatively used : 1) 10 mg
of 3,3' diaminobenzidine (Koch Light Laboratories) diluted in 50 ml
Tris-HCl buffer pH7.6, containing 0.01% H_2O_2) : 2) 40 mg of
4-chloro-1napthol in O.5. ml of 95% ethanol added to 100 ml Tris-
HCl buffer pH7.6, containing 0.01% H_2O_2. Melanoma cells or tissues
were stained for 5 to 12 minutes by one of the solutions.

Three immunocytochemical controls were performed by omitting
1) anti ∝-MSH ; 2) anti-∝MSH and GAR ; 3) anti-∝MSH, GAR and
R/PAP in the series of antibodies.

4. RESULTS

4.1 - Cell cultures receptivity to ∝-MSH.

Fig.1a) shows a positive immunocytochemical staining of the external surface in cultured metastatic malignant cells previously
incubated for 30 minutes in ∝-MSH 10^{-8}M. No molecules possessing
the immunoreactivity of the melanotropic hormone were found inside
the cells. Immunocytochemical controls were all negative, as shown

248

in Fig 1/b)Cells which were not preincubated in ∝-MSH failed to present any membrane fixation when submitted to the complete immuno-cytochemical reaction. If those cells were incubated in ∝-MSH after methanol fixation, binding was observed. This indicates that mela-noma cells fixed with methanol retain their hormonal receptivity.

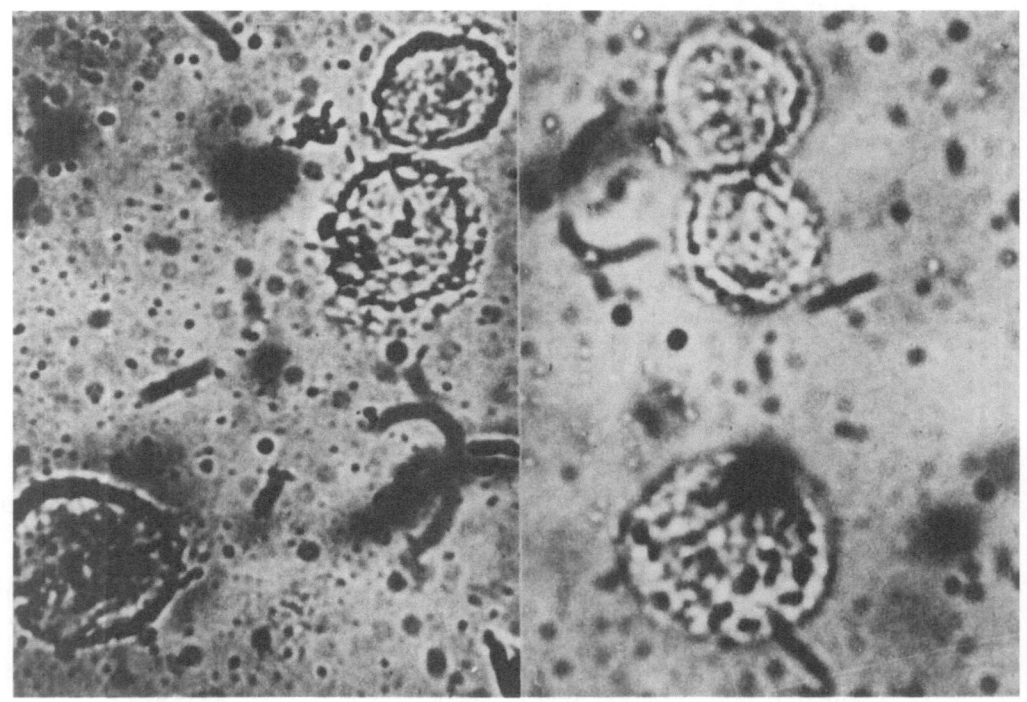

Fig. 1. Visualization of ∝ -MSH binding to cultured malignant cells from a subcutaneous human melanoma metastasis (x 1250) ; a - Hormo-nal fixation to the external surface ; b - Immunocytochemical control (No anti-MSH).

Not all the cells from the same redifferentiated culture bind ∝-MSH. A heterogeneity regarding hormonal receptivity was observed in all cultures where part of the cells bind the hormone to their external surface.

In addition, redifferentiated cultures derived from some melano-ma metastatic tumours did not exhibit any hormonal receptivity.

4.2.   MSH binding to metastatic tumours.

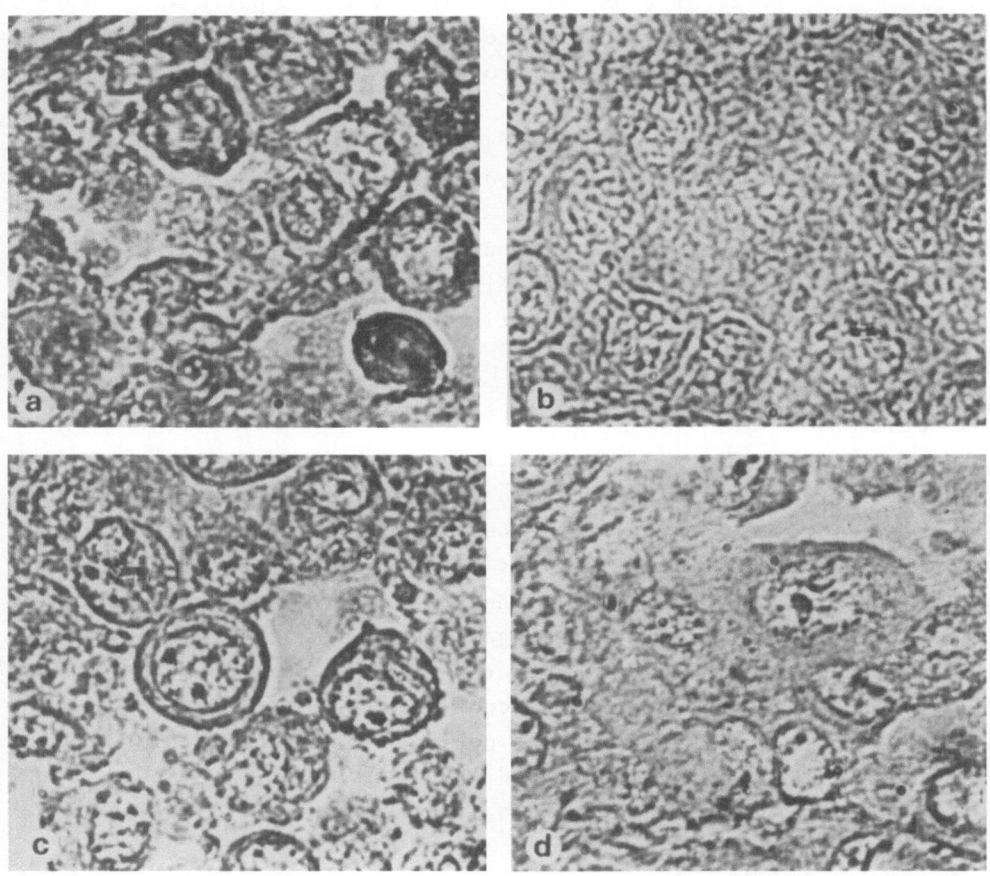

Fig.2 - ∝-MSH binding to malignant cells of a lymph node human melanoma metastasis ; a- Surface fixation to pigmented cells ; b -
Immunocytochemical control (No anti-MSH) ; c - Binding to unpigmented
cells ; d - Immunocytochemical control (No anti-MSH) (X 1250).

Fig.2a shows a positive immunocytochemical reaction on the external surface of malignant cells from a lymph node melanoma metastasis. Labeling was selectively located on heavily pigmented malignant
melanocytes. A less important number of slightly or non-pigmented
cells were receptive to the hormone (Fig.2c) . Labeling was always

on the external surface. These results indicate that malignant melanocytes from this metastasis   bind endogenous molecules possessing the immunoreactivity of ⍺-MSH originating from the patient. No further difference was observed when sections were preincubated in MSH fc $10^{-8}M$ Immunohistochemical controls were all negative, as indicated in Fig.2b and d.

Sub-cutaneous and hepatic metastases were also tested. Only a limited number of patients exhibited a plasma membrane hormonal fixation.

In all positive metastases, receptors to molecules possessing the immunoreactivity of ⍺-MSH were confined to malignant cells. Controls of receptive tumours were all negative. Controls of non-receptive tumours were all negative too.

5. DISCUSSION

We found that some malignant cells from a limited number of melanoma metastases bear receptors to molecules possessing the immunoreactivity of ⍺-MSH. This was observed on cultured cells as well as on solid tumours. Receptivity is not an overall feature of melanoma metastases, since it is confined to a limited number of cultures or tumours. We plan to investigate an eventual correlation between tissue sections and cell cultures from the same metastasis, that is between in vivo and in vitro receptivity.

Location of ⍺-MSH fixation.was confined to the external surface of malignant cells. This is in good agreement with established criteria of polypeptide hormone binding to receptive cells (Carpentier et al., 1979).

Heterogeneity of melanoma cells from the same metastasis regarding hormonal receptivity was observed in vivo as well as in vitro. In solid metastases, heavily pigmented melanocytes were selectively receptive, but unpigmented melanoma cells also showed MSH binding sites. It may be concluded that receptive cells possess a genotypic heterogeneity. Cells of the same metastasis may originate from genotypically different malignant melanocytes of the primary tumour. Alternatively, genotypically indentical cells from the primary tumour are able to metastasize but they differentiate into receptive and non receptive cells in the course of melanoma spreading.

Metastatic tumours do not behave identically regarding ⍺-MSH receptivity, since some   bind and others do not bind the hormone.

This must not be attributed to metastasis localization, since lymph node metastases from some patients are receptive while other ones are not. When several metastases from the same patient were studied, they all behaved in the same way. The meaning of this difference in hormonal receptivity among melanomas must be questioned keeping in mind the cytostatic effect of α-MSH on human malignant melanocytes (Legros et al., 1979). The heterogeneity of α-MSH receptivity in vivo and in vitro of malignant melanoma strongly suggests the existence of different malignant melanocytes populations. The relevance of this hypothesis to metastasization must be further investigated.

REFERENCES

Barnea, A., Oliver, C., and Porter, J.C., 1977. Subcellular localization of α-melanocyte stimulating hormone in the rat hypothalamus.J. Neurochem., 29: 619-624.
Carpentier, J.L., Gorden, P., Le Cam, A. and Orci, L., 1979. Relationship of binding to internalization of ^{125}I-insulin in isolated rat hepatocytes. Diabetologia, 17: 379-384.
Legros, F., Defleur, V., Doyen, A., Hanson, P., Massant, B., Rogister C., Van Tieghem, N., Vercamen-Grandjean, A., Frühling, J. and Lejeune, F., 1979. Modulation by α-MSH of human melanoma cell growth and differentiation. Cancer Treat.Rep., 63: 1199.
Remy, Ch. et Dubois, M.P., 1978. Identification par immunofluorescence des cellules corticotropes et mélanotropes de l'hypophyse d'Alytes obstetricans (Laur.) larvaire. C.R.Soc.Biol., 10-12: 1275-1279.
Swaab, D.F. and Visser, B., 1978. Immunocytochemical localization of α-melanocyte stimulating hormone (α-MSH)-like compounds in the rat nervous system. Neurosci. Letters, 7: 313-317.
Usategui, R., Oliver, C., Vaudry, H., Lombardi, G., Rozenberg, I.and Mourre, A.-M., 1976. Immunoreactive α-MSH and ACTH levels in rat plasma and pituitary. Endocrinology, 98:189-196.
Vaudry, H., Oliver, C., Jegou, S., Leboulenger, F., Tenon, M.-C., Delarue, C., Morin, J.-P. and Vaillant, R., 1978. Immunoreactive melanocyte-stimulating hormone (α-MSH) in the brain of the frog (Rana esculenta L.) Gen.Comp. Endocrinol., 34: 391-401.

METASTASES OF HUMAN TUMOURS IN THE NUDE MOUSE: THE BEHAVIOUR OF COLON CARCINOMA XENOGRAFTS*

B. Sordat, R.K. Lees, E. Bogenmann and G. Terres

1. INTRODUCTION

The congenitally athymic nude mouse which is defective in various T cell functions including xenograft rejection provides a potentially useful system for studying some aspects of tumour-host relationships when malignant cells of human origin are introduced into a xenogeneic recipient. The value of the model will be dependent on the extent to which the characteristics of the patient's tumour are maintained for the first or the subsequent transplants into this murine environment. The comparative analysis of morphological, kinetic, biochemical, functional and surface-associated characteristics between the original and the grafted tumour cells is currently evaluated. Reports on tumour xenografts have in fact drawn attention to their apparently benign behaviour with respect to local invasion and dissemination. Thus, in a large series of human tumour-grafted nude mice which have been examined histologically, Ueyama recently found an overall incidence of metastasis close to 6% (Sordat et al., 1980c). From numerous studies on the relative resistance to metastasis expressed by adult nude mice has emerged a spectrum of parameters which appear to determine the degree of xenogeneic malignancy. These include host factors, modes of inoculation and the nature of the tumour cells and they will be briefly reviewed here.

It has also been our experience that colorectal tumours demonstrate a high success rate in transplantation. Among the tumours growing in nude mice (14 out of 20 assayed), 4 have been analyzed in details and used in previous studies. Tumour cell cultures from the Co115 poorly-differentiated carcinoma were initiated in vitro and a permanent cell line was obtained and characterized (Carrel et al., 1976). In separate experiments the fate of Co115 inoculum was followed in vivo by labelling the injected tumour cells with ^{125}I-IUdR and

* Supported by grants from the Swiss Science Foundation 3.136-0.77, 470-0.79 and by NIH CA 22664.

measuring the extent of live tumour cell retention by whole body counting (Sordat et al., 1980). These studies have brought additional information on the initial tumour-host interactions particularly when various doses and nodes of inoculation are to be compared. Finally, preliminary results on the extent of metastasis following the surgical removal of the subcutaneous (sc) Co 15 graft will also be presented.

2. HOST FACTORS AND XENOGENEIC TUMOUR METASTASIS

2.1. Age of the host

The mechanism which prevents the development of metastases in adult nude mice was found to be absent at birth and during the post-natal period (Sordat et al., 1977; Lozzio et al., 1979). Tumour cells of various types and origins can now widely disseminate from the sc space into lungs, kidneys, liver, lymph nodes and spleen but the extent of this dissemination decreases when cells are injected shortly after birth. The age-dependence can vary from a tumour cell line to another. Moreover, in vitro maintained cells (leukaemic, lymphoblastoid but also carcinoma lines) appear to metastasize more readily than implanted solid carcinomas. It is assumed that the maturation of the resistance mechanism which takes place in the first two weeks after birth interferes rapidly with some characteristics of the tumour cells including kinetic and possibly surface-associated properties. Indeed 3 well-differentiated colon carcinomas grafted neonatally did not demonstrate histological evidence of metastasis when compared to 2 poorly-differentiated tumours which did metastasize in these conditions. The extent to which terminal differentiation pathways within grafted colon tumours may restrict their metastatic potential remains an open but attractive question.

2.2. Conditions of nude mice maintenance

A number of reports suggest that the maintenance conditions of the nude mouse colony can influence the tumour xenograft behaviour. Kameya et al. (1976) showed that the take rate of a human choriocarcinoma was increased in specific-pathogen-free (spf) nude mice when compared to conventionally-raised animals. Moreover the presence of a mouse hepatitis infection can account for variability in the success rate of transplantation (Kyriazis et al., 1979). It may be pertinent to mention here that metastases of various sc-grafted tumours which have been recently documented (Hata et al., 1978; Ueyama et al., 1978; Duke, 1980) were observed in spf nude mice. In this context, recent studies indicate that immunodepression of nude mice by anti-mouse interferon may result in the dissemination of various grafted tumours (Reid et al., 1980). Since several cell-mediated activities can be depressed by anti-host interferon antibody, these interesting results do not yet clarify which cell type(s) may actually control the metastatic potential of a xenogeneic tumour. Viral, bacterial, possibly alimentary immunogens may alter the resistance of the nude mouse colony, a factor which should be taken into consideration when tumour growth and metastasis are analysed.

In a previous study (Sordat and Bogenmann, 1980), we investigated the extent of metastasis of 4 colon carcinomas grafted sc into conventionally-maintained and pathogen-protected mice. In contrast with the conventional animals, pathogen-protected Col15-grafted nude mice had a higher incidence of regional (lymph nodes) and pulmonary dissemination. The 3 other colon tumours, of a differentiated type, did not metastasize in the two groups of animals. The incidence of Col15 metastasis in spf BALB/c nude mice has been recently reevaluated. The results that have been obtained on semi-serial sections of plastic-embedded material are presented in

TABLE 1.

INCIDENCE OF METASTASES IN SPF BALB/c NUDE MICE GRAFTED SC
WITH Col15 COLON CARCINOMA
(22 MICE) *

TIME INTERVAL	METASTASES			
(DAYS)	REGIONAL LYMPH NODES	LUNGS		
		ISOLATED TUMOUR CELLS	MICRO - · MACROMETASTASES	
20 - 22	1 / 3	5 / 5	2 / 5	0 / 5
24 - 26	4 / 5	5 / 5	5 / 5	2 / 5
32 - 36	0 / 2	3 / 4	3 / 4	2 / 4
38 - 41	3 / 5	5 / 5	5 / 5	3 / 5
45 - 54	3 / 3	3 / 3	3 / 3	3 / 3
OVERALL	11 / 18	21 / 22	18 / 22	10 / 22

* AS THE NUMBER OF MICE WITH MORPHOLOGIC EVIDENCE OF METASTASIS
PER GROUP OF MICE INVESTIGATED

Isolated tumour cells (1 to 3 cells) can be detected in the lungs throughout the observation period (20 to 54 days following tumour grafting). This
possibly reflects tumour cell circulation and embolization within the lung capillaries. The incidence of micro- (aggregates of 10 to 30 cells) and macrome-
tastases (as detected also by the aid of the dissecting microscope) appears to
increase with the length of host exposure to the tumour graft. This overall
high incidence of Coll5 metastases led us to study the fate of the tumour deposits after surgical removal of the graft (see section 4).

3. TUMOUR CELL SURVIVAL IN NUDE MICE

The ability to induce an ascitic form was found to be dose-dependent and
some experimental results indicated that a large proportion of the inoculum
could die soon after injection. This possibility was tested by labelling Coll5
cells with ^{125} or ^{131}I-IUdR and following tumour cell survival by whole-body
measurements of retained radioactivity (Sordat et al., 1980a). Mice given relatively low cell doses, not able to induce an ascites, showed considerable individual variations in the rate of label excretion. A large part of the radioactivity was excreted early indicating that a high percentage of the injected
cells in fact died within the first 24 hrs. In contrast, the retention curves
of mice given a high dose of tumour cells ip (10^6) showed little individual
variation and only a small percentage of the label was lost at an accelerated
rate. However when the same dose was injected intravenously, the rate of iodine
excretion incicated that the tumour cells were killed almost immediately.
Additional results have been obtained following the sc route : they demonstrate
a marked lag period for iodine excretion suggesting either a slower diffusion
equilibrium or an improved initial survival of tumour cells within this anatomical compartment. It was found in separate experiments that comparatively
small doses (5.10^4 to 10^5) of cells are required to induce a sc tumour. Part
of the results obtained by IUdR labelling and wholebody counting have been recently published in an abstract form (Sordat et al., 1980b).

4. REMOVAL OF THE TUMOUR GRAFT

The length of host exposure to a sc tumour graft proved to increase the
incidence of metastases in spf nude mice. The presence of the metastatic tumour cells can be demonstrated histologically. In addition, autoradiography
following ^{3}H-thymidine pulse labelling can establish that a good proportion of
these metastatic cells are cycling and, furthermore, the lung colony assay

in vitro demonstrates that clonogenic cells can be recovered from distant sites. Surgical removal of the sc graft can now introduce two conditions, i.e. whether or not recurrences occur locally or regionally. Preliminary results obtained with a limited number of mice are presented here in **TABLE 2.**

TABLE 2.

INCIDENCE OF METASTASES FOLLOWING SURGICAL REMOVAL
OF SC-GRAFTED Col15 TUMOUR *

	NO RELAPSE	LOCAL/REGIONAL RELAPSE
TIME INTERVAL AFTER SURGERY (DAYS) **	22 - 150	22 - 92
METASTASES IN		
- REGIONAL LYMPH NODES	1 / 8	11 / 13
- LUNGS :		
- TUMOUR CELLS	1 / 8	9 / 13
- MICROMETASTASES	2 / 8	10 / 13
- MACROMETASTASES	2 / 8	6 / 13

*   21 MICE ANALYSED AFTER SURGERY
** PRIMARY TUMOUR GROWTH PERIOD : 18 - 24 DAYS

In the absence of recurrence and by comparing to the results in TABLE 1 , it can be seen that the incidence of tumour deposits can actually decrease with the graft removal. Although a number of animals still exhibit metastases, it would be pertinent to follow the rate of tumour cell disappearance and to know whether these animals can stay free of residual disease. Tumour recurrence exposes the host to a second cycle of growth which increases again the frequency of the metastases. In some animals of this group, lung metastases can be massive and mediastinal lymphatic localizations are frequent. Additional results are required to understand these tumour-host interactions which take place in xenogeneic metastatic deposits.

5. CONCLUSIONS

Colon carcinomas of human origin exhibit a wide range of differentiation grades among which poorly-differentiated tumours constitute only a small proportion (approx. 5%). In current studies, the emphasis has been placed upon the analysis of a poorly-differentiated colon tumour, the Col15, which proved to be metastatic in the spf nude mouse. Dissemination can take place both from a subcutaneously grafted transplant and from the peritoneal cavity in which this tumour has the ability to grow in ascitic form. Lymph nodes and lungs are the main sites where Col15 tumour deposits can be detected and recovered. Although the in vitro colony forming assay gives only a minimal estimate of the number of tumour cells present at these sites, it provides quantitative informations on metastatic and clonogenic Col15 cells. The results based on the functional assay appear to parallel those obtained by morphology when semi-serial sections of lungs or lymph nodes are prepared and analysed. As demonstrated previously and discussed above (section 3.), the rate of initial tumour cell elimination in the nude mouse appears to be influenced both by the dose and the route of inoculation. Tumour cell survival under various experimental conditions can therefore be evaluated by IUdR labelling and wholebody measurements of retained radioactivity. The results demonstrate different survival kinetics when the cells are introduced into various anatomical compartments such as the subcutaneous space, the peritoneal cavity and the venous blood. These differences possibly relate within the nude mouse to some levels of resistance which could relatively influence the outcome of circulating and embolized tumour cells. In this context, mechanisms which participate to the various steps of the metastasis process such as the extent of cell detachment from a tumour graft or the interactions of endothelial and tumour cells within a target organ are still poorly understood. To further analyse the fate of Col15 tumour cells which spontaneously migrate out of the sc graft, the tumour mass can be surgically removed and the extent of metastatic deposits evaluated. Local and/or regional recurrences appear to increase the frequency of these deposits. Whether this is due to the increased length of exposure to the proliferating tumour cell load or to tumour-associated products shed and prone to interact with the host resistance requires additional investigations. This condition of residual disease after tumour removal may represent an in vivo situation in which the issue of a tumour deposit can be experimentally modulated.

REFERENCES

Carrel, S., Sordat, B. and Merenda, C. 1976. Establishment of a cell line
(Col15) from a human colon carcinoma transplanted into nude mice. Cancer
Res. 36: 3978-3984.
Duke, D.I., 1980. Establishment of a metastasizing human carcinoma of the
gall bladder in nude mice. In: Bastert, G. and Schmidt-Matthiesen, H. (Edi-
tors), Thymusaplastic nude mice and rats in clinical oncology, Gustav
Fischer Verlag, Stuttgart/New York, in press.
Epstein, A.L., Herman, M.M., Kim, H., Dorfman, R.F. and Kaplan, H.S., 1976.
Biology of the human malignant lymphomas. III. Intracranial heterotrans-
plantation in the nude, athymic mouse. Cancer (Philad.) 37: 2158-2176.
Giovanella, B.C., Stehlin, B.S. and Williams, L.J., 1974. Heterotransplanta-
tion of human malignant tumors in nude thymusless mice. II. Malignant
tumors induced by injection of cell cultures derived from solid tumors.
J. Natl. Cancer Inst. 52: 921-930.
Hata, J.H., Ueyama, Y., Tamaoki, N., Furukawa, T. and Morita, K., 1978. Human
neuroblastoma serially transplanted in nude mice and metastases. Cancer 42:
468-473.
Helson, L., Das, S.K. and Hadju, S.I., 1975. Human neuroblastoma in nude mice.
Cancer Res. 35: 2594-2599.
Hirohashi, S., Shimosato, Y., Nagai, K., Koide, T. and Kameya, T., 1976. Human
breast cancer serially transplantable in nude mice in ascites form. Gann 67:
431-436.
Kameya, T., Shimosato, Y., Tumuraya, M., Ohsawa, N. and Nomura, T., 1976.
Human gastric choriocarcinomas serially transplanted in nude mice. J. Natl.
Cancer Inst. 56: 325-329.
Kyriazis, A.P., DiPersio, L., Michael, G.T., Pesce, A.J. and Stinnet, J.D.,
1978. Growth patterns and metastatic behavior of human tumors growing in
athymic mice. Cancer Res. 38: 3186-3190.
Kyriazis, A.P., DiPersio, L., Michael, G.T. and Pesce, A.J., 1979. Influence of
the mouse hepatitis virus (MHV) infection on the growth of human tumors in
the athymic mouse. Intern. J. Cancer 23: 402-409.
Lozzio, B.B., Machado, E.A., Lair, S.V., and Lozzio, C.B., 1979. Reproducible
metastatic growth of K-562 human myelogenous leukemia cells in nude mice.
J. Natl. Cancer Inst. 63: 295-299.
Reid, L.M., Minato, N., Jones, C., Bloom, B. and Holland J., 1980. Rejection
of virus persistently infected tumor cells and its implications for regulation of tumor growth and metastasis in athymic nude mice. In: Proc. 3rd
Int. Workshop on Nude Mice, Gustav Fischer, New York, in press.
Sordat, B., Merenda, C., and Carrel, S., 1977. Invasive growth and dissemina-
tion of human solid tumors and malignant cell lines grafted subcutaneously
to newborn nude mice. In: Proc. 2nd intern. Workshop on Nude Mice, University of Tokyo Press, Tokyo, pp. 313-325.
Sordat, B. and Bogenmann, E., 1980. Metastatic behaviour of human colon carcinoma in nude mice. In: Immunodeficient Animals in Cancer Research, London,
Macmillan's, pp. 145-158, in press.
Sordat, B., Lees, R.K., Bogenmann, E. and Terres, G., 1980a. The behavior of
Col15 human colon carcinoma in nude mice. In : Proc. 3rd Intern. Workshop
on Nude Mice, Gustav Fischer, New York, in press.
Sordat, B., Lees, R.K., Bogenmann, E. and Terres, G., 1980b. Metastatic be-
havior of a human colon carcinoma (Col15) in nude mice. Proc. AACR, in press.

Sordat, B., Ueyama, Y. and Fogh, J., 1980c. Metastasis of tumor heterotrans-
plants in nude mice. In: The Nude Mouse in Experimental and Clinical Research. vol. II, Academic Press, N.Y., in press.
Ueyama, Y., Morita, K., Ochiai, C., Ohsawa, J., Hata, J. and Tamaoki, N., 1978.
Xenotransplantation of a human meningioma and its lung metastasis in nude
mice. Br. J. Cancer 37: 644-647.

IMMUNE REGRESSION OF METASTASES FOLLOWING HYPERTHERMIC TREATMENT OF PRIMARY TUMOURS

J.A. Dickson, S.K. Calderwood, S.A. Shah and A.C. Simpson

In the present renewal of interest in the use of hyperthermia (temperatures $\geqslant 42^{\circ}$C) for the treatment of cancer, a striking finding has been the disappearance of established metastases with host cure following effective heating of the primary tumour. This was first reported by Strauss for the Brown-Pearce carcinoma in the rabbit, and we have confirmed the occurrence of this phenomenon (the 'abscopal' response) for 3 different rat tumours and 2 strains of rabbit tumour, encompassing both allogeneic and syngeneic systems (Table 1).

TABLE 1. Primary tumours with sites of metastases at time of heating. The VX2 tumour grows in the muscles of the hind leg, and was heated at 15 - 20 ml volume; the rat tumours grow s.c. on the dorsum of the hind foot, and were heated at 1.0 - 1.5 ml. Figures in brackets are p᾽ centage host cure rates obtained with the degree of heating specified.

Tumour	Metastases	Heat Sensitivity	Reference
VX2 carcinoma, London strain (allogeneic, rabbit)	regional and distant lymph nodes, lungs	42.5°/180 min (50%)	Muckle & Dickson (197.
VX2 carcinoma, Oxford Strain	regional and distant lymph nodes, lungs	47° / 30 min (75%)	Shah & Dicks᾽ (1978)
D23 carcinoma (syngeneic, rat)	regional nodes	45° / 60 min (50%)	Dickson (197{
MC7 sarcoma (syngeneic, rat)	regional and distant nodes, lungs	43° /120 min (72%)	Shah & Dicks᾽ (1980)
Yoshida sarcoma (allogeneic, rat)	regional and distant nodes	42° / 60 min (100%)	Dickson & Ellis (1976)

Regression of tumour subsequent to heating a similar tumour at a distal site has also been observed directly in hamsters with bilaterally imp-lanted pouch tumours (Goldenberg & Langner, 1971), in rats with a tumoi on both hind feet (Dickson et al., 1977), and in rabbits with tumour ii

the abdomen and testis (Strauss, 1969). Similar regression of metastases has occurred following hyperthermic perfusion of limb tumours in
humans (Cavaliere et al., 1967; Stehlin et al., 1977). This paper exa-
mines the possible mechanisms involved in the abscopal response and
its relevance to the thermotherapy of human tumours.

Role of the Immune System

Following curative heating in the rabbit, VX2 tumour regression
was accompanied by a marked and sustained increase in delayed hypersensitivity skin reactions to 3M KCl extract of VX2 and to DNCB, and
there was a 100-fold increase in anti-tumour and anti-BSA antibody
levels in the host serum. Animals with tumours that were not cured by
heat treatment (25%) showed a progressive decrease in the response to
skin tests and in antibody titres to $^1/10$ or less, findings similar to
those in untreated tumour-bearing rabbits (Shah & Dickson, 1978).
Similarly in rats, curative heating of the MC7 sarcoma ($43^{\circ}/2$ hr) was
accompanied by an increase in both specific (skin response to KCl tumour
extract) and non-specific (skin response to DNCB and anti-BSA antibody
titre) host immune competence. When cellular and humoral immune competence was depressed in VX2 bearing rabbits by total body heating ($42^{\circ}C/$
1 hr x 3 at 24 hr intervals), or in rats with MC7 tumours by X-irradiation (150 rads x 3 at 48 hr intervals) plus cortisone (60 mg/kg body
wt. x 4 at 48 hr intervals) tumour regression did not occur and host
cure was reduced from 75% (rabbit) and 72% (rat) to zero.

Following tumour heating, cured hosts became immune to tumour
inoculation. Cured rabbits withstood challenge with 30 x 10^6 VX2 cells
(1 x 10^6 cells led to death in 10 weeks in untreated hosts) and 50%
of cured rats tolerated 2.5 x 10^6 MC7 cells (this challenge killed
90% of untreated rats). When cured rabbits or rats were immunosuppressed by total body irradiation plus cortisone, there was a decrease
in measured host immune competence and a 100% death rate when the
animals were challenged with previously innocuous doses of VX2 or MC7
tumour cells.

Role of the Mononuclear Phagocyte System

In 1971 Muckle and Dickson emphasized the intense macrophage
infiltration of VX2 carcinomas regressing after heating. In rats with
MC7 sarcoma treated at $43^{\circ}C/2$ hr, i.p. injection of silica (1 mg/g
body wt.), a macrophage toxin, impaired the clearance rate of colloidal
carbon from the blood, and led to a decrease in cure rate of the host
rats from 72% to 43%. Moreover, all the cured animals produced tumours

when challenged with 2.5 x 10[6] MC7 cells; 50% of the cured rats not injected with silica consistently rejected this challenge dose. Suboptimal heating of the MC7 sarcoma (43°C/1.5 hr) gave a cure rate of 31%. This was increased to 65% by injection (i.v.) of the macrophage stimulant, C. parvum, 1 - 4 days before hyperthermia; C. parvum by itself had no curative effect on this tumour.

Role of Tumour Blood Flow

In the tumours listed in Table 1, tumour blood flow was inhibited by glucose loading of the host. Normal tissue blood flow remained unaffected or was increased. At a blood glucose level of 50 mmol/l (1000 mg %) there was a rapid and complete inhibition of tumour blood flow (Fig. 1). That this inhibition was 100% was evidenced by failure of exchange of substances such as water, chloride, glucose and organic acids between the tumour and host, and by tumour angiograms obtained before and after glucose loading (Calderwood & Dickson, 1980).

When tumour blood flow was inhibited for 12 hr by hyperglycaemia and the rat tumours subjected to curative heating (Table 1), tumours re gressed as in normoglycaemic hosts but the animals died from metastases

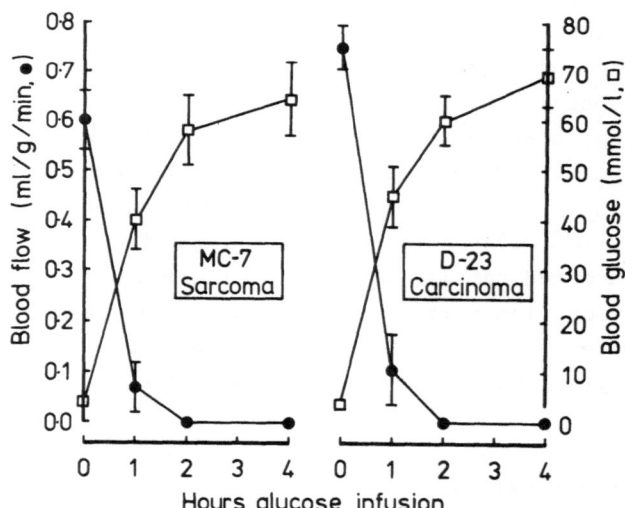

Inhibition of blood flow in the MC7 sarcoma and D23 carcinoma at elevat blood glucose levels. Hyperglycaemia was achieved by infusion of 20% glucose into the femoral vein. Blood flow was measured by fractional distribution of [86]Rubidium in the tissues (Sapirstein, 1958) 40 sec aft injection of 100 uCi isotope in 0.1 ml of 0.9% NaCl into the femoral vein. Blood glucose and blood flow values are means (± 1 S.D.) derived from 5 - 7 animals

Generation of the Anti-tumour Host Response

This was investigated by examining the interstitial fluid of tumours for changes in composition following heating. Samples of fluid were obtained from small plexiglass Millipore membrane chambers embedded in growing tumours on the flank by a modification of the method of Gullino et al. (1964). The profiles of labelled proteins obtained on gel electrophoresis of interstitial fluid show a shift from a predominantly high molecular weight pattern in untreated MC7 and D23 tumours to one in which the major component(s) after curative tumour heating is in the low molecular weight region (Fig. 2). This change was not seen after curative X-irradiation of the tumours. The profiles in Fig. 2 are also different to those obtained with normal rat serum, before or after heating.

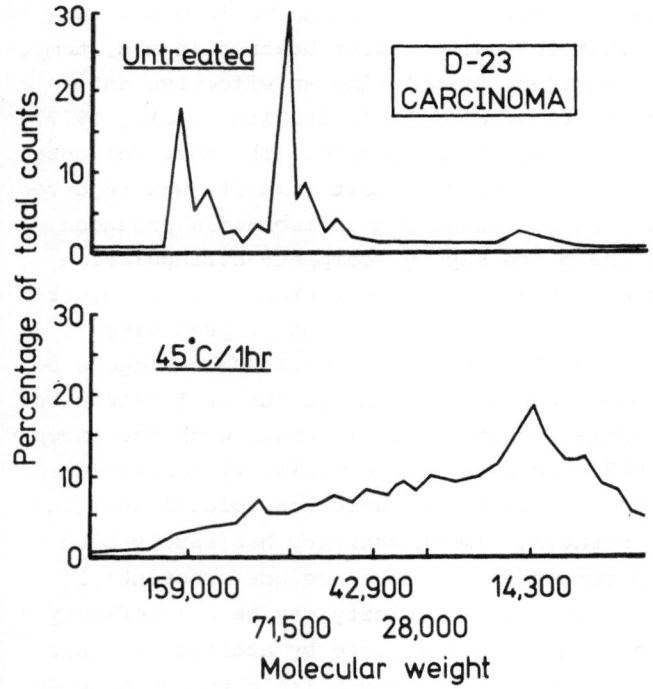

Electrophoretic patterns of iodinated proteins from D23 tumour inter-stitial fluid following treatment. Each pattern represents 1 ul of interstitial fluid labelled with [125]I (Salacinski et al., 1979) before electrophoresis on phosphate buffered 8.5% polyacrylamide gel at 5 mA for 16 hr. The origin is on the left with the bromophenol blue front marker on the right. Mobilities of the molecular weight markers (B.D.H.) used to calibrate the gels are shown on the abscissa. Similar patterns were obtained after electrophoresis of iodinated samples of interstitial fluid from MC7 tumours, before and after heating.

Discussion

The present results confirm that curative heating of animal tumours can lead to a host response that destroys established metastases; the response also renders the animal immune to a previously letha tumour challenge. An intact host immune system would appear to be necessary for the response, but the evidence for a specific and effective tumour directed immune response is not impressive, especially in view of recent work showing that the presence of tumour specific antiserum may not be related to the ability of a host animal to reject tumour (Dennick et al., 1979). The findings are more suggestive of a non-specific host response comprising both cellular and humoral immune components and a major macrophage involvement. The response may be elicited by tumour breakdown products, possibly low molecular weight proteins, entering the bloodstream and/or subsequent entry of lymphocytes and macrophages into the tumour area to be 'armed'. Although it has been claimed that following tumour heating in man, tumou degradation products act as antigens stimulating an effective anti-tumour immune response (Cavaliere et al., 1967; Stehlin et al., 1977) definitive evidence for this postulate is lacking. The host response described is not unique to tumour heating. Host immunity was reported many years ago in mice and rats following tumour ischaemia produced by incompletely ligaturing the blood supply; complete strangulation inhibited the response (Foley, 1953; Lewis & Aptekman, 1962). Hyper-thermia may therefore be simply a convenient method of producing tumour damage and breakdown, and hyperglycaemia would be analogous to tumour strangulation. A common denominator in the tumour ligature wor and in the data on hyperthermia reported here is that, with the exception of the virus-induced VX2 carcinoma, the experiments concerned chemically induced animal tumours in which tumour associated antigens have been most easily demonstrated. Immunogenicity has rarely been demonstrated in spontaneous tumours, and there are now substantial grounds for believing that tumour immunogenicity may be a laboratory artifact largely restricted to neoplasms induced by artificial means (Moore, 1978). On this basis, it may seem unrealistic to envisage an abscopal response occurring after heating human tumours. However, the proteins released from heated tumour cells are unlikely to be native surface antigen as currently believed (Currie, 1974) to be continuousl shed by tumour cells. In support of this point is the reported molecular weight of the D23 and MC7 tumour associated antigens of 50 - 60 $\times 10^3$ daltons (Baldwin et al., 1973), well in excess of the moiety (15 $\times 10^3$ daltons) detected after hyperthermia (Fig. 2).

References

Baldwin, R.W., Harris, J.R. and Price, M.R., 1973. Fractionation of plasma membrane-associated tumour-specific antigen from an aminoazo dye-induced rat hepatoma. Int. J. Cancer, 11: 385-397.

Calderwood, S.K. and Dickson, J.A., In press. Effect of hyperglycemia on the blood flow, pH and response to hyperthermia of the Yoshida sarcoma in the rat. Cancer Res.

Cavaliere, R., Ciocatto, E.C., Giovanella, B.C., Heidelberger, C., Johnson, R.O., Margottini, M., Mondovi, B., Moricca, G. and Rossi-Fanelli, A., 1967. Selective heat sensitivity of cancer cells. Cancer, 20: 1351-1381.

Currie, G.A., 1974. Cancer and the Immune Response. Ed. Arnold, London.

Dennick, R.G., Price, M.R. and Baldwin, R.W., 1979. Modification of the immunogenicity and antigenicity of rat hepatoma cells. II. Mild heat treatment. Brit. J. Cancer, 39: 630-636.

Dickson, J.A., 1978. The sensitivity of human cancer to hyperthermia. In: W.L. Caldwell and R.E. Durand (editors), Proc. Conf. Clinical Prospects for Hypoxic Cell Sensitizers and Hyperthermia. Univ. of Wisconsin Press, Madison, Wisconsin, pp. 174-193.

Dickson, J.A., Calderwood, S.K. and Jasiewicz, M.L., 1977. Radio-frequency heating of tumours in rodents. Eur. J. Cancer, 13: 753-763.

Dickson, J.A. and Ellis, H.A., 1976. The influence of tumor volume and the degree of heating on the response of the solid Yoshida sar-coma to hyperthermia (40 - 42°C). Cancer Res., 36: 1188-1195.

Foley, E.J., 1953. Antigenic properties of methylcholanthrene-induced tumors in mice of the strain of origin. Cancer Res., 13: 835-840.

Goldenberg, D.M. and Langner, M., 1971. Direct and abscopal antitumour action of local hyperthermia. Z. Naturforsch, 26b: 359-361.

Gullino, P.M., Clark, S.H. and Grantham, F.H., 1964. The interstitial fluid of solid tumors. Cancer Res., 24: 780-797.

Lewis, M.R. and Aptekman, P.M., 1952. Atrophy of tumours caused by strangulation and accompanied by development of tumour immunity in rats. Cancer, 5: 411-413.

Moore, M., 1978. Antigens in experimentally induced neoplasms: a conspectus. In: J.E. Castro (Editor), Immunological Aspects of Cancer. MTP Press Ltd., Lancaster, England, pp. 15-50.

Muckle, D.S. and Dickson, J.A., 1971. The selective inhibitory effect of hyperthermia on the metabolism and growth of malignant cells. Brit. J. Cancer, 25: 771-778.

Salacinski, P., Hope, J., McLean, C., Clement-Jones, V., Sykes, J., Price, J. and Lowry, P.J., 1979. A new simple method which allows theoretical incorporation of radioiodine into proteins and peptides without damage. J. Endocrinol., 81: 131.

Sapirstein, L.A., 1958. Regional blood flow by fractional distribution of indicators. Amer. J. Physiol., 193: 163-168.

Shah, S.A. and Dickson, J.A., 1978. Effect of hyperthermia on the immunocompetence of VX2 tumour-bearing rabbits. Cancer Res., 38: 3523-3531.

Shah, S.A. and Dickson, J.A., 1980. Effects of immunosuppression on the response of animal tumours to hyperthermia. In preparation.

Stehlin, J.S., Giovanella, B.C., DeIpolyi, P.D., Muenz, L.R., Anderson, R.F. and Gutierrez, A.A., 1977. Hyperthermic perfusion of extremi-ties for melanoma and soft tissue sarcomas. Recent Results Cancer Res., 59: 171-185.

Strauss, A.A., 1969. Immunologic Resistance to Carcinoma Produced by Electrocoagulation. Based on Fifty-Seven Years of Experimental and Clinical Results. Chas. C. Thomas, Springfield, Illinois.

CLONAL TUMOR CELL VARIANTS ARISING BY ADAPTATION

K. Bosslet and V. Schirrmacher

SUMMARY

The experiments to be presented will demonstrate a new type of tumor variant which can arise with high frequency even within carefully cloned tumor cell lines. Cloned lines of a metastasizing chemically induced tumor (ESb) will be shown to loose their tumor-associated transplantation antigen (TATA) in adaptation to a T cell mediated anti-tumor immune response. This changed phenotype enables the tumor cells to escape immune destruction and to grow even in lymphoid organs such as the spleen. The loss of tumor antigen seen in our system differs from the phenomenon of antigenic modulation as described for thymus-leukemia (TL) antigens (Boyse et al., 1967) in that it is more stable and inherited to many subsequent cell generations. We therefore suggest as a basis for the changed phenotype a genetic (gene regulation type) rather than an epigenetic mechanism.

INTRODUCTION, MATERIALS AND METHODS

As model system we chose the chemically induced DBA/2 lymphoma L5178Y with the two sublines Eb and ESb (Parr, 1972). We previously described morphological, functional and antigenic differences between the parental line Eb and its spontaneous variant ESb which arose in 1968 and had highly increased metastatic capacity (Schirrmacher et al., 1979a). In spite of these differences the tumor lines could be shown to be closely related (Schirrmacher and Bosslet, 1980a). Tumor immunization experiments revealed the presence of TATA's on both Eb and ESb tumor cells. These TATA's of Eb and ESb were shown to be distinct and non-cross reactive and could be detected in vitro with the help of tumor specific syngeneic cytotoxic T lymphocytes (CTL) (Bosslet et al., 1979).

These tumor-specific CTL were obtained by culturing spleen cells from tumor-immune animals (animals inoculated twice at weekly intervals with 10^7 irradiated tumor cells) for five days in vitro in the presence of mitomycin treated autologous tumor cells. Large batches of such cells with high and

specific cytolytic activity in a 4 h ^{51}Cr release test were aliquoted,
frozen in liquid nitrogen, and used - just like tissue typing sera - for
typing tumor cell lines for expression of their individually-specific
TATA's.

RESULTS AND DISCUSSION

Table 1 summarizes the results of experiments in which the expression of
TATA was followed during the metastatic process of twice cloned s.c.
inoculated ESb tumor cell lines. Cloning was done by growing single cells
in suspension culture in micro-titer plates. More than 99.9% of the
starting cell populations (ESb clone 18.1 and clone 32.2) could be lysed by
anti ESb CTL thus demonstrating the homogeneity of the starting cell
populations with regard to TATA expression.

After s.c. transplantation of 10^5 of these cells into syngeneic DBA/2
mice, the outgrowing tumor cells were isolated from the local tumor and
from internal organs. This was done either 12 days (in case of the quickly
metastasizing clone 18.1) or 25 days (in case of the slower metastasizing
clone 32.2) after inoculation. The tumor cells were grown out first in vivo
(i.p.) and then in tissue culture to remove possible contaminating host
cells and factors. They were then tested with the above CTL for expression
of TATA. While tumor cells from the locally growing tumor and from most
internal organs or tissues were effectively lysed by anti ESb CTL, those
isolated from the spleens could not be lysed (Table 1). This resistance to
lysis of spleen derived metastasizing ESb tumor cells was reproducibly
found independent of whether we started with s.c. inoculation of cloned or
uncloned tumor cell populations.

Different results were obtained when the tumor cells were inoculated
directly into the spleens of normal mice. These tumor lines could be
specifically lysed by anti ESb CTL even after several spleen passages
(Table 2). A lysis resistant line was only obtained when small numbers of
ESb-Cl 18.1 cells were inoculated into the spleen of ESb immune animals
(Table 2).

When ESb-Cl 18.1 cells were inoculated s.c. into ESb immune animals, those
tumor cells which eventually grew out (after 4 weeks) were always resistant
to lysis by anti ESb CTL, whether isolated from the local tumor, the liver or
the spleen (Table 3).

TABLE 1

Expression of tumor antigen (TATA) on cloned ESb tumor lines during the metastatic process.

Isolation of tumor cells from	ESb-Cl 18.1		ESb-Cl 32.2	
	% Spec.Cytotoxicity		% Spec.Cytotoxicity	
	anti-Eb (control)	anti-ESb (experimental)	anti-Eb (control)	anti-ESb (experimental)
(control ascites line)	6	78	5	47
local. tumor	1	45	nd.	20
lung	2	63	2	42
brain	1	45	nd.	63
liver	1	60	2	2
spleen	2	4	0	7

12 days after s.c. transplantation of 10^5 ESb-Cl 18.1 cells and 25 days after s.c. transplantation of ESb-Cl 32.2 cells the local tumor and internal organs were removed from one mouse each, cell suspensions prepared and transplanted i.p. into normal DBA/2 recipients in order to expand the tumor cell number; the ascites tumor cells were adapted to growth in tissue culture, labeled with ^{51}Cr and then tested as target cells for anti-tumor CTL in a 4 h cytotoxicity test; ratio of CTL to target cells 40:1; values indicate % specific ^{51}Cr release; nd. = not done.

TABLE 2

Expression of tumor antigen (TATA) on cloned ESb tumor lines inoculated directly into the spleen.

Host	Tumor	Dose	No.of passages in spleen[1]	% Specific cytotoxicity of CTL[2]		
				anti-Eb	anti-ESb	anti-H-2^d
DBA/2 normal	ESb-Cl 32.2	10^5	2 x	1.8	67	68
	"	10^5	3 x	9.6	60	73
	"	10^3	2 x	1.2	60	71
	"	10^3	3 x	1.2	64	72
DBA/2 ESb immune	ESb-Cl 18.1	10^5	1 x (day 8)	4.6	44	65
		10^4	1 x (day14)	0.0	0	52

[1] For direct inoculation of tumor cells into the spleen anaestesized animals were carefully operated;

[2] % specific ^{51}Cr release after 4 h coincubation of the indicated tissue culture adapted ^{51}Cr labeled tumor lines with the indicated cytotoxic T lymphocytes (CTL) at an effector to target cell ratio of 40:1. The anti H-2^d CTL were generated in a mixed lymphocyte culture of C57Bl/6 spleen cells as responder and DBA/2 spleen cells as stimulator cells.

TABLE 3

Expression of tumor antigen (TATA) on ESb-Cl 18.1 cells after s.c. inoculation
into normal or ESb immune DBA/2 mice.

Isolation of tumor cells from	normal % cytotoxicity		immune % cytotoxicity	
	anti ESb	anti H-2	anti ESb	anti H-2
local tumor	45	64	7	65
liver	69	74	0	59
spleen	4	49	2	73

For details see footnotes to Table 1 and 2.

In Table 4 we have summarized our evidence that the resistance to lysis
of the clonal tumor variants is due to a decreased expression or even loss
of TATA's on their cell surface.

TABLE 4

Evidence for loss of TATA by clonal tumor variants

1. Cells are not generally resistant to lysis;
   they can be killed by anti H-2 CTL (see Table 2,3,5);

2. Cells don't bind to anti-TATA CTL;
   see cold target competition experiment (Schirrmacher and Bosslet, 1980b);

3. Variants could not induce CTL's;
   they do not express a changed TATA;

4. No effect of enzyme treatments (trypsin and neuraminidase);
   the antigens are not covered up.

The loss of TATA by the clonal variants was a rather stable type of changed
phenotype: Spleen-derived antigen negative tumor variants passaged for prolonged periods (ten and more passages) in tissue culture remained antigen
negative. This means that the reduced expression or loss of TATA was inherited
to thirty or more subsequent cell generations. We therefore suggest that
the antigenic changes observed are not due to "antigenic modulation" which
is of short duration but rather to a genetic mechanism.

The disappearance of the tumor antigen is suggested to be due to a process
of adaptation of the tumor cells to a T cell mediated anti-tumor immune
response by the host, a process which could be termed "immuno-adaptation".
The evidence that this process is dependent of and influenced by T
lymphocytes is summarized in Table 5:

TABLE 5

Evidence for immunomodulatory role of T lymphocytes

		% Specific cytotoxicity with CTL[3]		
		anti-Eb	anti-ESb	anti-H-2^d
1. nu/nu	ESb control	3	53	79
versus	ESb-SPL, DBA/2 4x	3	8	85
normal[1]	ESb-SPL, nu/nu,4x	0	35	72
2. addition of CTL	Local tumor, control	1	45	64
in Winn assay (WA)[2]	" , WA	0	0	65
	ESb-Liv, control	1	60	64
	" , WA	0	0	62
	ESb-SPL, control	0	10	63
	" , WA	0	6	65

[1] Spleen localizing tumor cells were selected by s.c. inoculation of uncloned
ESb cells, isolation of tumor cells from the spleens and repeated s.c.
inoculation. This process was repeated 4 times; the tumor lines were then
passaged 2x in tissue culture; recipients were either normal DBA/2 or BALB/c
nude (nu/nu) mice;

[2] 10^5 ESb-Cl 18.1 cells were inoculated s.c. either alone or in a Winn assay
after mixture with 10^7 irradiated anti ESb CTL; 4 weeks later tumor cells
were removed from the local tumor, liver and spleen of the WA mouse,
which had a local tumor of 8 mm in diameter; tumor lines were isolated
as described in Table 1;

[3] See footnote of Table 2.

The evidence is twofold: Firstly, a comparison of spleeen-derived tumor lines
from T cell deficient nude (nu/nu) and normal mice revealed that the
antigen loss was only observed on the lines isolated from normal mice. Even
four repeated passages (s.c.——> spleen) through nude mice did not lead to
a loss of TATA. Secondly, the direct addition of anti ESb CTL in a Winn
type assay led to a loss of TATA on tumor cells isolated eventually (after
4 weeks) from the s.c. site and from internal organs.

The evidence that the changed phenotype is due to immunoadaptation by the tumor cells rather than to a selection by the host of a potential preexisting antigen-negative variant can be summarized as follows: (i) > 99.9% of the original clones could be lysed by anti ESb CTL when presented in excess (500:1) in a 4 h cytotoxicity test, (ii) shifts in antigen expression were occasionally observed in our cloned tumor lines during one in vitro passage (manuscript in preparation). Since such changes occured in less than 3 cell generations they could hardly be explained by the outgrowth of a preexisting minority subpopulation, (iii) a clonal analysis of the original ESb population revealed a homogenous positive antigen phenotype. From 30 clones tested none was antigen negative.

We assume that the changes in antigen expression by the tumor cells are not brought about by mutation of the structural genes coding for the tumor antigen because the changes can be reproduced with too high a frequency. On the other hand, the ability of the tumor cells to express their distinct TATA has been a constant characteristic over a period of more than ten years (Schirrmacher and Bosslet, 1980a). We rather suggest that the clonal tumor variants represent gene regulatory variants. The antigen negative variants could have arisen during a process of immunoadaptation where T cells reacting against the TATA might have signaled to the tumor cell to repress the biosynthesis of the antigen. Adaptive behavior of tumor cells may not only explain a new type of immune escape mechanism. It could also have a more general biological significance for tumor cell behavior, in particular during the complex process of metastasis.

REFERENCES

Bosslet, K., Schirrmacher, V. and Shantz, G., 1979. Tumor metastases and cell-mediated immunity in a model system in DBA/2 mice. VI. Similar specificity patterns of protective anti-tumor immunity in vivo and of cytolytic T cells in vitro. Int.J.Cancer 24: 303-313.

Boyse, E.A., Stockert, E. and Old, L.J., 1967. Modification of the antigenic structure of the cell membrane by thymus-leukemia (TL) antibody. Proc.Natl.Acad.Sci. 58: 954-957.

Parr, I., 1972. Response of murine lymphomata to immunotherapy in relation to the antigenicity of the tumor. Brit.J.Cancer 26: 174-182.

Schirrmacher, V., Shantz, G., Clauer, K., Komitowski, D., Zimmermann, H.-P., and Lohmann-Matthes, M.L., 1979. Tumor metastases and cell-mediated immunity in a model system in DBA/2 mice. I. Tumor invasiveness in vitro and metastases formation in vivo. Int.J.Cancer 23: 233-244.

Schirrmacher, V. and Bosslet, K., 1980a. Tumor metastases and cell-mediated immunity in a model system in DBA/2 mice. X. Immunoselection of tumor variants differing in tumor antigen expression and metastatic capacity. Int.J.Cancer, in press.

Schirrmacher, V. and Bosslet, K., 1980b. Loss of tumor antigen by spleen metastasizing tumor cell variants - an example of immuno-adaptation by cloned tumor lines. Nature, submitted.

REVERSIBILITY OF IMMUNOLOGICAL AND ANTITUMORAL EFFECTS PRODUCED IN VIVO BY PARTICULATE β1-3 GLUCANS

F.J. Lejeune, A. Vercammen-Grandjean, R. Arnould, A. Libert, G. Atassi

β1-3 glucan, an insoluble polysaccharidic extract isolated from Saccharomyces cerevisiae zymosan, was shown to share the immuno modulatory properties of bacterial vaccines (such as BCG, C.parvum). In contrast to the latter, β1-3 glucan preparations are partially purified and biochemically defined, they are not toxic when administered systemically in animals, and the resulting hyperplasia and hyperfunction on the immune system are reversible (Riggi S.J. and Di Luzio, N.R. 1961 - Lejeune F.J. et al., 1978, 1979).

Since glucan preparations are particulate, they are taken up not only by macrophages of the reticulo-endothelial system (Riggi and Di Luzio 1961) but also by tumour macrophages (Lejeune et al., 1978).

The aim of this work was to investigate the effects of particulate β1-3 glucan on B16 mouse melanoma and to study the changes occurring in lymphocytes and macrophages.

MATERIALS AND METHODS

Glucans : B1-3 glucan glucan preparations were gifts from Gist-Brocades, Delft, The Netherlands (glucan GB) and from N.R. Di Luzio, New Orleans LA, USA (glucan DL).

Mice: C57BL/6 (C57BL x DBA/2) F_1 (BDF$_1$) and Balb/C mice were purchased from Charles River Inc. (USA) via the NCI Liaison Office of the Institut J. Bordet, Brussels.

Peritoneal macrophages were studied for activation: acid phosphatase, spreading, cytolysis and inhibition of H_3 TdR uptake tests were performed according to already published methods (Lejeune and Evans 1972, Lejeune et al, 1978).

Spleen lymphocyte mitogenic response to PHA (Wellcome) and to LPS (Difco) was assessed as published previously (Lejeune et al, 1980).

Thymidine (TdR) detection in macrophage supernatants:
macrophages were cultured for 72 hours in MEM (Gibco) medium without serum.   Supernatants were studied by thin layer chromatography,
on cellulose layers in methanol/HCl 1,18/water (70/20/10, v/v) -
(K. Randerath, E. Randerath 1967).

RESULTS

B16 melanoma immunotherapy

10 different batches of glucan GB were used in immunotherapy
experiments.   C57Bl/6 mice were s.c. injected with 10^6 B16 cells
in suspension on day O. Glucans were administered i.v. at a dose
of 7.5, 15 cnd 30 mg/kg on days 1,5, 9 and 13 after tumour transplantation.

Results shown on Table 1 are those obtained with 15 mg/kg
glucan, which was found to be the optimal dose. The results are
expressed as increase in lifespan of treated mice over control
(ILS) and as inhibition of tumour growth over control.   ILS was
slightly increased but no treatment produced a significant 40%
prolongatior of survival, according to the NCI requirements.

Tumour growth was most significantly inhibited on day 12 -
5/10 batches of glucan had at least 80% inhibition -; on days 16
and 19, the effect became gradually weaker since 3/10 and 0/10
batches of glucan had an 80% inhibition of the B16 melanoma growth
respectively.

Spleen cells response to glucan

Groups of BDF_1 mice received a single i.v. injection of 40 mg/
kg glucan DL on day O. DNA synthesis was measured by H_3 TdR uptake
either withcut any mitogen in vitro or in presence of PHA or LPS.
Table 2 shows the results expressed in % after 3,6 and 12 days.
Glucan induced in vivo DNA synthesis in spleen cells, which other-
wise showed a depression of T (PHA) and B (LPS) mitogenic indexes
in vitro This effect was insensitive to indomethacin (results not
shown).

Peritoneal macrophages activation

On day 3 after single i.p. injection of glucan DL 40 mg/kg, peritoneal macrophages were found to be activated (Table 3). The percentage of acid phosphatase positive macrophages increased, spreading index augmented and there was a significant increase of macrophage specific cytolysis (chromium release).

In contrase, the inhibition of H_3 TdR uptake, by target mitogen stimulated spleen cells, exhibited by normal macrophages, was not significantly changed. This inhibition is equivalent to the effect of $4.10^{-6}M$ TdR (Vercammen-Grandjean and Lejeune 1977) on a reference curve in HM6 melanoma cell line.

Batch N°	I.L.S.(1) (%)	Inhibition of tumor growth (% of control) on day		
		12	16	19
BO1	25	82 **	50.8	67.6 *
BO2	27	83.7 **	86.1 **	62.0 *
BO3	29	94.2 **	86.2 **	62.0 *
BO4	27	14.9	68.8 *	54.8
BO5	20	88.7 **	79.8 **	74.7 *
BO6	29	79.3 **	50.7	69.2
BO7	15	0	45.8	38.5
BO8	20	74.4	72.0	71.5
BO9	16	56.8	77.8	42.5
BO10	23	86.0	71.6	64.5

Table 1 : Antitumour effect of β1-3 glucans on B16 melanoma.
GB glucans were administered i.v. at the doses of 15, mg/kg on days 1,5,9 and 13 after tumourtransplantation.
(1) I.L.S. = increase in lifespan of treated mice over controls
  * <80%, ** > 80 % tumour growth inhibition.

Day	DNA synthesis without mitogen	Mitogenic index	
		PHA	LPS
0	100	100	100
3	156	55	63
6	190	28	84
12	73	87	131

Table 2 : Spleen cells response to β 1-3 glucan 40 mg/kg i.v.

TdR release by peritoneal macrophages

In order to evaluate whether glucan activated macrophages
could release cold TdR, supernatants of normal resident macrophages
and glucan activated macrophages were assayed. Thin layer chromatography for nucleosides was performed on 72 hours 10^6/ml macrophages supernatants.

Table 4 indicates that all normal and glucan activated
macrophages released detectable amounts of TdR. None of the supernatants contained detectable UdR, CdR or GdR.

Day	Acid phosphatase	Spreading	Cytolysis (1)	Inhibition of H_3 TdR uptake PHA	LPS
0	100	100	0	55	45
3	395	152	15	54	56
6	127	168	1	NT	42

Table 3 : Peritoneal macrophage activation by β1-3 glucan 40 mg/kg i.p. (1) spe-
cific chromium release by melanoma cells (2). Normal spleen cells stimulated with
PHA or LPS in the presence of macrophage supernatants incubated for 24 hours.
Results expressed as % of control.

	Normal resident peritoneal macrophages			Glucan activated peritoneal macrophages
	C 57 B1	BDF$_1$	Balb/C	Balb/C
TdR	+	+	+	+
UdR	0	0	0	0
CdR	0	0	0	0
GdR	0	0	0	0

Table 4 : TdR release in peritoneal macrophages supernatants. Thin layer chromatography for nucleosides.

DISCUSSION

Our results clearly indicate that antitumour effects of some
batches of β1-3 glucans are reversible, eventually after repeated
i.v. inoculations. This was not noted by others (Cook J.A. et
al 1978) who only reported punctual experiments. The reversibility
of the antimelanoma effect was well correlated with parallel hyper-
trophy of spleen and liver (Lejeune et al 1980) due to the in vivo
mitogenic effect of β1-3 glucan. The latter phenomenon might explain
the reduced response to T & B mitogens in vitro (Lejeune et al 1980).

In addition, we could that macrophage activity was only detected on day 3 after glucan administration, at least in 2 out of 3 tests and that it had disappeared by day 6.

Since macrophage and lymphocyte functions appear to be modulated by β1-3 glucan, it is tempting to ascribe to it, the reversibility of the antitumour effects. Prolonged schedules of β1-3 glucan administration are needed in order to find out whether a plateau of stimulation could be reached.

Besides the immunomodulatory effects of glucans, the finding that glucan activated or elicited macrophages can release consistent amounts of TdR is of interest.

TdR released by macrophages can produce a DNA synthesis blockade (Stadecker et al, 1977) in tumour cells. Since B1-3 glucan induces a strong recruitment of macrophages in liver - which is a target organ for metastasis - and in tumours (Cook et al, 1978 - Lejeune et al 1978), it can be expected that this phenomenon should increase the local TdR concentration. That such a mechanism would be relevant to inhibition of tumour growth and metastasis is being currently investigated. (FRSM grant No. 3.4520.79 and NCI contract No. NO1-CM-57040.

REFERENCES

Cook, J.A., Taylor, D., Cohen C., Rodriguez, J., Malshet V. and Di Luzio, N.R. Comparative evaluation of the role of macrophages and lymphocytes in mediating the antitumour action of glucan. In: Immuno Modulation and Control of Neoplasia by Adjuvant Therapy. Edited by Chirigos. Raven Press N.Y. pp183-194 1978.

Lejeune, F. and Evans, R. Ultrastructural, cytochemical and biochemical changes occurring during syngeneic macrophage-lymphoma interaction in vitro. Eur.J.Cancer 8, 549-555, 1972

Lejeune, F.J., Beaumont, E., Garcia, Y., Regnier, R. Peritoneal macrophages cytotoxicity induced by serum in vitro. Biomedecine 28, 48-54. 1978

Lejeune, F.J., Song, M., Delville, J., Stadtsbaeder, S., Gillet, J. and Jacques, P.J. Effects of the yest polysaccharide glucan in transplanted colon carcinoma of the rat and experimental infectious diseases. In: Gastrointestinal tumors: A clinical and experimental approach. Ed. A. Gérard. Eur.J.Cancer.Suppl.1, pp 127-134. 1978

Lejeune, F.J., Vercammen-Grandjean A., Mendes da Costa, P., Bron, D., Defleur, V. Suppressor cell induction and reticuloendothelial cell activation produced in the mouse by B1-3 glucan. In: Macrophages and Lymphocytes. Part A. Eds. M.R. Escobar and H. Friedman. Plenum Publishing Cpn. pp 235-244. 1980.

Randerath, K., Randerath, E. Thin-layer separation methods for nucleic acid derivatives. Methods Enzym 12, 323-347. 1967.

Riggi, S.J. and Di Luzio, N.R. Identification of a reticuloendothelial agent in Zymosan. Am. J. Physiology 200, 297-300. 1961.

Stadecker, M.J., Calderon, J., Karnovsky, M. and Unaneu, E.R. Synthesis and release of thymidine by macrophages. Journal of Immunology 119, 1738-1743. 1977

Vercammen-Grandjean, A.F. and Lejeune. Production and mode of action of macrophages secretions that interfere with the in vitro incorporation of radioactive DNA precursors by tumour cells. In: The Macrophage and Cancer. Eds. K. James, B. McBride, A. Stuart. Edinburgh pp 50-59. 1977

MODULATION OF TUMOR GROWTH AND METASTASIS BY AN ACUTE INFLAMMATION

D. Nolibe, I. Florentin, M. Pelletier, R. Masse and J.P. Giroud

1. INTRODUCTION

Many studies have led to the conclusion that macrophage can contribute in a variety of ways to host resistance against tumors. Non immune inflammation represents the major mechanism by which indirect activation of macrophages occurs in vivo. This process induces proliferation (GIROUD et al., 1977) and activation (KIGER et al., 1978) of macrophages which render them cytotoxic against tumor target cells in vitro (POSTE, 1979). On the other hand, in vivo, FAUVE and HEVIN (1977) had shown that an inflammatory reaction, induced by inoculation of talc embedded in calcium phosphate gel, was able to inhibit the growth of spontaneous metastases in the lungs. The purpose of the present work is to study the effect of a non immune acute inflammation on the growth and metastasis processes in different tumors models. Further mechanisms by which inflammation could modify tumor dissemination are tested.

2. MATERIAL AND METHODS

2.1. Non immunological acute inflammation (NIAI) induction

NIAI was induced in C 57 B1/6 mice (OLAC, Bicester, England) by intrapleural injection of 0.5 ml 12% dextran (MW 40000), or of 1 ml 1% calcium pyrophosphate in rats of a Wistar inbred strain (CNRS, Orléans la Source, France).

2.2. Tumors

(i) Lewis lung carcinoma (3LL) tumor cells were isolated from lung metastatic foci and cultured in vitro during 3 days before inoculation ; 5×10^4 viable tumor cells were inoculated into the footpad and the animals sacrificed 30 days later.

(ii) Calibrated pieces of lung hemangiosarcoma (C 433), initially radio-induced in Wistar AG rats (NOLIBE, in prep.), were s.c grafted in syngeneic animals.

(iii) An in vitro, established cell line of a malignant fibrohistyocytoma (P 77) also induced by irradiation (NOLIBE, in prep.) was used for induction of artificial metastasis.

2.3. In vivo tests

(i) Primary tumor growth and number of visible metastases on organs were recorded, for each model.

(ii) Tumor cell arrest in lungs was measured with P 77 cells labelled by ^{125}IUdR according to FIDLER (1978).

2.4. In vitro immunological tests

(i) Assay for peritoneal macrophage mediated cytostasis against L 1210 tumor cells was performed in mice according to the method described in detail previously (KIGER et al. 1978).

(ii) Natural killer (NK) activities of mouse spleen and peritoneal cells were tested against YAC-1 lymphoma cell line as described by HERBERMANN et al., 1975.

3. RESULTS

3.1. Influence of acute inflammation on tumor growth and spontaneous metastasis

Tumor growth was recorded in 4 groups of 3 LL Lewis grafted mice and in 4 groups of hemangiosarcoma grafted rats. For each model, 3 groups received NIAI at different times with regard to tumor inoculation, and one group was kept as control. In mice, inflammation induced 3 days after tumor grafting did not significantly

TABLE 3.1.

Influence of an acute inflammation on spontaneous metastases

Day of inflammatory stimulus *	Mean n° of lung metastases per animal (± S.E)		Total n° of organs with metastases
	3 LL	C 433	C 433
− 3	33 ± 7**		
0	25 ± 7**	11 ± 1**	8
+ 3	17 ± 3		
+ 7		22 ± 3	3
+ 14		63 ± 11**	2
controls (No inflam.)	11 ± 3	19.5 ± 3	14

* Day 0 = day of tumor inoculation (10 animals per group)

** Significantly different from controls

modify tumor growth. A significant acceleration of tumor development was observed when the inflammation was applied 3 days before or at the same time as tumor cell inoculation. This phenomenon was detectable from day 10 to day 15 after tumor grafting, after this time the rate of tumor growth was similar in all groups. However the tumor size at sacrifice in groups treated at day − 3 (800 ± 40) and day 0 (765 ± 45) was significantly higher than in control group (660 ± 24). In contrast, in hemangiosarcoma bearing rats, tumor growth rate and tumor size at death were not significantly modified by NIAI.

In mice, a significant increase in the number of lung metastases was only observed in the groups treated 3 days before and on the same day as tumor grafting (table 3.1). In rats, when inflammation and tumor graft were performed on the same day, the number of lung metastases significantly decreased. In contrast, metastases increased if inflammation was induced 14 days after tumor graft. No effect was observed at day 7 (table 3.1). Currently, hemangiosarcoma-bearing rats presented a limited (less than five) number of macroscopically visible metastases in other organs than lungs, this metastatic process was inhibited in all groups submitted to inflammatory stimulus (table 3.1).

In another experiment, the hemangiosarcoma was excised on day 14 and NIAI was induced on day 11 or 14. A maximal increase in the number of lung metastases was observed when NIAI was applied on the same day as surgery i.e when a large number of tumor cells was released in the blood stream. A model of artificial metastasis was used to test a possible enhancing effect of metastatic process by NIAI when a large number of cells is present. Three parameters were measured : trapping of tumor cells in the lung one hour after injection, number of viable cells after one day and number of metastases after 4 weeks. No modification of tumor cell arrest and of the number of metastases in the lung was observed when NIAI was applied 3 days before tumor cell inoculation (table 3.2).

TABLE 3.2.
Pulmonary distribution and pulmonary metastases after IV injection of 10^5 ^{125}IUdR Labeled P 77 tumor cells.

Time of application of inflammatory stimulus	Lung distribution of P 77 tumor cells		Mean number of pulmonary metastases
	N° 1 hr after	N° after 24 hrs	
controls* (no inflammation)	70 558 ± 9507	1316 ± 390	30 ± 30
- 3 days*	76 172 ± 12 370	1168 ± 297	27 ± 20
- 1 hour*	83 934 ± 6571	2718 ± 965	75 ± 71

* 10 animals per group

When inflammation was induced only one hour before tumor cell injection, a slight but not significant, increase of cell trapping in the lung was detected. Moreover, in similarly treated animals but sacrificed one day later a significant increase of surviving tumor cells in lungs was observed suggesting that

NIAI may induce a defect in some antitumoral cytotoxicity mechanism. This hypothesis was reinforced by the observation of an increase in the mean number of
lung metastases, although this increase was apparently not significant, a mathematical analysis has shown that two subpopulations could be individualized in
this group of animals, one (70%) with a large number of metastases (110 ± 58)
and the other (30%) with a low number (13 ± 2).

3.2. Influence of acute inflammation on non specific cytotoxicity mechanisms

(i) Natural killer activities of spleen and peritoneal cells were measured
at different times after induction of NIAI in normal mice (table 3.3). A decrease
in the NK activity occured very rapidly after the intrapleural injection and this
effect was still detectable 3 days after.

TABLE 3.3.

Effect of inflammation on natural killer (NK) activity

| Effector cells | Controls | Percent specific cytotoxicity ± S.E. | | | | |
| | | Time after application of inflammatory stimulus | | | | |
		12 H	1 D	2 D	3 D	4 D
Spleen cells	21.2	15.4	15.7	16.3	12.6	22.5
	± 0.6	± 0.9	± 0.7	± 0.1	± 0.2	± 0.5
Peritoneal cells	3.1	3.1	2.6	1.5	1.7	–
	± 0.05	± 0.1	± 0.2	± 0.05	± 0.2	

* The effectors to target cells ratio was 50 : 1

(ii) NIAI, when applied to normal mice, markedly increased the cytostatic activity of peritoneal macrophages for tumor cells. This stimulatory effect was detected as early as 1 hour after inflammation and was maximal on day 3 (table 3.4).

TABLE 3.4.

Effect of inflammation on peritoneal macrophages cytostatic activity

| | Time after application of inflammation stimulus | | | | |
	1 H	1 D	2 D	3 D	5 D
Percent inhibition (3 H – TDR incorporation into tumor cells	38	45	50	58	65

* Macrophages to tumor cells ratio was 20 : 1

4. DISCUSSION

It appears from the present work that an acute non immune inflammation was able to modulate tumor growth and metastasis development. According to the scheduled times between inflammation induction and tumor grafting, an enhancement or an inhibition of the metastatic process could be observed.

Moreover, at the same time, opposite results could be obtained according to the tumor model. In fact our models differed widely. a) by the nature of inoculum (cell suspensions or explants). b) by the histologic growth patterns and the metastatic kinetics (Lewis tumor is encapsulated while hemangiosarcoma tumor cells have a large direct access to bloodstream). c) by the nature and functional properties of tumor cells due to different ontogenesis. Additional comparative studies between the tumor models are needed to clarify these points, especially dealing with the capacity of the different tumors to release inflammatory mediators.

Moreover, individual variation of the animal response to the inflammatory stimulus could also explain, in some cases, the opposite effect of NIAI. Indeed in the model of artificial metastasis, we were able to individualize two subpopulations in similarly treated rats : one responding by an increase and the other one by a decrease in metastatic development.

We have observed that NIAI, in normal mice, stimulated macrophage mediated cytotoxicity for tumor cells but decreased NK cell activity. These results show that NIAI is able to modulate immune mechanisms which are known to play a role in tumor resistance. However we did not observe an increase in tumor cell killing in the lung 24 hours after i.v injection of tumor cells in inflamed animals. This suggests that activated macrophages could not exert their cytotoxic properties in vivo. We are presently testing this hypothesis by measuring, in vivo, the antitumoral activity of inflammatory macrophages mixed with tumor cells. On the other hand there is some evidence that mediators released during an inflammatory reaction could affect tumor development. For example bradikinin was shown by KOPPELMAN et al. (1978) to exert suppressive effect on tumor growth. Conversely VAN DEN BRENK et al. (1974) described that a tumor growth promoting factor is associated to acute inflammation. Prostaglandins were reported by LUPULESCU (1978) to be active in enhancing tumor growth but they also may act as modulators of immune functions (DROLLER et al. 1978).

In conclusion, the present work suggests that inflammation mediators and other host defense mechanisms may compete in determining the ultimate number of surviving tumor cells.

REFERENCES

Droller, M.J., Schneider, M.U. and Perlmann, P., 1978. A possible role of prostaglandins in the inhibition of natural and antibody-dependent cell mediated cytotoxicity against tumor cells. Cell Immunol., 39: 165-177.
Fauve, R.M. and Hevin, M.B., 1977. Inflammation et résistance antitumorale. Ann.
  Immunol. Inst. Pasteur, 128C: 923-928.
Fidler, I.J., 1970. Metastasis : quantitative analysis of distribution and fate
  of tumor emboli labeled with 125I-5-iodo-2'-deoxyuridine. J. Natl. Cancer Inst.,
  45: 775-782.
Giroud, J.P., Pelletier, M. and Girre, C., 1977. Pouvoir mitogène de sérums de
  rats porteurs d'une inflammation aiguë vis à vis de macrophages en culture.
  C.R. Acad. Sci. Paris, série D, 285: 1143-1145.
Herberman, R.B., Nunn, M.E. and Lavrin, D.H., 1975. Natural cytotoxic reactivity
  of mouse lymphoid cells against syngeneic and allogeneic tumors. I. Distribution of reactivity and specificity. Int. J. Cancer, 16: 216-229.
Kiger, N., Pelletier, M., Florentin, I., Mathé, G. and Giroud, J.P., 1978. Effects
  of an non specific acute inflammatory stimulus on a macrophage and antibody
  dependent cellular cytotoxicity. Eur. J. Rheumatol. Inflam., 1: 321-325.
Koppelman, L.E., Moore, T.C. and Porter, D.D., 1978. Increased plasma kallikrein
  activity and tumor growth suppression associated with intralesional bradykinin
  injection in hamsters. J. Pathol., 126: 1-10.
Lupulescu, A., 1978. Enhancement of carcinogenesis by prostaglandins. Nature,
  272: 634-636.
Nolibe, D., (in preparation) Tumeurs pulmonaires radioinduites chez le rat.
Poste, G., 1979. The tumoricidal properties of inflammatory tissue macrophages
  and multinucleate giant cells. An. J. Pathol., 96: 595-610.
Van Den Brenk, H.A., Stone, M. and Kelly, H., 1974. Promotion of growth of tumor cells in acutely inflamed tissues. Brit. J. Cancer, 30: 246-260

ENHANCEMENT OF PULMONARY METASTASES INDUCED IN MICE BY CYCLOPHOSPHAMIDE: ROLE OF THE IMMUNE SYSTEM

B. Malenica and L. Milas*

INTRODUCTION

Host factors, both local and systemic, play an important role in formation of tumor metastases. They can be modified to promote or to restrict metastasis formation. For example, local thoracic irradiation predisposes the lung to the development of metastases by tumor cells injected intravenously (iv) (Withers and Milas, 1973). Enhancement of tumor nodule formation in the lung can also be produced by pretreatment of animals with chemotherapeutic agents (Carmel and Brown, 1975; Peters and Mason, 1977; van Putten, et. al., 1975). One of the most potent agents in this respect is cyclophosphamide (CY), which increases formation of lung metastases by factors of up to 1000 (van Putten, et. al., 1975). Mechanisms that underly this phenomenon have not been established, and most authors agree that the effect is primarily nonimmunologic, resulting most likely from local damage of the lung that led to increased retention of tumor cells in that organ. Our studies on this subject revealed that destruction of lymphoid cells by CY greatly participate in the development of this phenomenon (Milas, et. al., 1979). This paper describes our major findings.

MATERIALS AND METHODS

Experiments were performed with a methylcholenthrene-induced fibrosarcoma (FSa), syngeneic to CBA mice. This tumor is weakly immunogenic (Malenica and Milas, 1979). To obtain tumor metastases in the lung, tumor cells were injected iv, and metastases were counted 14 days later. CY (Bosnalijek, Sarajevo, Yugoslavia) was given to mice intraperitoneally (ip) at a dose of 180 mg/kg body weight. Immunosuppression of mice was achieved by whole body irradiation (WBI) with 450 rad X-rays or by thymectomy, WBI and reconstitution with bone marrow (TIR procedure). Reconstitution of CY-treated mice was achieved by bone marrow and spleen cells transplanted iv. Immunization of mice was performed by injecting mice ip with 2×10^7 heavily irradiated (10000 rad) tumor cells one week prior to iv injection of viable tumor cells. Similarly, Corynebacterium parvum (CP) (Wellcome Research Laboratories, Beckenham, England), in the dose of 0.25 mg per mouse, was given ip one week prior to tumor cell injection. All of the above procedures are described in detail elsewhere (Milas and Mujagic, 1973;

*Present address: Department of Experimental Radiotherapy, The University of Texas System Cancer Center, M. D. Anderson Hospital and Tumor Institute, Houston, Texas, U.S.A.

Milas, et. al., 1974; Milas, et. al., 1979). Mann-Whitney U̲ test was used for statistical evaluation of results.

RESULTS

Effect of CY in immunosuppressed animals

Mice were exposed to 450 rad WBI and two days later to CY. One day after treatment with CY they were injected iv with 10^4 FSa cells. Given separately, both WBI and CY increased the number of lung metastases; CY was more effective in this respect (Fig. 1A). In addition, CY induced a further increase in the number of metastases in WBI mice. Fig. 1B shows that CY induced enhancement of lung colony formation equally well in normal and T-cell depleted mice.

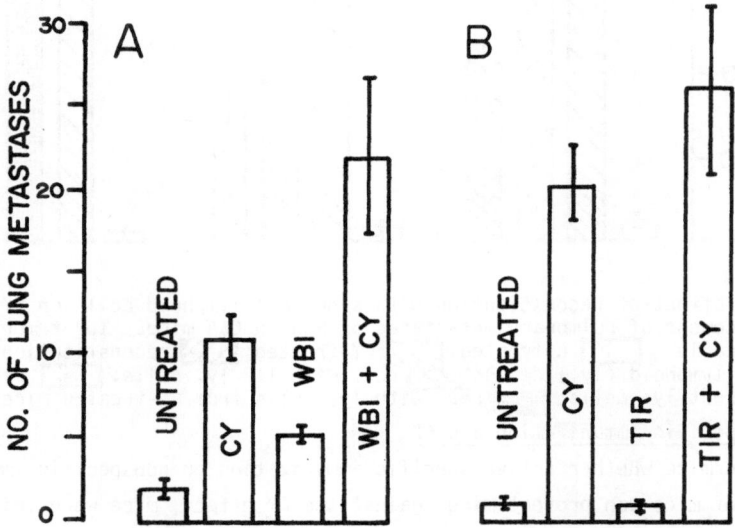

Fig. 1 The effect of CY on the number of artificial pulmonary metastases of FSa in WBI (A) and in T cell-deficient CBA mice (B). 10^4 tumor cells were injected iv.

Reconstitution with lymphoid cells

The effect of reconstitution with lymphoid cells was investigated in the following way. Mice were treated with CY, two days later injected iv with 10^8 spleen and bone marrow cells and one day after injection with lymphoid cells inoculated iv with 10^4 FSa cells. Lymphoid cells were from either normal or TIR mice. Fig. 2A shows that cells from normal mice abolished 44% and cells from TIR mice 63% of the CY activity. Results presented in Fig. 2B show that removal of adherent cells (macrophages) from the TIR lymphoid cell suspension did not alter the reconstituting capacity of such suspension. In contrast,

10^8 spleen cells derived from mice that had been treated with CY three days earlier were not capable of counteracting the effect of CY on metastases (Fig. 2C).

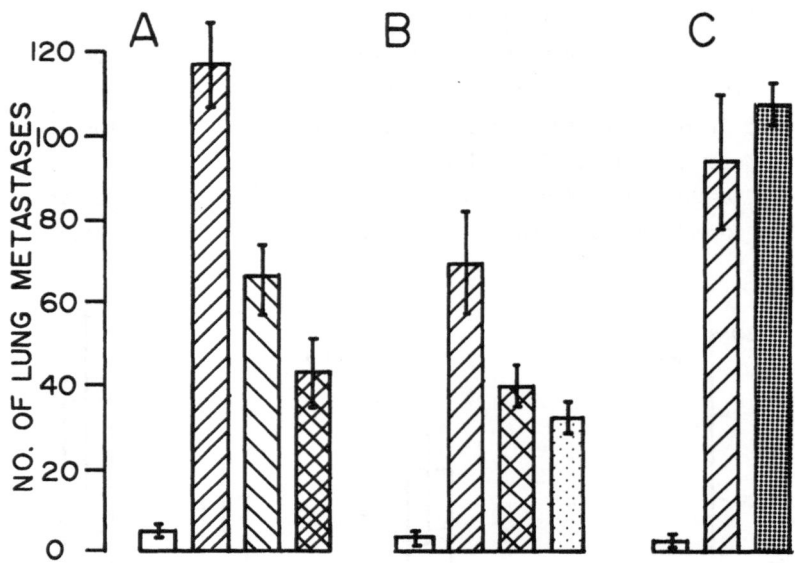

Fig. 2 The effect of reconstitution with syngeneic lymphoid cells on CY-induced enhancement of pulmonary metastases of FSa in CBA mice. 10^8 tumor cells were injected iv. ☐ untreated; ▨ CY-treated; ☒ reconstitution (rec.) with normal lymphoid (ly.) cells; ▧ rec. with TIR ly. cells; ▥ rec. with TIR nonadherent ly. cells; ▦ rec. with ly. cells from CY-treated mice.

Effect of specific immunization and CP

To determine whether active specific immunization or nonspecific immuno-modulation of mice can protect mice against the CY effect, mice were injected ip with 2×10^7 heavily irradiated FSa cells or treated with CP 6 days before treatment with CY. One day after CY treatment mice were injected iv with 10^5 FSa cells. Figure 3 shows that both treatments greatly reduced the effect of CY. CP was particularly effective. It reduced the number of metastases below that in untreated control mice.

DISCUSSION

Considerations that CY-induced enhancement of tumor nodule formation in the lung is a nonimmunological phenomenon were based on the following observations: CY promotes metastasis formation of nonimmunogenic tumors (Carmel and Brown, 1977; van Putten, et. al., 1975), it is effective in immunosuppressed animals (Carmel and Brown, 1977; Peters and Mason, 1977) and CY increases early retention of tumor cells in the lung (de Ruiter, et. al., 1976, Peters and

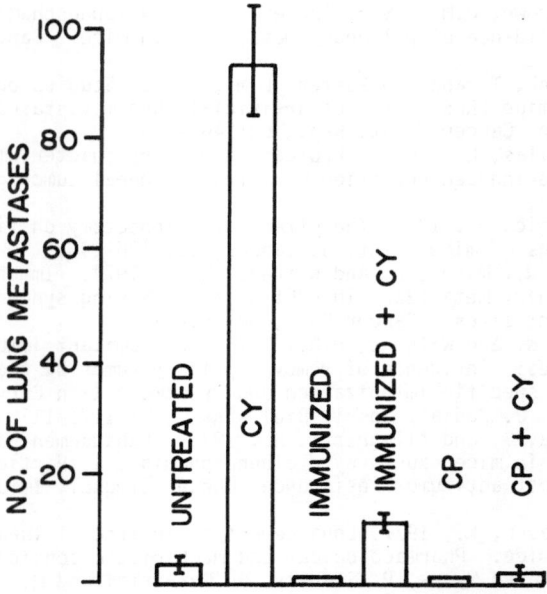

Fig. 3 The effect of active specific immunization and CP on the CY-induced enhancement of pulmonary metastases of FSa in CBA mice. 10^5 tumor cells were injected iv.

Mason, 1977). Our data on the effect of CY in WBI and TIR mice are in concordance with above considerations. However, ability of lymphoid cells from normal mice to reduce, upon transfer, the effect of CY by nearly 50%, implies that suppression of antitumor resistance plays a significant role in the CY-induced promotion of lung metastases. This is further supported by the inability of spleen cells from CY-treated mice to transfer antitumor resistance. Ability of lymphoid cells, unseparated or macrophage depleted, from TIR mice to confer such protection shows that CY did not act through the elimination of T-lymphocytes or macrophages but rather through the elimination of non- T-lymphocytes. At present we have no evidence whether cells eliminated by CY are conventional B-cells or other non- T-lymphocytes. Findings that specific immunization reduced the effect of CY to a great extent and that treatment of mice with CP abolished it entirely are examples of further evidence that CY acted through a suppression of the immune system. Still about 50% of the CY effect can be attributed to non-immunological factors, most likely to the damage afflicted directly to the lung tissue.

REFERENCES

Carmel, J.R. and Brown, J.M., 1977. The effect of cyclophosphamide and other drugs on the incidence of pulmonary metastases in mice. Cancer Res., 37: 145-151.

de Ruiter, J., Smink, T. and van Putten, L.M., 1976. Studies on the enhancement by cyclophosphamide (NCS-26271) of artificial lung metastases after labeled cell inoculation. Cancer Treat. Rep., 60: 465-470.

Malenica, B. and Milas, L., 1979. Protection by Corynebacterium parvum against cyclophosphamide-induced promotion of intraperitoneal tumor growth. Period. Biol., 81: 15-18.

Milas, L. and Mujagić, H., 1973. The effect of splenectomy on fibrosarcoma metastases in lungs of mice. Int. J. Cancer, 11: 186-190.

Milas, L., Hunter, N., Mason, K. and Withers, H.R., 1974. Immunologic resistance to pulmonary metastases in C3Hf/Bu mice bearing syngeneic fibrosarcoma of different sizes. Cancer Res., 34: 61-71.

Milas, L., Hunter, N. and Withers, H.R., 1976. Concomitant immunity to pulmonary metastases: Influence of removal primary tumor by radiation or surgery, of active specific immunization and treatment with Corynebacterium granulosum. Int. J. Radiat. Oncol. Biol. Phys., 1: 1171-1176.

Milas, L., Malenica, B. and Allegretti, N., 1979. Enhancement of artificial lung metastases in mice caused by cyclophosphamide. I. Participation of impairment of host antitumor resistance. Cancer Immunol. Immunother., 6: 191-196.

Peters, L.J. and Mason, K., 1977. Enhancement of artificial lung metastases by cyclophosphamide: Pharmacological and mechanistic consideration. In: S.B. Day, W.P. Laird Myers, P. Stansly, S. Garattini and M.G. Lewis (Editors) Cancer invasion and metastasis: Biologic mechanisms and therapy. Raven Press, New York, pp. 397-410.

van Putten, L.M., Kram, L.K.J., van Dierendenck, H.H.C., Smink, T. and Fuzy, M., 1975. Enhancement by drugs of metastatic lung nodule formation after intravenous tumor cell injection. Int. J. Cancer, 15: 588-595.

Withers, H.R. and Milas, L., 1973. Influence of preirradiation of lung on development of artificial pulmonary metastases in mice. Cancer Res., 33: 1931-1936.

ANTIMETASTATIC EFFECTS OF INTRAPLEURALLY INJECTED CORYNEBACTERIUM PARVUM

I. Basic, B. Malenica, D. Eljuga and L. Milas

INTRODUCTION

Since McKneally et al. (1976) have reported encouraging results concerning intrapleural (ipl) administration of BCG to patients with resected lung cancer there has been a great interest in the ipl application of biological response modifiers such as BCG and Corynebacterium parvum (CP) in experimental (Baldwin and Pimm, 1978; Basic et al., 1979; Scott and Decker, 1978) and clinical studies (Ludwig Lung Cancer Study Group, 1978). It has been reported that these bacteria given ipl effectively suppress intrapleural or intrapulmonary growth of several tumors in experimental animals. Antimetastatic effects of ipl administered CP against spontaneous lung metastases of murine and rat tumors have also recently been described (Malenica et al., 1980). This paper summarizes our studies undertaken to define the antitumor efficacy of ipl administered CP in experimental murine tumors and the antitumor mechanism(s) engaged. The antitumor effects of ipl CP have been compared with those resulting from CP injected intravenously (iv).

MATERIALS AND METHODS

Male and female C3Hf/Bu and CBA inbred mice from our conventional colony were used. In all experiments mice were of the same sex and all animals were approximately 3 months old at the initiation of each experiment.

Three syngeneic murine tumors were used: C3Hf/Bu and CBA methylcholanthrene-induced fibrosarcoma (FSa), and CBA spontaneously developed mammary carcinoma (MCa). C3Hf/Bu FSa is fairly immunogenic, and CBA FSa and MCa are weakly immunogenic tumors. Tumor cell suspensions were prepared by the methods described elsewhere (Basic et al., 1979). The tumor nodules in the lung were produced by iv injection of 10^4 or 10^5 tumor cells suspended in 0.5ml Medium 199. Mice were killed 14 days after inoculation of FSa cells or 17 days after iv inoculation of MCa cells. Their lungs were removed, fixed in Bouin's solution, and the number of tumor nodules on their surface were counted. Subcutaneous (sc) tumors were generated by an injection of 5×10^5 viable tumor cells in 0.2 ml of Medium 199 inoculated into the sc tissue of the flank of mice.

Pleural cells were harvested at different time intervals after ipl or iv injection of 0.25 mg CP (lot CA 528B, Wellcome Research Laboratories, England)

and then resuspended in 0.5 ml Hanks' solution. Ipl administration of CP and collection of the cells from the pleural cavity of mice were performed as described elsewhere (Basic et al., 1979). To asses whether CP stimulation macrophages are involved in the in vivo antitumor resistance of ipl injected CP mice, animals were given an ipl injection of 0.5 mg carrageenan (Marine Coloids, Inc, Springfield, N.Y.). Corrageenan was disolved in Hanks' solution by heating to 100°C for 15 min in water bath.

The results were statistically evaluated by Student's t test; differences between groups were considered significant if the P value of comparison was 0.05 or smaller.

RESULTS
Effect against tumor deposits in the lung

C3Hf/Bu and CBA mice were inoculated iv with syngeneic 10^5 FSa and 10^4 MCa cells, respectively, and 2 or 7 days thereafter they were given 0.25 mg CP ipl or iv. Results presented in Fig. 1 show that ipl administration greatly reduced the number of FSa nodules in the lung, and the effect was more pronounced than that produced by iv CP. However, reduction of MCa metastases was observed only

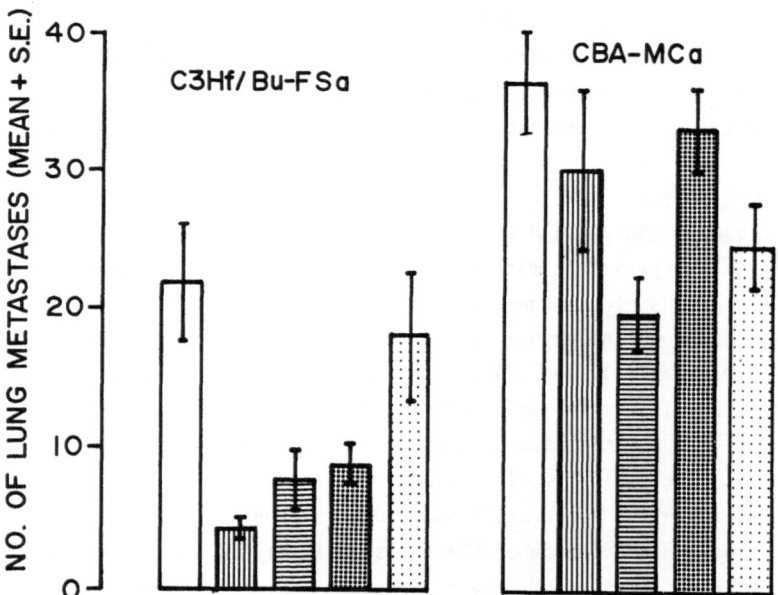

Fig. 1. Effect of ipl and iv injection of 0.25 mg CP against C3Hf/Bu FSa or CBA MCa tumor nodules in the lung by iv injection of 10^5 C3Hf/Bu FSa or 10^4 CBA MCa cells. CP was given 7 days after tumor cell inoculation. ☐ untreated; ▥ CP ipl on day 2; ▤ CP ipl on day 7; ▦ CP iv on day 2; ⬚ CP iv on day 7.

in mice that received CP 7 days after tumor cell inoculation. Again, ipl route
of injection was more efficient. Multiple injections of CP were more effective
than single injection (Basic et al., 1979).

Effect against sc tumor growth

C3Hf/Bu mice were injected sc with 5×10^5 syngeneic FSa cells, and 3 days
later ipl or iv with CP (Table 1). All untreated and treated animals developed
tumors. However, in contrast to the progressive growth of tumors in untreated
mice, 69% and 28% of tumors underwent complete regression if mice received CP
iv and ipl, respectively.

TABLE 1

Effect of ipl and iv injection of CP against sc growth
of FSa in C3Hf/Bu mice[a]

| Treatment[b] | Tumor take | | % of tumors rejected |
	Initial	Final	
None	17/17	17/17	0
CP ipl	18/18	13/18	28
CP iv	13/13	4/13	69

[a]Data from Basic et al., 1979.
[b]Mice received 0.25 mg CP 3 days after sc injection of 5×10^5 tumor cells.

Effect of iv injected tumor cells on pleural macrophages in mice treated with CP

Ipl injection of CP causes a significant increase in the number of macrophages in the pleural cavity of CBA mice (Table 2). To investigate whether an
iv or sc injection of tumor cells influences the number of macrophages in the
pleural cavity, CBA mice were given ipl injection of CP one day before they received 2×10^6 CBA FSa cell iv or sc. Already at one day after iv tumor cell
injection the number of macrophages in the pleural cavity decreased significantly.
This decrease was especially pronounced at the third day after tumor cell inoculation; the number of macrophages in the pleural cavity of mice that received iv
injection of tumor cells was still higher than that in mice receiving no CP.
Seven days after tumor cell inoculation the number of macrophages in the pleural
cavity was similar to that in mice that received CP only. Sc growing tumor,
however, did not influence the number of pleural macrophages.

Abolition of antitumor activity of ipl CP by carrageenan

To evaluate whether CP-stimulated macrophages were responsible for the
in vivo antitumor resistance CBA mice received iv 10^4 CBA MCa cells. Seven
days thereafter, they received 0.25 mg CP ipl. One day after CP injection mice

TABLE 2

Effect of an iv injection of CBA FSa cells on the number
of macrophages in the pleural cavity of CBA mice treated ipl with CP

Treatment	No of macrophages (Mean ± S.E. x 10^6) at days after CP treatment			
	1	2	4	8
None	1.2±0.3			
CP[a]	5.3±0.6	5.3±0.5	6.0±0.4	2.8±0.3
CP and TCiv[b]		3.4±0.7	1.9±0.6	3.4±0.1
CP and TCsc[b]		5.6±0.4	5.9±0.7	3.1±0.2

[a]Mice received 0.25 mg CP ipl one day before tumor cells inoculation. Groups contained 9 - 10 mice each.

[b]2×10^6 tumor cells.

received an ipl injection of 0.5 mg carrageenan, a specific macrophage poison, dissolved in 0.5 ml Hanks' solution. Table 3 shows that carrageenan entirely abrogated the effect of CP on the growth of tumor nodules in the lung. Furthermore, mice that were treated ipl with CP survived significantly longer than untreated mice. Treatment of mice with carrageenan, however, completely abolished this effect of CP.

TABLE 3

Abrogation by carrageenan of effects of ipl CP on the number of
tumor nodules in the lung and survival of CBA mice injected iv
with 10^4 CBA MC cells

Treatment[a]	Lung nodules		Survival	
	Mean per lung±SE	Range	Mean survival time (days)±SE	survivors/ total mice
None	15.3±1.6	5-27	19.2±0.3[b]	0/10
CP ipl on day 7	3.1±0.9[b]	0-7	27.9±1.2[b]	2/9
CP ipl on day 7+C[c]	17.8±1.4	11-26	18.8±1.0	0/14

[a]Mice received 0.25 mg CP. Groups contained 8-11 mice each.

[b]$p<0.001$; t-test.

[c]Carrageenan (0.5 mg/kg) was given 24 hours following treatment with CP.

DISCUSSION

Our results demonstrate that ipl application of CP can reduce the number of tumor nodules generated in the lung of C3Hf/Bu and CBA mice by iv injection of corresponding syngeneic FSa or MCa cells. The effect was more pronounced against fairly immunogenic C3Hf/Bu FSa than against poorly immunogenic CBA MCa.

If compared with the iv route of administration, ipl treatment appears to be more effective

In contrast to the more pronounced activity against tumor deposits in the lung, ipl CP was less effective in inducing complete regressions of sc tumors than iv CP. This suggests that antitumor effects of the ipl CP are mainly confined to the thoracic area. Findings of our previous studies (Basic et al., 1979) along with the present investigation lead to this conclusion. Ipl administration of CP induces accumulation of macrophages in the pleural cavity and increases the lung weight (Basic et al., 1979; Table 2) more so than iv CP. However systemic effects of ipl CP, as determined by the stimulation of the reticuloendothelial system, are small (Basic et al., 1979). Results presented in Table 2 also indicate that iv, but not sc, inoculation of tumor cells that followed ipl treatment with CP reduced accumulation of macrophages in the pleural cavity. Although the reasons for this are as yet uncertain, it is probably that CP-activated macrophages, in order to cope with tumor cells, left the pleural cavity and migrated into the lung in which iv injected tumor cells became arrested. Dominant role of activated macrophages in the activity against tumor deposits in the lung produced by ipl CP is well established by our previous findings that pleural macrophages from ipl injected mice exhibit strong in vitro destruction of tumor cells (Basic et al., 1979) and by present observation (Table 3) that the in vivo effect of ipl CP can be entirely abolished by treatment of mice with carrageenan.

To conclude, ipl administration of CP is effective against murine tumor deposits in the lung. The effect seems to be limited mainly to the thoracic area, and is mediated by activated macrophages. Ipl administration of biological response modifiers may, therefore, appear to be an efficient way of immunotherapeutic treatment of patients bearing malignant tumors in the lung.

REFERENCES

Baldwin, T.W. and Pimm, M.V., 1978. BCG in tumor immunotherapy. Adv. Cancer Res., 28: 91-147.
Basic, I., Malenica, B. Vujicic, N., and Milas, L., 1979. Antitumor activity of Corynebacterium parvum administered into the pleural cavity of mice. Cancer Immunol. Immunother. 7: 107-115.
Ludwig Lung Cancer Study Group, 1978: Search for the possible role of "immunotherapy" in operable bronchial non-small cell carcinoma (stage I and II): A phase I study with Corynebacterium parvum intrapleurally. Cancer Immunol. Immunother. 4: 69-75.
McKneally, M.F., Maver, C., Kausel, H.W., 1976. Regional immunotherapy of lung cancer with intrapleural BCG. Lancet 1: 377-379.
Malenica, B., Basic, I. and Milas, L., 1980. Effect of intrapleurally administered Corynebacterium parvum on spontaneous pulmonary metastases. Period. Biol., In press.
Scott, M.T., Decker, J., 1978. The distribution and effects of intrapleural Corynebacterium parvum. Cancer Immunol. Immunother. 5: 85-91.

DOES C. PARVUM TREATMENT AFFECT TUMOUR BLOOD FLOW AND HENCE METASTASIS?

P.D.E. Jones and R.T. Mathie

ABSTRACT

The blood flow of the Lewis lung carcinoma was determined at 7,10,12 and 14 days after its subcutaneous implantation in C57Bl mice, from the rate of clearance of an intratumour injection of ^{133}Xe dissolved in saline. Tumour tissue perfusion (ml/100g/min) was reduced by day 10 in mice receiving C.parvum (466ug) intravenously on day 0 or 7. Tumour growth was impaired after C.parvum treatment; consequently the reduction in total tumour blood flow (ml/min) was even more dramatic. Most of the observed inhibition of metastasis after C.parvum given on day 0 could be explained by the reduced volume of blood flowing through tumour tissue during the period of 7 to 14 days; however the inhibition of metastasis after C.parvum given on day 7 could not be explained in this way.

INTRODUCTION

The retardation of tumour development in experimental animals after systemic administration of Corynebacterium parvum is generally attributed to increased macrophage activity (Milas and Scott, 1978). However, C.parvum also causes a sustained disseminated intravascular coagulation (Lampert et al., 1977). A reduced blood flow to body and tumour tissues might therefore be expected, with a consequent decrease in metastases.

MATERIALS AND METHODS

Mice. Age-matched adult, female C57Bl/10ScSn mice (OLAC Southern Ltd.) were randomised into groups of 8.

Tumour. The Lewis lung carcinoma, which originated spontaneously in the lung of a female C57Bl mouse in 1951 (Sugiura and Stock, 1955) was implanted subcutaneously (s.c.) as a 0.1ml homogenate in the lower flank. Tumour size was determined thrice weekly from the mean of 2 diameters measured at right angles. Tumour mass was estimated from the same tumour diameters (mm):

Tumour mass in mg (assuming unit density) = length x (width)^2/2

which is the equation for the volume of a prolate ellipsoid with the short axes equal, if π is approximated to 3.

The tumour, when implanted s.c., metastasises to the lungs (Simpson-Herren et al., 1974). Macroscopic surface lung metastases were counted 21 days after tumour implantation, after staining the lungs with Indian ink and fixation in

Fekete's solution (Wexler, 1966). All tumours in the study arose from the same tumour homogenate preparation. The diameters and blood flow of the occasional tumour which ulcerated were not recorded.

Blood flow measurements. Tumour tissue perfusion was determined on days 7, 10, 12 and 14 after tumour implantation from the rate of clearance of intra-tumour injections of ^{133}Xe dissolved in 30 ul of normal saline (Kallman et al., 1972) in unanaesthetised but restrained mice. Radioactivity was detected with a lead-collimated $\frac{1}{2}$ inch sodium iodide crystal and photomultiplier connected to a pulse height analyser and ratemeter (Nuclear Enterprises SR 5) and linear chart recorder (Smiths RE 511.210).

$$\text{Tumour tissue perfusion (ml/100g/min)} = (\ln 2.100.\lambda)/T_{\frac{1}{2}}$$

where λ (=0.891; Kallman et al., 1972) is the partition coefficient for Xenon between tumour tissue and blood. The $T_{\frac{1}{2}}$ was determined from the logarithmic plot of the clearance curve obtained from each injection, and is the time (in minutes) for the measured activity to decrease to half its value. After an initial rapid decay, most of the curves showed a subsequent monoexponential clearance whose $T_{\frac{1}{2}}$ could be assessed for flow calculation. However, about 20% of the curves showed no initial component, and were monoexponential throughout the detection period of 20 minutes.

The total tumour blood flow was estimated from:

$$\text{Total tumour blood flow (ml/min)} = \text{tumour tissue perfusion} \times \text{tumour mass}$$

For each individual tumour, the area under the curve of total tumour blood flow against time after tumour implantation was used to estimate its total blood flow for days 7 to 14.

RESULTS

Tumour tissue perfusion was reduced after treatment with C.parvum, and was lowest, between days 7 and 14, in mice treated at the time of tumour implantation (Fig. 1). Tumour growth was also impaired after C.parvum treatment. Up to day 17, mice treated on day 0 had smaller tumours than those treated on day 7, but by day 21 the position was reversed. The act of measuring tumour tissue perfusion did not significantly affect either tumour growth or the antitumour action of C.parvum (Fig. 2). Total tumour blood flow was similarly reduced after treatment and lowest in mice treated on day 0 (Fig. 3).

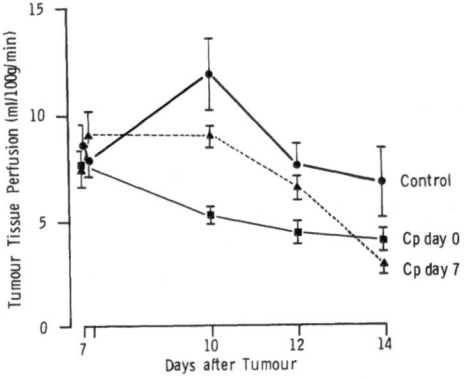

Fig. 1 Effect of C.parvum on
tumour tissue perfusion.
(Mean $\pm$ standard error)

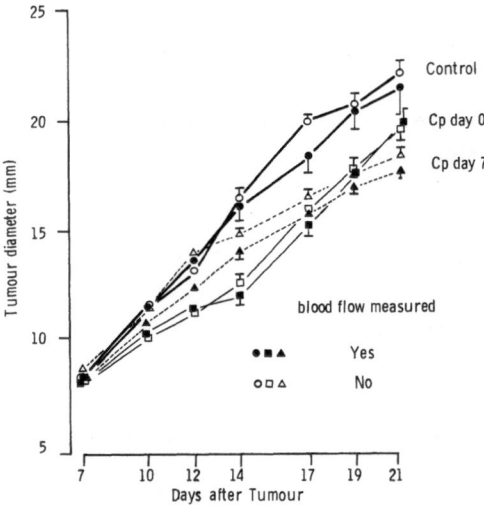

Fig. 2 Effect of C.parvum and
blood flow measurements on
tumour growth.
(Mean $\pm$ standard error)

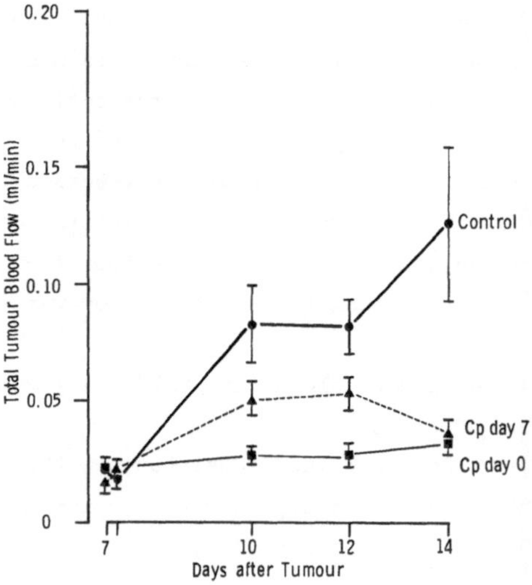

Fig. 3 Effect of C.parvum on
total tumour blood flow.
(Mean $\pm$ standard error)

The effect of C.parvum and blood flow measurements on metastasis is shown
in Table 1. C.parvum inhibited metastasis and least metastases were found in
mice treated on day 7. Blood flow measurements caused a small but significant
($p < 0.05$; 2 way analysis of variance) increase in metastasis but did not affect
the antimetastatic action of C.parvum.

The relationship between total tumour blood flow for the period of
7 to 14 days and metastasis is shown in Fig. 4. Mice treated with C.parvum
on day 0 showed the same direct relationship between tumour blood flcw and
metastasis, as the controls. This relationship was not apparent in those
treated on day 7. The ratio of the number of metastases to the total tumour
blood flow for days 7 to 14 was similar for the control and C.parvum day 0
treated mice, but was significantly (p<0.01; Student's t test) less in those
treated on day 7 (Table 2).

TABLE 1.

Effect of C.parvum and blood flow measurement on metastasis.

| Treatment | Number of Metastases (mean ± S.E.) | |
	Blood Flow Measured.	Blood Flow Not Measured.
Control	26.2 ± 6.1	17.3 ± 2.6
C.parvum day 0	11.3 ± 1.9*	6.7 ± 1.3*
C.parvum day 7	3.3 ± 0.7*	2.6 ± 1.1*

*Significance by Student's t test p<0.05.

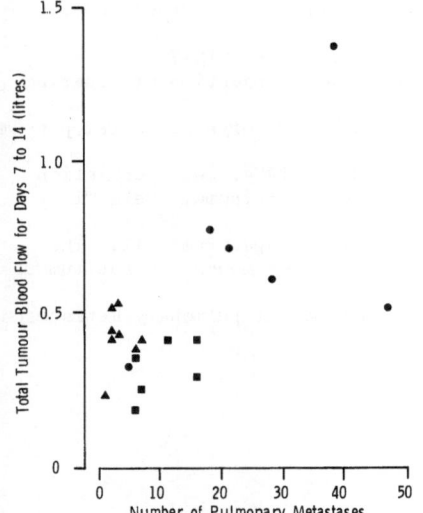

Fig. 4 Relationship between
total tumour blood flow for
days 7 to 14 and number of
pulmonary metastases.
● Control; ■ C.parvum day 0;
▲ C.parvum day 7.

TABLE 2.

Ratio of number of metastases
to total tumour blood flow
for days 7 to 14.

Treatment	Metastases per litre blood flow (Mean ± S.E.)
Control	39.1 ± 11.4
C.parvum day 0	33.2 ± 5.3
C.parvum day 7	7.9 ± 1.9*

*Significance by Student's t test
p<0.01

DISCUSSION

C.parvum treatment caused a reduction in tumour tissue perfusion, probably as a consequence of the sustained disseminated intravascular coagulation (Lampert et al., 1977) and also inhibited tumour growth. The combined effect was a marked reduction in total tumour blood flow.

Most of the metastases countable at day 21 arose from cells released from the primary tumour between days 7 and 14 (unpublished). Metastasis is likely to be dependent upon the total tumour blood flow, and indeed a direct relationship between total tumour blood flow for days 7 to 14 and numbers of pulmonary metastases was seen in control mice and those treated with C.parvum on day 0. Moreover, the ratio of metastases to total tumour blood flow was similar in these two groups, suggesting that the inhibition of metastasis after C.parvum treatment on day 0 is mainly due to the effects of C.parvum on blood flow. However, mice treated on day 7 had the fewest metastases and did not show any relationship between blood flow and metastases, suggesting that in this regimen another factor must be involved.

REFERENCES

Kallman, R.F., DeNardo, G.L. and Stasch, M.J., 1972. Blood flow in irradiated mouse sarcoma as determined by the clearance of Xenon-133. Cancer Res., 32: 483.
Lampert, I.A., Jones, P.D.E., Sadler, T.E. and Castro, J.E., 1977. Intravascular coagulation resulting from intravenous injection of C.parvum in mice. Br. J. Cancer, 36: 15.
Milas, L. and Scott, M.T., 1978. Antitumour activity of Corynebacterium parvum. Adv. Cancer Res., 26: 257.
Simpson—Herren, L., Sanford, A.H. and Holmquist, J.P., 1974. Cell population kinetics of transplanted and metastatic Lewis lung carcinoma. Cell Tiss. Kinet., 7: 349.
Sugiura, K. and Stock, C.C., 1955. Studies in a tumour spectrum: III. The effect of phosphoramides on the growth of a variety of mouse and rat tumours. Cancer Res., 15: 38.
Wexler, H., 1966. Accurate identification of experimental pulmonary metastases. J. Natn. Cancer Inst., 36: 641.

RETICULOENDOTHELIAL SYSTEM FUNCTION IN CANCER PATIENTS TREATED WITH C. PARVUM

H.D. Mitcheson, Adele Nicolas, N. Bowley and J.E. Castro

INTRODUCTION:

The anti-tumour effect of C. parvum (C.p.) in rodents is generally regarded as being mediated by non-specific activation of macrophages (reviewed by Milas and Scott, 1978). The phagocytic index in mice is increased and massive hepatosplenomegaly occurs (Halpern et al, 1963; Adlam and Scott, 1973). Numerous phase II clinical studies of C.p., evaluating its efficacy in specific malignant diseases, are currently in progress but few have reported on the mechanisms of resistance to tumour growth. We have measured the reticuloendothelial system (RES) function of patients entered in a prospective randomised study of C.p. treatment for inoperable bronchial carcinoma.

PATIENTS AND METHODS:

Patients: 15 patients with inoperable bronchial carcinoma were studied. 8 had squamous cell, 3 oat cell and 4 carcinomas of other types. All 15 patients received radiotherapy. 3 had no other treatment and acted as controls; 12 after giving informed consent were additionally treated with C.p. (Wellcome strain CN 6134, 7 mg dry wt/ml) given at a dose of $10mg/m^2$ by intravenous infusion at monthly intervals to a planned total of 4 infusions for each patient. Patients were examined and venous blood samples taken immediately before, 1h., 24h., 3, 7 and 14 days after each infusion. 10 patients had clearance studies with autologous heat-damaged erythrocytes, 4 with sulphur-colloid, and 1 had both. Liver and spleen volumes were measured in 9. 3 patients had clearance studies and organ volume measurements immediately before and 3, 7 and 14 days after the first infusion; 6 others were studied immediately before and after 14 days. 8 healthy volunteers acted as controls.

Clearance Studies with radiolabelled autologous heat-damaged erythrocytes: A modified version of the method of Bowring et al, (1976), was used. Blood (10 ml) was collected into heparin and the samples centrifuged at 1500g for 5 minutes. The packed red blood cells were then heat-damaged at $49.5^{\circ}C$ for exactly 20 minutes and, after washing, labelled with 1 mCi ^{99m}Tc. A freshly prepared 1% solution of stannous chloride was then added and the mixture allowed to stand for 5 minutes. The cells were then washed twice in NaCl 9 g/l, resuspended with an equal volume of saline, and injected. Blood samples were taken at 3,8,13,18 and 23 minutes and the radioactivity per unit volume of whole blood subsequently measured. Results were plotted on semi-log paper and the time taken to clear half of the cells from the circulation (T/2) calculated.

Clearance studies with sulphur-colloid: Similarly the T/2 was calculated for sulphur-colloid labelled with 1 mCi ^{99m}Tc.

Quantitative scanning: The activity of the ^{99m}Tc - labelled heat-damaged erythrocytes or sulphur-colloid was measured before injection together with a standard of similar activity and volume.   The residue after injection was also recorded together with the same standard.   The patient was seated back to a large field-of-view gamma camera which viewed the lungs, liver and spleen. Data were recorded onto magnetic tape and serial polaroid photographs of the distribution produced.   A whole body quantitative scan was performed after 1h. Uptake and clearance curves were obtained of the areas of interest.

Ultrasonic determination of liver and spleen volumes: These were measured as described (Kardel et al, 1971).

Circulating immune complexes (CIC):   The Clq-binding assay for detecting CIC was performed as described (Pussell et al, 1978).

Haptoglobins were measured as described (Palmer and Schueler, 1976).

RESULTS

Heat-damaged erythrocytes studies:
11 patients had heat-damaged erythrocyte clearance studies before treatment (Fig.1.).   The T/2 clearance was normal in 4 (8-14 minutes), slightly delayed in 2 and considerably delayed in 5.   8 of the 11 had impaired splenic uptake (normal range > 50% of the injected dose 1h. after injection).   1 patient had normal splenic uptake at 1 hour despite having a delayed clearance.

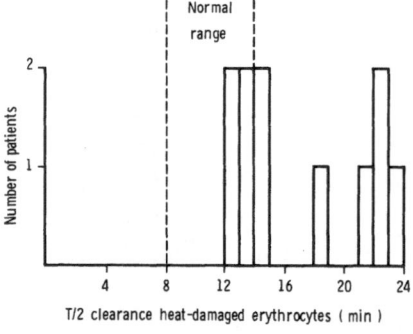

Fig. 1

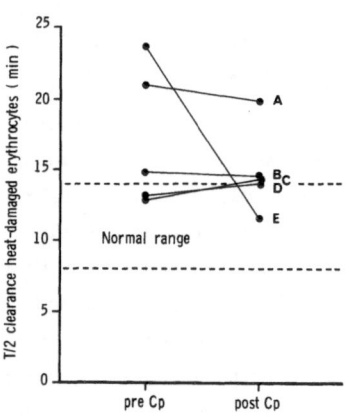

Fig. 2

clinical studies of C.p. evaluating its efficacy in specific malignant diseases are currently in progress but there are few reports of its effects on the mechanisms of resistance to tumour growth.   Increase in spleen size has been reported (Morahan et al, 1977), and Attie (1975) investigated phagocytic activity in a small number of patients treated with BCG, C.p. poly IC and cortisone but his results were inconclusive.   This paucity of information applies to many methods of RES stimulation that have been recommended or attempted in cancer patients (Magarey and Baum, 1970).

We found that 10 of 15 lung cancer patients had impaired RES function.   Of the 11 patients who had RES function determined by heat-damaged erythrocyte studies, 7 had delayed clearance and 8 had impaired splenic uptake.   4 others were given sulphur-colloid and 2 had delayed clearance.   CIC were detected in 4 of the 9 with prolonged clearance times and in 2 of the 6 with normal clearances.

C.p. treatment did not significantly affect the clearance or organ uptake of either heat-damaged erythrocytes or sulphur-colloid.   Hepatosplenomegaly did not occur.   CIC and haptoglobins were not altered.   The discrepancy between the effect of C.p. on the RES of rodents and its lack of effect in man may be because the usual rodent dose (related to surface area) is much greater than the human dose (Mitcheson et al, 1980).   We conclude that intravenous C.p. treatment does not affect the impaired RES function of lung cancer patients.

REFERENCES

Adlam, C. and Scott, M.T., 1973.
Lymphoreticular stimulatory properties of Corynebacterium parvum and related bacteria.
J. Med. Microbiol. 6,261.

Attie, E., 1975.
Action of Corynebacterium parvum on the phagocytic activity of the reticuloendothelial system in cancer patients.
In: Corynebacterium parvum.   Applications in experimental and clinical oncology.
Ed. by B. Halpern, New York. Plenum Press, p.341.

Blamey, R.W., 1968.
Experiments in tumour immunology.
Br. J. Surg. 55, 769.

Bowring, C.S., Glass, H.I. and Lewis, S.M., 1976.
Rates of clearance by the spleen of heat-damaged erythrocytes.
Journal of Clinical Pathology, 29, 852.

Halpern, B.N., Biozzi, G., Stiffel, C and Mouton, D., 1966.
Inhibition of tumour growth by administration of heat-killed Corynebacterium parvum.
Nature, London, 212, 853.

Halpern, B.n., Prevot, A.R., Biozzi, G., Stiffel, C., Mouton, D., Morard, J.C., Bouthillier, Y. and Decreusefond, C., 1963.
Stimulation de l'activite phagocytaire du systeme reticuloendothelial provoquee par Corynebacterium parvum.
J. Reticuloendoth. Soc., 1,77.

302

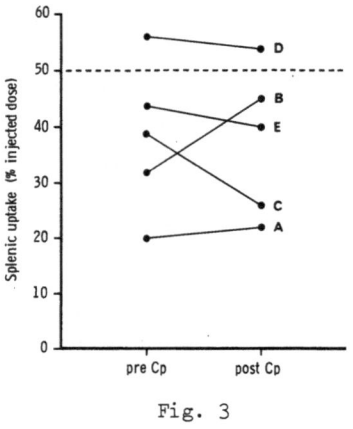

Fig. 3

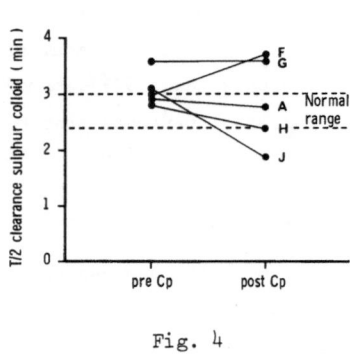

Fig. 4

5 patients were studied before and 14 days after the first C.p. infusion
(Figs. 2 and 3).   Patient E's grossly prolonged clearance before treatment
became normal but his splenic uptake remained impaired.   C.p. did not
significantly alter either the clearance rate or splenic uptake.   Liver and
lung uptakes were unchanged.

Sulphur-colloid studies:
5 patients were studied before and 14 days after the first C.p. infusion.   The
T/2 clearance (Fig.4) and organ uptakes were not significantly altered.

Liver and spleen volumes: All patients had normal liver volume (median = 437 ml
range 310-578 ml) and spleen volume (median = 80 ml, range 54-163 ml) and these
were not altered by C.p.

Circulating immune complexes:
CIC were detected in 4 of the 9 patients who had prolonged clearance times of
heat damaged erythrocytes or sulphur-colloid and in 2 of the 6 who had normal
clearance times.   C.p. treatment did not affect CIC.

Haptoglobins:
Serum haptoglobin levels were elevated in most patients, median = 412, range
114-944 mg/100 ml (normal range 30-190 mg/ml).   Levels were unaltered by C.p.

DISCUSSION
There is a strong correlation between resistance to tumours and RES function
as determined by phagocytic activity in laboratory animals and humans (Blamey
1968; Magarey and Baum, 1970).   C.p. inhibits the growth of a variety of primary
and metastatic rodent tumours (Halpern et al, 1966; Sadler and Castro, 1976)
and non-specific activation of macrophages is generally regarded as mediating
the anti-tumour effect (reviewed by Milas and Scott, 1978).   Numerous phase II

Kardel, T., Holm, H.H., Rasmussen, S.N. and Mortensen, T., 1971.
Ultrasonic determination of liver and spleen volumes.
Scand. J. clin. lab. Investig. 27, 123.

Magarey, C.J. and Baum, M., 1970.
Reticulo-endothelial activity in humans with cancer.
Br. J. Surg., 57, 10, 748.

Milas, L. and Scott, M.T., 1978.
Antitumour activity of Corynebacterium parvum.
Advances in Cancer Res., 26, 257.

Mitcheson, H.D., Sadler, T.E., and Castro, J.E., 1980.
Single versus multiple human equivalent doses of C. parvum in mice :
neutralisation of the anti-metastatic effect.
Br. J. Cancer, 1980.

Morahan, P.S., Glasgow, L.A., Crane, J.L. Jr. and Kern, E.R., 1977.
Comparison of antiviral and antitumour activity of activated macrophages.
Cell. Immunol. 28, 2, 404.

Palmer, W.G. and Schueler, R.L., 1976.
Association between macrophage activity and serum haptoglobin levels.
Biomedicine, 25, 88.

Pussell, B.A., Scott, D.M., Lockwood, C.M., Pinching, A.J. and Peters, D.K., 1978.
Value of immune-complex assays in diagnosis and management.
Lancet, 2, 359.

Sadler, T.E., and Castro, J.E., 1976.
Abrogation of the antimetastatic effect of Corynebacterium parvum by
antilymphocyte serum.
Br. J. Cancer, 34, 291.

INHIBITION OF PULMONARY METASTASIS OF LEWIS LUNG TUMOR BY NOCARDIA RUBRA-CELL WALL SKELETON OR SCHIZOPHYLLAN

E. Tsubura, T. Yamashita, K. Kagawa and T. Yamamoto

Tumor metastasis depends on the interaction of tumor cells with their host. This phenomenon is complex and affected by many host factors. The host immune defense mechanism, involving possible stimulation and/or inhibition of tumor growth (Vaage et al., 1971) and metastasis (Deodhar and Crile, 1969) is of great importance. Apparent facilitation of pulmonary metastases was recognized in immunologically impaired animals. Restoration of the immune competence of these animals by transfer of lymphoid cells or reimplantation of the thymus reduced metastases (Carnaud et al., 1974). Therefore, host manipulation may be useful in preventing the development of metastasis.

Immunotherapy with various agents which stimulate the lymphoid system, is being increasingly employed in the therapy of animal and human cancers. The inhibitory effect of Nocardia rubra-cell wall skeleton (N-CWS) or a glucan, Schizophyllan (SPG), on pulmonary metastases in syngeneic mice bearing Lewis lung tumor (3LL) was studied.

MATERIALS AND METHODS

Animals and Tumor: Male C57BL/6 mice of 6 to 8 weeks old, weighing 20 to 25g were used. 3LL has been maintained by serial biweekly subcutaneous passage in the same strain of mice. The tumor fragments were stirred in RPMI 1640 medium containing 0.2% trypsin at $37^{\circ}C$ for 30 min. The isolated tumor cells were washed twice, suspended in fresh RPMI 1640 medium and counted in a hemocytometer.

CWS of N. rubra: CWS prepared from N. rubra (Azuma et al,1974, a generous gift from 3rd Dept. of Int. Med., Osaka University, Osaka, Japan) was given to mice as a cholesterol-attached preparation disolved in saline.

Schizophyllan: Purified $\beta(1-3)$ glucan, SPG isolated from the culture filtrate of Schizophyllum commune Fries, is a saline soluble polysaccharide with a rather low molecular weight ($1-8 \times 10^4$Mw).

Assay of Pulmonary Metastases: Subcutaneous implantation of 5×10^5 to 10^6 3LL cells into foot pads of mice led to progressive growth of local tumor. When the primary tumor had become 5 to 6mm in diameter 9 to 10 days after tumor implantation, the tumor-bearing legs were amputated by the cautery clamp technique. Mice were autopsied 14 days after removal of primary tumors. Pulmonary metastases were estimated by counting the numbers of metastatic nodules on the pulmonary surface.

Assay of In Vitro Cytostatic Activities of Peritoneal or Lung Macrophages: The cytostatic activities of peritoneal or lung macrophages were tested by assay of terminal ^{3}H-thymidine labelled target cells which survived after interaction with effector cells (Schechter et al., 1976). Peritoneal macrophages were collected by washing the peritoneal cavity with RPMI 1640 medium and adhering the cells to glass plates. Lung macrophages were isolated following the method of Howard et al (1969). Mixtures of effector cells and 3LL cells were incubated at 37°C for 24 hr. in an atmosphere of 5% CO_2 in air. The percentage of cytostatic activity was calculated as follows;

$$\frac{\text{cpm in control group} - \text{cpm in test group}}{\text{cpm in control group}} \times 100$$

RESULTS

Inhibition of Pulmonary Metastases by N-CWS or SPG : As shown in Table 1, N-CWS or SPG was injected intravenously or intraperitoneally into mice after removal of primary tumors. In experiments examining various doses and times of injection, maximal inhibitory effects on pulmonary metastases were obtained at the dose of 2.5mg/kg of N-CWS or 20 mg/kg of SPG.

Combined Effect of N-CWS or SPG and Cyclophosphamide on Pulmonary Metastases: The effect of combined therapy with N-CWS or SPG and cyclophosphamide on pulmonary metastases was observed. As shown in Table 2, each treatment alone inhibited the development of pulmonary metastases and a combined therapeutic effect was also observed. The survival of mice bearing pulmonary metastases was prolonged by combined therapy, but not by N-CWS or SPG alone.

TABLE 1
Dose dependency on inhibition of pulmonary metastases by N-CWS or SPG

Tumor of 5x10⁵cells		Removal of primary tumor		Assay of pulm. metastases

N-CWS i.v.
SPG i.p.

Day 0   10   16   21

Exp. group	Dose (mg/kg)	No. of pulmonary surface nodules (mean ± S.E.)	Incidence of pulmonary metastases
Control		43.6 ± 6.1	10/10
N-CWS	0.5	35.8 ± 4.3	10/10
	2.5	15.1 ± 3.6 ($p<0.01$)	10/10
	10.0	28.1 ± 6.4 ($p<0.05$)	10/10
Control		21.2 ± 5.0	10/10
SPG	10.0	11.8 ± 3.0 ($p<0.05$)	9/10
	20.0	3.9 ± 1.4 ($p<0.01$)	7/10
	50.0	5.3 ± 1.2 ($p<0.01$)	9/10

TABLE 2
Combined effect of N-CWS or SPG and cyclophosphamide on pulmonary metastases

Exp. group	Dose N-CWS or SPG (mg/kg)	CY (mg/kg)	No. of pulmonary surface nodules (mean± S.E.)	Incidence of metastases	T/C (%)
Control			31.0 ± 5.0	9/9	100
N-CWS	2.5x3		18.1 ± 2.8 ($p<0.05$)	9/9	118
CY		50x1	4.8 ± 1.9 ($p<0.01$)	7/9	134 ($p<0.001$)
N-CWS + CY	2.5x3	50x1	1.9 ± 1.0 ($p<0.001$)	5/9	>184 ($p<0.001$)
Control			33.4 ± 5.6	10/10	100
SPG	20.0x7		5.1 ± 1.3 ($p<0.001$)	10/10	102
CY		50x1	4.8 ± 2.8 ($p<0.001$)	7/10	128 ($p<0.001$)
SPG + CY	20.0x7	50x1	1.2 ± 0.8 ($p<0.001$)	3/10	142 ($p<0.001$)

Inocula of 5 x 10⁵ cells were injected into foot pads of mice.
A daily dose of 2.5 mg/kg of N-CWS or 20 mg/kg of SPG was injected
intravenously or intraperitoneally 3 or 7 times after removal of
primary tumor, respectively. Significance of differences of values
from that of control by Student's t-test. T/C: Mean survival time
of treated mice (T) as a percentage of that of control mice (C).

In Vitro Cytostatic Activity of Peritoneal or Lung Macrophages:

The cytostatic activity of peritoneal or lung macrophages was examined against 3LL cells. Effector cells were harvested 5 days following intravenous or intraperitoneal injection of 5 mg/kg of N-CWS or 20 mg/kg of SPG, respectively. The cytostatic activity of peritoneal macrophages from N-CWS-treated mice was 53.0% (E/T 5:1), whereas that from untreated mice was 16.1%. That from SPG-treated mice was 78.3%, compared with 13.4% from untreated mice. The cytostatic activity of lung macrophages in mice treated with N-CWS was 56.4% (E/T 10:1), compared with -8.2% from untreated mice. On the other hand, the cytostatic activity in mice treated with SPG was 51.5%.

Inhibition of Pulmonary Metastases by Intravenous Transfer of Activated Peritoneal Macrophages:

Peritoneal macrophages activated by N-CWS or SPG as described above were transferred into mice after removal of primary tumors. As shown in Table 3, significant reduction of pulmonary metastatic nodules was observed in the mice inoculated with activated peritoneal macrophages.

TABLE 3
Inhibitory effect of transferred peritoneal macrophages activated with N-CWS or SPG on pulmonary metastases

Exp. group	No. of pulmonary surface nodules (mean ± S.E.)	Incidence cf pulmonary metastases
Control	25.9 ± 3.9	10/10
Normal peritoneal macrophages	21.9 ± 6.2	9/10
N-CWS-activated peritoneal macrophages	14.3 ± 3.4 ($p < 0.05$)	10/10
SPG-activated peritoneal macrophages	14.2 ± 3.5 ($p < 0.05$)	9/9

5×10^5 peritoneal macrophages were transferred into the mice with pulmonary metastases. Significance of differences of values from that of control by Student's t-test.

DISCUSSION

The inhibiting and prevention of cancer metastasis is one of the main problems of cancer research. It may be possible to inhibit micrometastasis although it is difficult to inhibit overt metastasis or primary tumor growth. There are several reports that metastasis can be inhibited by immunological modulation of

the host and we attempted to inhibit micrometastasis by such stimulation of the host.   We used Lewis lung tumor as a suitable
experimental model of spontaneous pulmonary micrometastases.   Based
on our previous experience, we found that pulmonary micrometastases
developed 5 days after tumor implantation into foot pads of C57BL/6
mice.   It is thought that our experimental model of pulmonary
metastases excluded influences of primary tumors on metastases by
removal of the local tumor, it suitable for investigating the effect
of host modulation on metastases.   We tested N-CWS and SPG as a
host modulator.   N-CWS is the effective component extraction from
Nocardia rubra.   Inhibitory effects on metastases by these substances greatly depended on the dose and time of their injection.
For instance, 3 injections of 2.5 mg/kg of N-CWS or 7 injections of
20 mg/kg of SPG significantly inhibited the development of pulmonary
metastases only when it was given after removal of primary tumors.
These results indicated that these substances inhibit the developmen
of micrometastases in the lung.

        We considered the possibility that macrophages were involved
in the antimetastatic activity of these substances.   Peritoneal or
lung macrophages activated by N-CWS or SPG showed cytostatic activit
against 3LL cells.   Intravenous transfer of activated peritoneal
macrophages played a role in the inhibition of pulmonary metastases
under some conditions.   However in the future we have to investigat
killer T cells and regulation of macrophage functions by lymphoid
cells which may be concerned in the inhibition of metastasis.
Combined therapy with an anticancer agent caused not only the inhibition of metastases but also the prolongation of survival.   These
results imply that our approaches might be useful for the inhibition
of micrometastases in clinical medicine.

SUMMARY

        N-CWS or SPG was found to have antimetastatic activity, which
depended on the dose and time of the injection of these substances.
Combined thereapy with these substances and cyclophosphamide
significantly prolonged the survival in mice with pulmonary metastases.   The cytostatic activity of peritoneal or lung macrophages

increased in mice treated with these substances.   Intravenous

transfer of peritoneal macrophages activated with these substances

inhibited the development of pulmonary metastases.

REFERENCES

Azuma, I., Ribi, E.E., Meyer, T.J. and Zbar, B., 1974. Biologically
active components from mycobacterial cell walls. I. Isolation
and composition of cell-wall skeleton and component P_3. J. Natl.
Cancer Inst., 52: 95-101.
Carnaud, C., Hoch, B. and Trainin, N., 1974. Influence of immunologic
competence of the host on metastases induced by the 3LL Lewis
tumor in mice. J. Natl. Cancer Inst., 52: 395-399.
Deodhar, S.D. and Crile, G., Jr., 1969. Enhancement of metastases
by antilymphocyte serum in allogeneic murine tumor system. Cancer
Res., 29: 776-779.
Howard, J.G., Christie, G.H., Boak, J.L. and Kinsky, R.G., 1969.
Peritoneal and alveolar macrophages derived from lymphocyte
populations during graft-versus-host reaction. Br. J. exp. Path.,
50: 448-455.
Schechter, B., Treves, A.J. and Feldman, M., 1976. Specific cytotoxicity in vitro of lymphocytes sensitized in culture against
tumor cells. J. Natl. Cancer Inst., 56: 975-979.
Vaage, J., Chen, K. and Merrick, S., 1971. Effect of immune status
on the development of artificially induced metastases in different
anatomical locations. Cancer Res., 31: 496-500.

MINIMAL RESIDUAL DISEASE MAY BE TREATED BY CHESSBOARD VACCINATION WITH VIBRIO CHOLERAE NEURAMINIDASE (VCN) AND TUMOR CELLSS

H.H. Sedlacek, H.J. Bengelsdorff, R. Kurrle and F.R. Seiler

SUMMARY

Vibrio cholerae neuraminidase (VCN) has been shown to have an adjuvant effect predominantly for the cellular immune response when admixed with a variety of antigens. On the basis of these findings, the therapeutic effect of specific immunotherapy with the use of VCN was evaluated on the growth of metastases of Lewis lung adenocarcinoma in C57Bl/6 mice. Tumor immunotherapy was performed after complete excision of the primary tumor graft and after an adapted chemotherapy (cyclophosphamide) by intradermal injection of increasing numbers of tumor cells (10^5 - 10^7) mixed with increasing amounts of VCN (0-65 mU). This procedure has already been described as "chessboard vaccination".

Such treatment reduced the number of animals that died due to metastasis. In contrast, subcutaneous injection of VCN-treated but subsequently washed tumor cells had no effect. In therapeutic studies in dogs suffering from spontaneous breast tumors, the s.c. injection of VCN-treated cells had, depending on the cell dose, either a therapeutical effect or no effect at all (low dose), or even an enhancing effect on tumor growth (high dose). With the chessboard vaccination procedure, however, a therapeutic effect could be seen which was not cell dose dependent. Thus, chessboard vaccination, which has less risk of inducing tumor enhancement, may be recommended for tumor immunotherapy.

INTRODUCTION

Specific tumor immunotherapy with VCN-treated cells has been tried in very different experimental tumors in mice, rats and dogs. The results which have been achieved up to now are controversial. Besides significant therapeutic effects, either no change of the tumor growth or even tumor enhancement could be found, and positive results could sometimes not be confirmed (review: Sedlacek and Seiler 1978 Subsequent experiments revealed that the number of VCN-treated cells injected into the tumor bearer is of the utmost importance for gaining the therapeutical effect (Wilson et al. 1974, Sedlacek et al. 1975). As the cell number which will be effective for the treatment of a tumor cannot be pre-evaluated by simple in vitro test systems, VCN-treated cells have to be blindly injected into the tumor bearer, that is, without knowing whether this treatment will harm the patient. Thus, the use of VCN-treated cells in tumor immunotherapy has to be considered as considerable risk for the patient.

As an alternative to the injection of VCN-treated cells, chessboard vaccination has been proposed and developed on the basis of cell membrane binding studies and immunizing experiments (Seiler and Sedlacek 1978). It had been shown in those experiments that after treatment of cells with VCN, enzymatically active VCN remains firmly attached to the cell surface membrane and it had been demonstrated that enzymatically active VCN is a strong adjuvant for cellular, bacterial, viral and protein antigens (reviewed in Sedlacek and Seiler 1978). This chessboard vaccination consists of intradermal injection into the tumor bearer of various cell numbers mixed with various amounts of VCN. Chessboard vaccination was first performed in mongrel dogs suffering from autochthonous mammary tumors. So far data in this tumor system has revealed that chessboard vaccination is more effective and there is a lower risk of it being ineffective or even enhancing tumor growth than the subcutaneous injection of VCN-treated cells (Sedlacek et al. 1979). Consequently, the specificity of chessboard vaccination is now being evaluated in a three-part random study in mongrel dogs with mammary tumors. Although the experiments in dogs are so far hopeful, it is still unclear whether chessboard vaccination is also effective in other experimental tumor systems. The data presented in this paper show that, under certain conditions, chessboard vaccination has an effect on the growth of spontaneous metastases in the Lewis lung adenocarcinoma of C56Bl/6 mice.

MATERIAL AND METHODS

Cell preparations

Red blood cells from sheep (SRBC) were isolated from heparinized fresh blood by at least 4 washings in PBS pH 7.2 and stored at 4°C for a maximum of 14 days.

The Lewis lung adenocarcinoma (LL) was maintained in syngeneic C56Bl/6 mice (De Fries, Denmark) as a subcutaneous tumor. For cell preparation, the primary tumor grafts were surgically excised and mechanically (scalpels) and enzymatically (collagenase, trypsin diluted in PBS pH 7.4) disintegrated (for details: Sedlacek et al. 1975). Cells from the supernatants were washed three times with PBS and incubated with mitomycin (100 µg/10^7 cells/ml, 60 min. 37°C). This treatment completely stopped the in vitro and in vivo growth of the LL cells.

After two washings the cells were treated with purified (Schick and Zilg 1978) VCN (Behringwerke AG, Marburg, FRG; 150 mU/5 x 10^7 cells/ml PBS containing 0.84 M $CaCl_2$ x $2H_2O$ pH 7.2; 30 min., 37°C) of very low toxicity and immunogenicity (Ronneberger 1978). The VCN preparation (1 ml) was proven to be free of endotoxins according to the European Pharmacopoeia (Ronneberger 1978). The enzymatic activity of 1 ml of this preparation is 5000 international milliunits (5000 mU = 5U). After a second washing, such treated cells were stored for a maximum of 6 h at 4°C without any demonstrable change of the various effects induced by VCN treatment (Seiler and Sedlacek 1974).

For chessboard vaccination various numbers of mitomycin-treated LL cells (0, 1 x 10^5, 1 x 10^6, 1 x 10^7) were resuspended in PBS, pH 7.2, supplemented with various amounts of VCN (0, 0.65, 6.5, or 65 mU) to give a final volume of about 0.1 ml. These mixtures were prepared within 30-60 min. before use, i.e. before intradermal injection of all the various combinations into one animal.

Treatment of the animals

The model according to Mackaness et al. (1974) using SPF outbred (NMRI, Wiga inbred (C57Bl/6, Bom) mice was applied to evaluate the immunosuppressive dosage o· cyclophosphamide (Asta, Bielefeld, FRG). On average, 10 mice per group were injec intravenously with different numbers of SRBC (10^3, 10^4, 10^5, 10^6, 10^7, 10^8, 10^9) (suspended in 0.1 ml PBS. Five days later, a challenge injection of 2 x 10^8 SRBC · 0.05 ml was given into a hind footpad. Footpads were measured before the challeng injection and 24 hours afterwards, using a dial gauge calliper. An increase in fc pad thickness was expressed as a percentage of the thickness before challenge. At clinical examination mice were killed by exsanguination. Serum was collected, hea inactivated and tested for hemagglutinating and hemolytic activity. The degree of the delayed-type hypersensitivity (DTH) and of the antibody reaction was compared that of those mice that had been treated with various doses of cyclophosphamide.

To assess the tumor therapeutic effect of tumor cells and VCN, 1 x 10^6 liv· LL cells were injected into the footpad of C57Bl/6 mice. The growth of the resul1 tumor nodule was measured daily with a dial gauge calliper. When the tumor size I reached about 6.5 mm in diameter, 8(6-10) days after tumor cell transplantation, 1 tumor-bearing limb, together with the lymphonodus popliteus, was amputated in anas thesia. At this time, no metastases could be found microscopically. Under these conc tions all the animals died as a result of metastases about 23 days after amputation Metastases were predominantly located in the lung. Treatment of the animals to a1 the growth of metastases was mainly performed after excision of the primary tumor graft. The therapeutic effect of the various treatments was assessed by record: survival and mortality rates of the animals due to metastases.

RESULTS

Injection of 10^6, 10^7, or 10^8 VCN-treated tumor cells either s.c. or i.d. 24 hours before or after excision of the primary tumor graft had no effect on the sur vival period of the animals, nor did it change the mortality rate. Chessboard vac cination also had no significant therapeutic effect when given as an alternative VCN-treated cells. Even repeating the immunization two or three times every four did not improve the results.

Consequently, the application of either VCN-treated cells or chessboard vacci tion has to be regarded as having no effect whatsoever on the growth of LL metast‪

The effect of cyclophosphamide on the immune response against SRBC was evalua in the Mackaness system. As demonstrated in Fig. 1, cyclophosphamide does not imp but rather improves, the immune response, especially the DTH reaction when given intravenously in a dosage equal to or less than 200 mg/kg two days before immuniza tion with SRBC.

I.V. injection of 100 mg/kg body weight of cyclophosphamide into C57Bl/6 mice 24 hours after excision of the primary tumor graft reduced the mortality rate caused by metastases by up to 60% (Table 1). When chemotherapy was followed by chessboard vaccination 24 hours later, we were able to improve the therapeutic success further. We were even able to cure all the animals in this experiment when chessboard vaccination was repeated after two weeks. The therapeutic effect of chessboard vaccination seems to depend on the enzymatic activity of VCN, as chessboard vaccinations with the use of VCN, inactivated according to Schneider et al. (1979), did not improve the therapeutic effect of the chemotherapy to the same extent.

DISCUSSION

Therapeutic methods elaborated in experimental transplantation tumor models, which show spontaneous metastases, might, with the same justification, be transferred to the clinical situation, but some caution must also be exercised. The differences between tumor transplantation models and autochthonous tumor diseases in man should not be forgotten. A stimulating example for the utilization of results, gained in experimental tumor models, for clinical treatment are the results of Bekesi et al. (1979). The synergistic effect of the combination of chemotherapy and specific immunotherapy found in experimental leukemia in mice has led to treating patients with Acute Myeloid Leukemia with chemoimmunotherapy. And this has so far been successful (Bekesi et al. 1979).

Tumor immunotherapy consisted of the intradermal injection of VCN-treated tumor cells. This treatment was given in addition to a chemotherapy, the dose and the timing of which has been shown not to abrogate completely the capacity of the host to respond to the specific immunotherapy.

The same reasoning led to our experiments in the LL system, the results of which show that even in a very disastrous experimental tumor disease, characterized by early death due to metastases after excision of the primary tumor transplant, the animals may be cured by chemoimmunotherapy. This consists of a non-immunosuppressive, but rather immunostimulating, dose of cyclophosphamide and chessboard vaccination. Together with the results of the clinical trial with chessboard vaccination in dogs with autochthonous breast tumors, the experiments may stimulate investigations into the value of chessboard vaccination in clinical solid tumor diseases, either alone or combined with adequate chemotherapy. Prospective random studies are in fact already underway in prostate carcinoma, and colon carcinoma.

However, the results gained in the LL system should also be judged with caution. It is known, and this is borne out by our own experience, that high doses of cyclophosphamide, given after excision of the primary tumor transplants, may cure nearly all the animals from their minimal residual disease. Thus, in this respect this model is not very realistic when compared to the human situation. Therefore, experiments are already going on to evaluate the therapeutic effect of the combination of chemotherapy and chessboard vaccination in other experimental metastasizing tumor diseases, which cannot be treated as successfully as the LL by any known chemotherapy alone.

REFERENCES

Bekesi, J.G., Holland, J.F., 1979. In: R. Neth, R.C. Gallo et al. (Editors), Modern Trends in Human Leukemia III, Springer-Verlag, Berlin, pp. 79-87.

Mackaness, G.B., Lagrange, P.H., Miller, T.E., Ishibashi, T., 1974. In: W.H. Wagner, H. Hahn, R. Evans (Editors), Activation of Macrophages, Excerpta Medica, Amsterdam, pp. 193-209.

Ronneberger, H., 1978. Develop. biol. Standard. 38, 413-419.

Schick, H.J., Zilg, H. 1978. Develop. biol. Standard. 38, 81-85.

Schneider, D.R., Sedlacek, H.H., Seiler, F.R., 1979. In: R. Schauer, P. Boer, et al. (Editors), Glycoconjugates, G. Thieme Verlag, Stuttgart, pp. 354-355.

Sedlacek, H.H., Meesmann, H., Seiler, F.R., 1975. Int. J. Cancer 15, 409-416.

Sedlacek, H.H., Seiler, F.R., 1978. Cancer Immunol. Immunother. 5, 153-163.

Sedlacek, H.H., Weise, M., Lemmer, A., Seiler, F.R., 1979. Cancer Immunol. Immunother. 6, 57-58.

Seiler, F.R., Sedlacek, H.H., 1974. Behring Inst. Mitt. No. 55, 258-271.

Seiler, F.R., Sedlacek, H.H., 1978. Proc. Symp. Immunother. of Malignant Diseases, Schattauer-Verlag, Stuttgart, pp. 479-488.

Wilson, R.E., Sonis, S.T., Godrick, E.A., 1974. Behring Inst. Mitt. No. 55, 334-342.

TABLE 1: Treatment of Lewis lung adenocarcinomas with chemoimmunotherapy

Treatment	After excision of primary tumor graft	
	Metastases (Mortality %)	Survival (days, only dead animals)
No treatment	100	23 ± 2.7
10^6 tumor cells, VCN treated	100	22.9 ± 2.1
10^7 tumor cells, VCN treated	100	23.6 ± 3.6
10^8 tumor cells, VCN treated	100	23.3 ± 3.3
1x chessboard vacc. - VCN	100	26.2 ± 5.2
1x chessboard vacc. + VCN	100	26.4 ± 5.9
Cyclophosphamide (2 mg/ mouse) —	60	30 ± 20
Cyclophosphamide (2 mg/ mouse) 1x chessboard vacc. + VCN (6.5 mU)	33	31 ± 12
Cyclophosphamide (2 mg/ mouse) 2x chessboard vacc. + VCN (6.5 mU)	0	(>200)

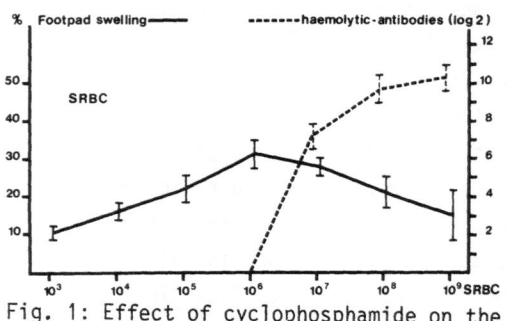

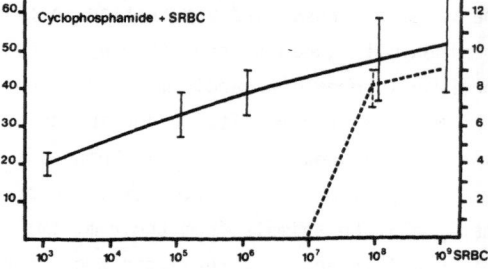

Fig. 1: Effect of cyclophosphamide on the immune response against SRBC in mice.

for details see Materials and Methods

APPLICATION OF THE LEUKOCYTE MIGRATION TEST (LMT) TO PATIENTS WITH METASTASES: EVIDENCE IN FAVOUR OF A CHANGE IN HOST RESPONSE

S. Matzku and M. Zöller

INTRODUCTION

A quantitative analysis of results obtained with in vitro test systems (e.g. LMT, LAI) reveals organ-related reaction specificity, e.g. leukocytes from patients with lung cancer "react" predominantly with lung cancer extracts and to a significantly lesser extent with extracts from other tumors. Similar reaction frequencies are observed with extracts of corresponding and non-corresponding fetal organs (S.Matzku, to be published). Leukocytes from patients with metastases "react" with primary tumor extracts, too, but with more or less decreased frequency. This raises the question, whether leukocytes from patients with metastases may or may not acquire novel reaction specificities and whether these may or may not relate to the organ of metastatic spread. Our approach toward an experimental resolution of the question consisted of testing leukocytes from patients awaiting thoracic surgery with lung cancer extracts. The group consisted of patients with different bronchogenic tumors, with benign lesions of the lung, and with lung metastases from non-lung primaries. After histological characterization of the specimen reaction frequencies obtained with lung cancer patients and with patients bearing metastases were compared in order to find out whether organ specificity of LMT reaction did extend to secondary tumors of the organ under investigation.

METHODS

The direct capillary tube assay was described in detail previously (Zöller et al., 1979). Tumor extracts were prepared by the 3M KCl method. Test evaluation: Migration index (MI) = migration area test (4 repl.) / migration area medium (12 repl.). MIs were considered as significant provided that a) $MI \leq 0.8$ or ≥ 1.2 and b) difference test area/medium area was significant by $p < 0.05$.

316

Positive reactivity with a panel of extracts was defined as the
occurrence of significant MIs with $\geqslant$ 3 out of 5 tumor extracts
tested (per patient).

The radioimmunoassay for CEA was purchased from CIS.

Patients

Fig.1 shows data from patients with colorectal cancer before
and after surgical removal of the primary tumor.[*] Tables 1 and 2
show data from patients awaiting thoracic surgery.

RESULTS

Fig.1 gives examples of different modes of LMT response observed with leukocytes from patients developing metastases after
removal of primary colorectal tumors. Tests were performed with a
panel of 5 colorectal tumor extracts. In addition, plasma CEA
levels were determined radioimmunologically. The organ of metastatic growth is indicated in abbreviated form.

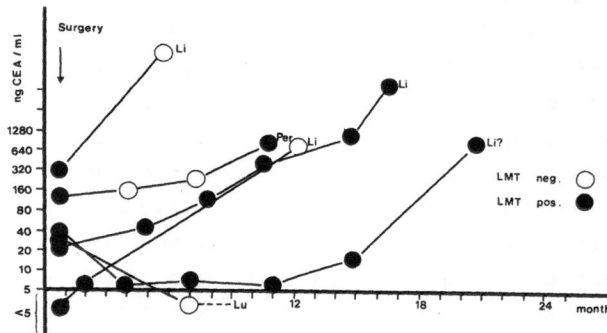

Fig.1. Growth of me-
tastases in the absence
of the primary colorec-
tal tumor. Influence on
the plasma CEA concen-
tration and LMT reacti-
vity. Organs of meta-
static growth are indi-
cated in the graph
(liver, lung, peri-
toneum).

While most patients reacted positively prior to the removal of
the primary tumor (and reacted negatively in the disease-free interval post op.; data not shown), a more complex situation was observed with patients developing metastases: some patients had a
positive LMT throughout; some of them returned to negative reactivity after surgery but got positive with metastatic growth (this
situation was regularly observed in patients with local recurren-

[*]We are grateful to Drs.U.Schulz, W.Dietze, H.D.Saeger, and
D.Zeidler for providing blood samples and giving access to patients'
data.

ces); some patients **lost** their positive reactivity when metastases were observed. Levels of circulating CEA did not ccrre-
late with LMT phenomena. Tab.1 illustrates the converse approach,
i.e. testing leukocytes from patients with metastases by using
extracts derived from either benign or tumorous tissue corresponding to the orcan of metastatic growth rather than extracts from
tissue corresponding to the organ of tumor origin. In this study,
lung tumor extracts and "normal" lung tissue extracts were tested,
lung cancer patients being the positive controls.

TABLE 1. REACTIVITY OF LEUKOCYTES FROM PATIENTS WITH PRIMARY AND
SECONDARY TUMCRS IN THE LUNG TO 3M KCL EXTRACTS FROM NORMAL AND
MALIGNANT LUNG TISSUE

| Leukocyte donor | Positive reactivities/total No of patients | | | Sign.MIs/total No of patients |
| | Histological type of the tumors extracted | | | Normal lung extract |
	Squamous cell Ca	Adeno Ca	Oat cell Ca	
Pulmonary cancer:				
Squamous cell carcinoma	52/73 (71%)	22/32 (69%)	27/36 (75%)	29/98 (30%)
Adenocarcinoma	11/13 (85%)	5/5 (100%)	4/5 (80%)	5/14 (30%)
Oat cell carcinoma	30/39 (77%)	12/15 (80%)	19/23 (83%)	21/53 (40%)
Other lung carcinoma	58/82 (71%)	15/16 (94%)	10/14 (71%)	23/61 (38%)
Non-pulmonary cancer:				
with lung metastases	14/24 (58%)	7/8 (88%)	5/7 (71%)	17/33 (52%)
without lung metastases	29/84 (35%)	0/1 (-)	18/38 (47%)	7/68 (10%)
Healthy controls	0/25 (0%)	0/17 (0%)	0/23 (0%)	0/40 (0%)

As expected, leukocytes from lung cancer patients showed a high
frequency of positive reactivity and this was not dependent on the
histologic type of the tumors used for extraction. A lower level
of reactivity was observed with "normal" lung tissue extract. In
the crucial group of patients with non-pulmonary tumors, two
different types of reactivity were observed. Patients with metastases to the lung exhibited a high frequency of positive reactivity
to lung tumor extracts (but also to "normal" lung extract!), while
patients without involvement of the lung showed relatively low
reaction frequencies with both "normal" lung and lung tumor extracts. Healthy donors proved to give the appropriate negative
control.

318

TABLE 2. SUMMARY OF TABLE 1

Leukocyte donors	Positive reactivity with lung tumor extracts/total No of pat.	%
Squamous cell carcinoma	101/141	72
Adenocarcinoma	20/23	87
Oat cell carcinoma	61/77	79
Other lung tumors	83/112	74
Non-pulmonary cancer with lung metastases	26/39	67
without lung metastases	41/123	38*

* significant difference to the above lines, χ^2-test, p 0.05

Data are summarized in Tab.2, no differentiation being made between different types of lung cancer extracts. It has to be emphasized that the reaction frequency of patients with lung metastases (26/39 = 67%) was not significantly different from the reaction frequency observed with lung cancer patients leukocytes. The opposite was true for patients without metastases of the lung. Patients with lung cancer having metastases in the opposite lobe did not show differences in LMT reactivity when compared to patients with primary lung cancer only (data not shown).

DISCUSSION

Fig.2 gives an impression of cross-reactivity patterns observed with our test system, emphasis being laid on the presence or absence of metastases and the reaction frequency with different categories of extracts. Since this figure is **meant** to illustrate the trend emerging from different studies, no attempt was made to perform a statistical analysis.

Patients bearing only primary tumors reacted predominantly with homologous tumor extracts and much less frequently with extracts of tumors from other sites (organ specificity). Once metastases appeared, reactivity with homologous (primary) tumor extracts decreased slightly, reactivity with irrelevant tumor extracts seemingly remained unchanged. However, a new type of reactivity appeared, which was directed toward some constituents of extracts related to the organ of metastatic spread. When metastases appeared

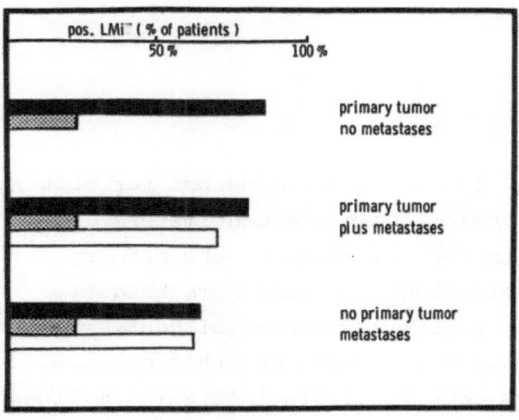

Figure 2. Synopsis of cross-reactivity data obtained with leukocytes from patients with or without metastases.

reactivity with primary tumor extract (stomach, colorectum, lung); reactivity with irrelevant tumor extracts; reactivity with extract related to the organ of metastatic growth.

■■■ primary tumour

▨▨▨ irrelevant tumour

☐ organ of 2° growth

after surgical removal of the primary, reactivity with primary tumor extracts declined even more, but reactivity with extracts related to the organ of metastatic growth was virtually unchanged. The decline in reactivity of leukocytes from patients with metastases toward extracts of the primary tumor is associated with the appearance of marked reactivity toward material related to the organ of metastatic growth.

It seems to be unlikely that the LMT actually reflects shifts of antigenic specificities possibly occurring during metastatic spread, unless one postulates an influence of the surrounding tissue on the expression of antigens on tumor cells. It rather is tempting to speculate that the LMT may monitor processes related to tissue decay, invasion and host cell infiltration.

REFERENCE

Zöller, M., Matzku, S., Schulz, U., and Price, M.R., 1979. Sensitization of leukocytes of cancer patients against fetal antigens: leukocyte migration studies. J.Natl.Cancer Inst., 63: 285-293.

COMPUTED TOMOGRAPHY IN THE STAGING OF MALIGNANCY

L. Kreel

Computed tomography is, by and large, a method for showing soft tissue mass lesions greater than two centimeters in diameter. Nevertheless, in the diagnosis of the primary tumour it has a limited role. Thus, in carcinoma breast, bronchus, kidney, thyroid, testis, prostate, bladder, stomach and colon, the initial diagnosis is made by other methods. Nor is computed tomography capable of distinguishing malignant from benign lesions. Thus, computed tomography has a very limited role in initial diagnosis or as a screening procedure.

Therefore, in the vast majority of cases, computed tomography has a limited role in the assessment in the size of the original tumour, with a few notable exceptions. In brain tumours, bladder carcinoma, pancreatic carcinoma, renal cell carcinoma, retroperitoneal sarcoma, especially lipo-sarcoma and gastro-intestinal lymphoma, the primary tumour mass can be delineated more accurately than by other methods.

However, the situation is quite different when considering spread of the tumour to lymph nodes or its distant haemo-togenous dissemination. Before considering the disseminated lesions, the associated factors influencing the assessment of a mass lesion on computed tomography should be reviewed.

Tumour Mass

The delineation of a soft tissue mass in radiology depends on the differential contrast between the lesion and the normal tissue, and in computed tomography is largely dependent on fatty tissue surrounding the tumour. In patients with poorly developed adipose tissue planes, such as children and wasted subjects, tumour delineation is difficult, but in most adult subjects presenting for assessment, abdominal tumours can be clearly visualised provided the bowel contains a contrast medium, such as 3% gastrografin given orally.

Computed tomography consists of axial sections, usually 1 cm thick and spaced at 2 - 3 cm intervals. For the accurate comparison of serial examinations, the level of the sections in the body must be matched precisely, which requires considerable care and attention to detail.

Once the position of the tumour has been demonstrated, adjacent or overlapping 1 cm sections provide the basis for accurate volumetric measurements of the tumour, which is occasionally crucial in determining growth or regression. The size of the mass and its internal relations can be very accurately measured, whereas with conventional radiography there is variable magnification. Thus, a surgical clip lying anteriorly in the abdomen can be projected to give the tumour almost a x 2 magnification. Furthermore, the surgical clip must be on the tangential border of the tumour, which is often impossible to achieve. Direct comparison of the conventional radiograph and C.T. is extremely difficult.

A further factor to be taken into account in serial comparison of mass lesions is their response to radiotherapy or chemotherapy. Apart from the possible initial enlargement due to tumour response, internal haemorrhage or necrosis may make the lesion appear larger. On C.T. haemorrhage or necrosis is indicated by internal low density (low tissue attenuation), which must also be taken into account in assessing tumour size. Liver metastases, after embolisation or chemotherapy, are particularly prone to necrosis and liquefaction. However, the low density of some lymph nodes prior to treatment is well recognised, especially in melanoma and is thought to be due to haemorrhage.

One other very important factor in considering tumour size is in the interpretation of residual mass lesions shown on C.T. There are at present no C.T. criteria for distinguishing between residual tumour and sterile tissue, short of serial examinations to show increase in size. Histology is still the only effective method of distinguishing residual tumour from 'sterile' tissue.

Position of the Tumour

There are a number of advantages in being able to show the exact position of a tumour inside the body, particularly in the abdomen. Using either computed tomography or ultra-sonography, the tip of a needle can be accurately placed inside a mass lesion to obtain material for cytology. This technique is now well established and almost routine in some centres. Using a fine needle, there appear to be no hazards, and an accuracy rate of 75 - 80% has been obtained in identifying malignant cells. Furthermore, in those cases where it is not clear whether the mass is solid or fluid or indeed, whether it is a cyst or abscess, needle puncture is almost obligatory. Not only can the abscesses and organism be identified, but it can be drained percutaneously, thus saving the patient a laparotomy.

While the relationship to other structures can usually be shown by computed tomography, unless a clear line of demarcation between the tumour and other organs is identified, it is not possible to distinguish infiltration from a pressure effect.

In hollow organs, such as the gastro-intestinal tract and the bladder, the extrinsic mass can be identified, and is particularly useful in showing lymphoma of the stomach and duodenum and in staging bladder carcinoma.

Local Spread of Malignancy

Thus, in the local spread of malignancy, whether from a primary tumour such as a bladder carcinoma, or from recurrent tumour such as colon carcinoma, accurate definition is possible. In the bladder, the tumour itself shows as a soft tissue mass delineated by the urine inside the bladder and the extrinsic adipose tissue. When there is infiltration of the bladder wall, the margin of the bladder becomes straightened and the bladder wall thickened. Penetration through the bladder is seen as a soft tissue convexity bulging outward from the bladder wall.

Enlarged lymph nodes can certainly be demonstrated by computed tomography, and indeed the demonstration of lymphadenopathy in testicular tumours and lymphoma is one of the major uses of this technique. In lymphoma it is particularly valuable because lymph node enlargement can be shown, which is not possible with lymphography, particularly in the upper abdomen above the level of L2. However, slightly enlarged nodes can be due to either malignant infiltration or reactive hyperplasia, and benign or inflammatory lymphadenopathy appears similar to malignant infiltration.

Once again, it must be stressed that, while C.T. is invaluable in the detection of lymphadenopathy, it is no substitute for histology.

Local infiltration of bone is clearly demonstrated, but adjacent infiltration of nerves and periosteum can only be inferred by the juxtaposition of the soft tissue mass. Occasionally peritoneal nodules are visible, but in most cases only the ascites is visible. Rarely, local peritoneal spread produces a loculated effusion, especially over the liver margin, which is readily visible on computed tomography and, using a bolus injection of contrast medium with rapid sequential scans and a fast scanner, venous tumour thrombus, particularly in the renal vein and inferior vena cava, is demonstrable. Thus, in the local spread of malignant disease there are a number of aspects where computed tomography can be extremely useful.

Tumour Recurrence

In the detection of tumour recurrence computed tomography is often the only effective method of diagnosis, especially in colon carcinoma and lymphoma. In a review of 50 cases of colon carcinoma examined for recurrence, tumour regrowth was detected up to twelve years after the original event. In the pre-sacral region, tumours down to 1.5 cm in diameter could be detected, size of the mass determined, bone and bladder involvement shown, and unsuspected metastases in the lung and liver demonstrated. Healing by new bone formation in the tumour, in response to radiotherapy, was shown in one case.

The distribution of the haematogenous metastates were of considerable interest. In nine cases there were pulmonary metastases, in nine cases liver metastases, but in only one case was there both liver and lung metastases. It would appear that the haematogenous spread occurs either by a break into the portal venous system or into the azygos inferior vena cava system, but rarely in both.

Similarly, both the response to treatment and the resurgence of lymphoma can be detected with computed tomography. The anatomical regions where computed tomography is particularly valuable are the upper abdomen, the retro-crural region and the mediastinum, especially the pre-cardiac and pre-vertebral regions.

Distant Metastases

The detection of lymphadenopathy and the associated problems have already been considered. Haematogenous spread to lung, liver, brain, bone and suprarenals can be detected at a pre-symptomatic stage, usually before being visible by other methods, apart from liver metastases, which can be detected by ultrasonography.

Pulmonary metastases are visible when only 2 - 3 mm in size and when not visible on conventional tomography. From post-mortem studies, it is clear that there are also much smaller metastases and even cellular permeation which cannot possibly be shown by computed tomography. Most pulmonary metastases are peripheral and sub-pleural, and these, in particular, are not visible on computed tomography.

Similarly, brain, bone and suprarenal tumours can be shown by computed tomography. In lung and bone, the problem is often that 1 - 2 mm nodules are visible, but it is not clear whether these are part of the tissue structure or pathological. In countries where histoplasmosis is endemic, granulomatous nodules in the lung are frequent and are indistinguishable from pulmonary metastases on computed tomography.

Summary and Conclusions

Computed tomography is, to date, the most reliable radio-logical method for diagnosing the presence and spread of tumour, because it produces the best anatomical resolution and all systems can be examined. Nevertheless, it has a relatively minor role in screening for malignancy and in the diagnosis of the primary tumour, but for the delineation of a mass for size, position and local spread, computed tomography is invaluable, though lack of fatty, soft tissue planes is a limiting factor. Serial measurements can be done and tumour volume calculated to monitor radiotherapy and chemotherapy.

Similarly, tumour recurrence can be diagnosed, lymph node enlargement can be accurately assessed, and bone infiltration, venous tumour thrombus and ascites clearly visualised. Computed tomography can also be used for percutaneous needle aspiration cytology and for aspirating abscesses.

Metastases to lung, liver, bone, brain and suprarenals can be shown at an early stage and earlier than with most other diagnostic methods. Nevertheless, there are a number of very notable deficiencies.

Benign and malignant masses cannot be distinguished, tumours and granulomas cannot be distinguished, and residual sterile tissue cannot be distinguished from active tumour except by serial examinations. This lack of tissue characterisation is an important limiting factor in the use of computed tomography.

In spite of the limitations inherent in computed tomography, the effective management of testicular tumours and lymphomas and the staging of bladder carcinoma is virtually impossible without computed tomography. It is, to date, the most reliable method for the early detection of pulmonary metastases.

SERIAL QUANTITATIVE SKELETAL SCINTIGRAPHY IN BREAST CANCER

S.P. Parbhoo, H. Alani, J.E. Agnew and B.A. Stoll

The skeleton is the commonest site of distant metastatic disease in breast cancer. Conventional methods such as radiography are relatively insensitive in picking up these lesions. In recent years the introduction of new isotopes such as Technetium – 99m Methylene Disphosphosphonate (99Tc MDP) has made high quality bone scans available, but their role in the detection and further management of bone deposits requires to be established.

The gamma camera picture gives reasonable resolution on polaroid film but visual inspection suffers from subjective bias and is often insensitive to early minor changes in the scan. In addition the variations in the scan image and background make optical comparison difficult. It is notoriously difficult to assess objective response to systemic therapy in the case of bone metastases. Inhibition of tumour activity cannot be assumed from relief of pain and associated symptoms, and the interpretation of small degrees of radiographic change is subject to considerable observer bias. In order to obtain earlier and more accurate assessment of bone secondary change, serial quantitative bone scanning has been advocated. The early attempts did not quantitate the serial scans by computer and it is only recently that this technique has been reported (Bull, et al 1977 and Pfannenstiel et al 1978).

METHODS:

Having established the sensitivity and reproducibility of our technique in a rat bone metastasis model (Williams et al 1980) we investigated the value of computer assisted serial scanning in patients with and without bone metastases from breast cancer in order to gather data on the possible variations in uptake, either in response to therapy or with the natural course of the tumour. The equipment used consisted of a gamma camera (ANGER, General Electric) interfaced with a digital computer (VARIAN 32-K).

Two different techniques of analysis were used. Firstly the profile technique of the thoracolumbar spine which measured isotope uptake fluctuations of the vertebrae under study. Secondly the region of interest (ROI) study which measured total counts within selected areas in patients without bone metastases – the bone to bone ratio and in those with secondaries – the metastasis to bone ratio.

This work was supported by Grant 165 from the Royal Free Hospital and School of Medicine Appeal Trust and the Jane Sinclair Memorial Trust.

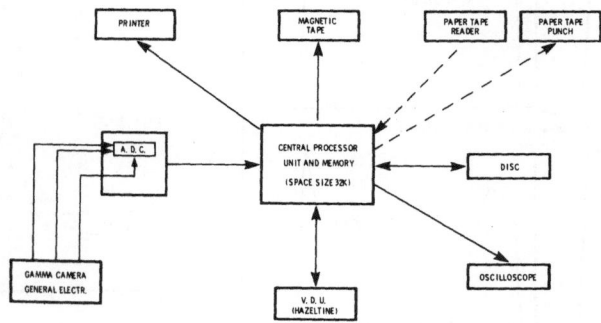

A BLOCK DIAGRAM OF THE ANGER GAMMA CAMERA CONNECTED TO
THE DIGITAL COMPUTER

Fig. 1

PATIENTS:

Serial quantitative bone scans were carried out in 2 groups of 11 and 15 women with breast cancer aged 31-87 years with a mean age of 57. The first group of 11 cases had had mastectomy for stage 1 - 3 breast cancer but showed no clinical or scan evidence of bone metastases at the time of scanning for the first time. The second group of 15 cases had overt bone secondaries with abnormal scans. Serial scans were carried out at intervals of between 1 and 8 months and the data stored on magnetic tape. Scans were carried out between 2 and 3 hours after intravenous injection of 15m Ci of 99 Tc MDP.

RESULTS:

Profile Studies of Thoracolumbosacral Spine

Profiles were constructed by computer measuring the counts in the matrix enclosing the width of the vertebral column (Fig 2). The large spikes at each end of the curve represent "hot" areas at the edge of the image, but are arte-facts since they are also demonstrable when imaging a uniform source. Each profile was analysed to determine a) the degree of fluctuations b) whether this was reproducible in a series of scans and c) whether this was different in patients with and without bone secondaries. The percentage fluctuations above minimum (% FAM) was based on the formula:

$$\%FAM = \frac{maximum\ count - minimum\ count}{minimum\ count} \times 100$$

The artefactual spikes at the edge of the profiles were omitted from the analysis.

Analysis of the profiles in a series of 11 patients without bone meta-stases who had more than 3 scans showed a %FAM of 35±10.4. This contrasts with a %FAM of 136±37 for the abnormal scans in patients with bone metastases.

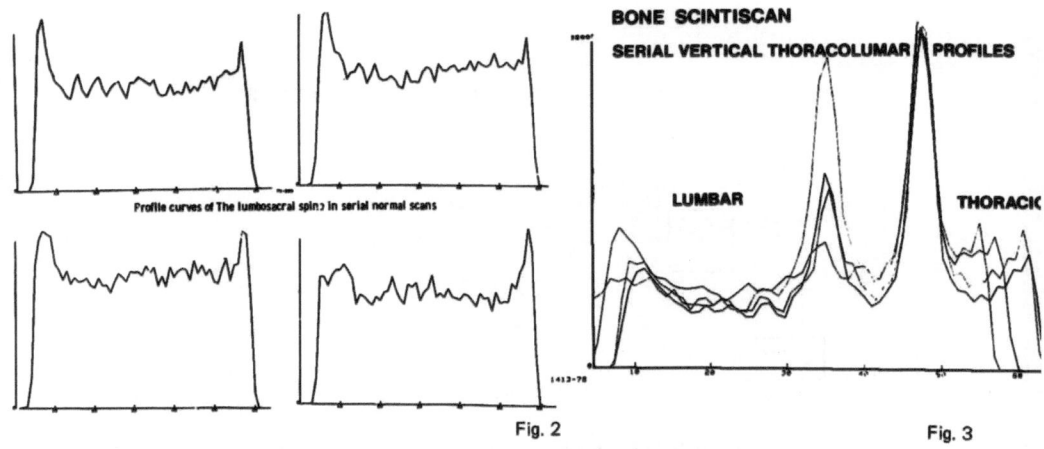

Fig. 2   Fig. 3

While the majority of profiles showed a high degree of reproducibility of the peaks and troughs, this comparison in the series required accurate visual superimposition of the curves. We found that the serial profile technique allowed the early detection of new deposits or recurrent disease. Profiles from a patient with a T_{10} lesion who developed a progressive lumbar deposit during the study followed by regression after radiotherapy are seen in Fig 3. Detailed agreement such as in Fig 3 was not seen consistantly. While the fluctuations could be due to development of multiple metastases we found that these fluctuations detracted from the value of the profile technique since it was based on super-imposition of the profiles liable to subjective bias. Other possible fluctuations are ascribed to difficulty in reproducing the exact setting of the patient under the gamma camera on each occasion and lastly to oblique positioning of the spine.

Region of Interest (ROI) Studies

In order to overcome the problems of the spine profile technique we used the region of interest (ROI) analysis. This also allowed us to study any suspicious area in the skeleton. The ROI represents a count over a defined area in a "hot spot" compared to a normal area of comparable size, used as a reference spot. Bone to bone ratios were calculated for each area and the background subtracted. In a series of 30 scans on 10 patients without bone metastases the ROI ratios were as follows:

SITE	MEAN ROI	ROI RANGE
T9/T11	1.06 $\pm$ 0.03	0.96 - 1.20
L2/L4	1.05 $\pm$ 0.2	0.88 - 1.19
R/L Upper $\frac{1}{3}$ of HUMERUS	1.07 $\pm$ 0.01	0.96 - 1.13
R/L SACRO ILIAC JOINT	1.03 $\pm$ 0.05	0.98 - 1.10
R/L Upper $\frac{1}{3}$ of FEMUR	1.03 $\pm$ 0.05	0.98 - 1.10

An initial ROI study of hot spots vs reference area in 34 scans in 12 patients showed a mean ratio of 1.73 ± 0.29. We have subsequently studied 15 patients with bone metastases who have had more than 3 serial scans. The average interval between studies was 3 months with a range of 1 - 8 months. A total of 49 hot spots were serially studied in these patients who had 72 bone scans. Thirteen patients showed progressive disease in 21 sites. In patients with rapidly advancing disease changes were seen early and progression was detected within the shortest interval (1 month) of repeat scanning. Table 1 shows the ROI data from an 80 year old patient who presented with a fungating breast cancer and was noted to have hot spots but no radiological evidence of secondaries. She later developed sacral pain due to progressive metastases which were treated with local radiotherapy. This table shows the progressive increase in uptake in all areas except the sacrum which was treated.

REGION OF INTEREST DATA   (A. D.)

Date	Sac/L5	D6/D8	D10/D8
18. 5. 79	1. 30	1. 62	1. 52
6. 7. 79	1. 49	1. 69	1. 53
17. 9. 79	1. 45	1. 70	1. 52
12. 11. 79	1. 48*	1. 87	1. 87
21. 1. 80	1. 31	2. 31	2. 39

* Radiotherapy to sacrum 10/79

Table 1

REGION OF INTEREST DATA IN RESPONSE TO OOPHORECTOMY*

Date	L1/L3	D8/D10	R.SIJ/L.SIJ
8. 9. 77	1. 45	1. 57	0. 98
14. 12. 77	1. 69	1. 61	1. 54
19. 6. 78	1. 40	1. 22	1. 92
13. 12. 78	1. 33	1. 20	1. 80
24. 5. 79	1. 23	1. 19	1. 31
17. 9. 79	1. 14	1. 09	1. 08
7. 2. 80	1. 05	1. 01	1. 09

* Sept. 1977   JS

Table 2

Response to oophorectomy may be seen in Tables 2 and 3. The 48 year old patient in Table 2 presented 4 years after radical mastectomy with skin, bone and pulmonary secondaries. The initial ROI ratios are clearly abnormal. Following oophorectomy in September 1977 the ROI ratio increased followed by a gradual fall to normal over 2 years. She has made an excellent clinical recovery. Table 3 shows the ROI ratios in a premenopausal patient who refused mastectomy in 1972 but had it in 1975 when recurrence was noted. She subsequently presented with lung and bone metastases. Following oophorectomy there was a delayed response on the ROI which is mirrored by her clinical response.

REGION OF INTEREST DATA IN RESPONSE TO OOPHORECTOMY

Date	Sac/Ilium	L4/L2	D10/D8
6. 7. 79	2. 23	0. 98	1. 28
23. 8. 79	2. 19	1. 15	1. 26
21. 9. 79	2. 43	1. 36	1. 24
13. 12. 79	2. 39	1. 35	1. 35
17. 1. 80	2. 67	1. 26	1. 32
8. 4. 80	2. 03	1. 12	1. 11

N. H.
Table 3

REGION OF INTEREST DATA IN RESPONSE TO RADIOTHERAPY*

Date	L1/L3	D10/D12
17. 8. 78	1. 70	3. 17*
21. 9. 78	1. 74	2. 45
12. 3. 79	1. 76	2. 41
9. 8. 79	2. 25	4. 20
25. 10. 79	4. 67**	4. 44
13. 12. 79	2. 47	4. 53
28. 2. 80	1. 25	2. 62

*July 1978   ** Sept. 1979   AM   Table 4

Development of further deposit despite oophorectomy is seen in Table 4. An initial improvement was seen at the site of laminectomy for spinal compression at T10. However symptomatic recurrence was noted together with development of a further deposit at L1 in July 1978. A second more extensive course of radiotherapy has resulted in clinical and quantitative scan improvement. Endocrine manipulation with anabolic steroids resulted in similar changes in the ROI ratios.

SUMMARY:

Quantitative bone scintigraphy is sensitive and reproducible. The use of a serial technique in the high risk patient picks up metastases early. The ROI is clearly more amenable to analysis than the profile technique. In our experience the changes in serial scans correlate well with the clinical response or deterioration. With all forms of treatment there is usually an increase in uptake prior to a fall if response is going to occur. It also allows the clinician to modify treatment without having to wait for radiological change.

REFERENCES:

Bull, U, Schuster, H, Pfeifer, J P, Tongendroff, J and Niendoff, H P: 1977 Bone-to-bone, Joint-to-bone and Joint-to-joint Ratios in normal and diseased skeletal states using region-of-interest techniques and bone-seeking radiopharmaceuticals, Nuklearmedizin 16 (3): 104 - 112.

Pfannenstiel, P, Semmler, U, Adam, W, Halbsguth, A, Bandilla, K and Berg D; 1978 Comparative study of quantitating radioactivity in sacroiliac scintigraphy. Presented at the 6th annual meeting of the British Nuc. Me. Society, Imperial College, London, April 17 - 19.

William D G, Parbhoo, S P, Agnew, J E, Stoll, B A, (1980) Serial quantitative bone scanning of metastatic tumour in rats.

FURTHER STUDIES ON THE EFFECT OF PROSTAGLANDIN SYNTHESIS INHIBITORS AND DIPHOSPHONATES ON TUMOUR-MEDIATED OSTEOLYSIS

C.S.B. Galasko, Stella Rushton, Eve Lacey and A.W. Samuel

Previous studies have shown that there are two main types of bone destruction that occur when tumour invades the skeleton (Galasko, 1976). The earlier phase, which quantitatively is probably the more important is mediated by osteoclasts. It has also been shown that the development of skeletal metastases is associated with the ability of malignant cells to form prostaglandin (PG) (Bennett et al, 1975, Voelkel et al, 1975, Galasko and Bennett 1976, Powles et al, 1976, Bennett et al, 1977), some prostaglandins, particularly PGE_2, stimulating osteoclast proliferation (Galasko and Bennett, 1976) but probably they are not the only osteoclast stimulating substances produced by cancer cells. Prostaglandin synthesis inhibitors of the non-steroidal anti-inflammatory group have been shown to inhibit hypercalcaemia and osteolysis in rats with the Walker tumour (Powles et al, 1973), hypercalcaemia in patients with various non-haematological tumours (Seyberth et al, 1975), and osteolysis and osteoclast proliferation in rabbits bearing the VX2 carcinoma (Galasko and Bennett, 1976). In the latter experiments the prostaglandin synthesis inhibitor indomethacin reduced the amount of prostaglandin-like material extracted from the VX2 carcinoma, osteoclast proliferation in the neighbourhood of the tumour and the amount of bone destruction. Further studies (Galasko et al, 1979) showed that the effect of prostaglandin inhibitors was dose dependent.

These non-steroidal anti-inflammatory drugs which inhibit prostaglandin activity indirectly affect bone resorption, which is directly inhibited by the diphosphonates (Fleisch and Felix, 1979). Dichloro-methylene diphosphonate (Cl_2MDP) is the most potent diphosphonate for inhibition of bone resorption and has less effect than ethane-hydroxy diphosphonate (EHDP) on mineralisation. The dose of EHDP that inhibits bone resorption is close to that inhibiting mineralisation (Fleisch and Felix, 1979) so that Cl_2MDP would seem to be the more promising as an inhibitor of bone resorption.

Our studies were designed to determine whether prostaglandin synthesis inhibitors had an effect on human mammary cancer as well as the VX2 carcinoma and whether the diphosphonates would inhibit the tumour osteolysis. A pilot study was carried out to determine whether these tumours could be examined in an organ culture system. The results (Galasko et al, 1980) indicated that human mammary cancers as well as the rabbit VX2 carcinoma could be cultured against mouse calvarium, that the tumour osteolytic activity could be measured by the amount of calcium released into the culture fluid and that the effect of non-steroidal anti-inflammatory agents and diphosphonates could be assessed by adding these compounds in varying concentrations to the culture fluid.

MATERIAL AND METHODS

One millimetre cubes taken from 17 mammary cancers were cultured with mouse calvarium.

The calvaria were obtained from neonatal mice and cultured in 2 millilitres of a modified Bigger's solution (Galasko et al, 1980) at 37° for 48 hours. The culture medium was removed and 2 ml. fresh culture medium introduced. Two one millimetre cubes of tumour were added to the second culture medium. Fifteen experiments were carried out on each tumour, the agents being added in 0.05 ml. aliquots, resulting in the following concentrations.

(a) Control
(b) EHDP 2.4 x 10^{-5} molar
(c) Cl_2MDP 2.4 x 10^{-5} molar
(d) Indomethacin 2.4 x 10^{-5} molar
(e) Indomethacin 2.4 x 10^{-6} molar
(f) Indomethacin 2.4 x 10^{-7} molar
(g) Indomethacin 2.4 x 10^{-5} molar + Cl_2MDP 2.4 x 10^{-5} molar
(h) Indomethacin 2.4 x 10^{-6} molar + Cl_2MDP 2.4 x 10^{-5} molar
 (i) Indomethacin 2.4 x 10^{-7} molar + Cl_2MDP 2.4 x 10^{-5} molar
(j) Ibuprofen 2.4 x 10^{-5} molar
(k) Ibuprofen 2.4 x 10^{-6} molar
(l) Ibuprofen 2.4 x 10^{-7} molar
(m) Flurbiprofen 2.4 x 10^{-5} molar
(n) Flurbiprofen 2.4 x 10^{-6} molar
(o) Flurbiprofen 2.4 x 10^{-7} molar

The calvaria were cultured for a further 48 hours, the culture fluid removed and the calcium content measured spectrophotometrically (Gindler and King, 1972). At the same time a parallel series of control cultures was established with calvarium and medium, the culture fluid being changed after 48 hours incubation.

The amount of tumour-induced osteolysis was obtained from the difference between the changes in calcium content in the test and control culture fluids using the formula :-

Amount of osteolysis (mg. calcium/dl.) = $(T - To) - (C - Co)$

where To = calcium content of the test fluid - first incubation
       T   = calcium content of the test fluid - second incubation
      Co = calcium content of the control fluid - first incubation
      C   = calcium content of the control fluid - second incubation

The results were analysed using the Wilcoxon Rank Test for non-parametric data and analysis of variance followed by Duncan's multiple range test.

RESULTS

The results are given in Tables I, II and III. When all the tumours were considered the osteolysis was significantly inhibited by the combination of indomethacin and Cl_2MDP, irrespective of the concentration of the non-steroidal anti-inflammatory agent. This combination produced the greatest reduction in osteolysis. The next most active agent was Ibuprofen in a concentration of 2.4 x 10^{-6} molar. The two higher concentrations of Flurbiprofen (2.4 x 10^{-5} molar and 2.4 x 10^{-6} molar) and the diphosphonate Cl_2MDP (2.4 x 10^{-5} molar) produced a similar effect. Indomethacin in a dose of 2.4 x 10^{-5} molar also produced a marked reduction in osteolysis but this just failed to reach significant levels. The other agents and doses used were less effective. Eleven of the 17 mammary cancers were osteolytically active, (calcium release more than 0.2 mg. calcium/dl.). The osteolytically active and osteolytically inactive tumours were analysed separately. The results obtained in the osteolytically active tumours were similar to those obtained for the entire group. The most active therapy was the combination of Cl_2MDP with a non-steroidal anti-inflammatory agent. The osteolysis was also significantly affected by Cl_2MDP (2.4 x 10^{-5} molar), indomethacin in its highest concentration (2.5 x 10^{-5} molar), Ibuprofen in a concentration of 2.4 x 10^{-6} molar and Flurbiprofen in all three test doses. None of the agents produced a significant alteration in calcium release in the osteolytically inactive tumours.

Table I. Effect of non-steroidal anti-inflammatory agents and diphosphonates on mammary carcinoma induced osteolysis - All tumours (n = 17)

Agent (See text)	a	b	c	d	e	f	g	h	i	j	k	l	m	n	o
Mean Osteolysis (all tumours) mg.Calcium/dl.	0.49	0.38	0.15	0.18	0.42	0.26	0.01	-0.09	0.09	0.23	0.10	0.33	0.15	0.16	0.24
S.E.M.	0.17	0.15	0.18	0.16	0.20	0.17	0.20	0.25	0.19	0.22	0.22	0.19	0.20	0.20	0.26
Rank Order (*$p<0.05$)(Duncan's Multiple Range Test)	-	13	6*	8	14	11	2*	1*	3*	9	4*	12	5*	7*	10

Table II. Effect of non-steroidal anti-inflammatory agents and diphosphonates on mammary carcinoma induced osteolysis - Osteolytically active tumours (n = 11)

Agent (See text)	a	b	c	d	e	f	g	h	i	j	k	l	m	n	o
Mean Osteolysis (Osteolytically active tumours) mg.Calcium/dl.	0.84	0.47	0.26	0.27	0.63	0.43	0.07	0.07	0.22	0.43	0.24	0.50	0.31	0.28	0.39
S.E.M.	0.17	0.16	0.19	0.13	0.24	0.19	0.23	0.23	0.19	0.25	0.27	0.22	0.24	0.21	0.30
Rank Order (*$p<0.05$)	-	12	5*	6*	14	11	2*	1*	3*	10	4*	13	8*	7*	9*

Table III. Effect of non-steroidal anti-inflammatory agents and diphosphonates on mammary carcinoma induced osteolysis - osteolytically inactive tumours (n = 6)
None of the agents produced a significant difference in osteolysis

Agent (See text)	a	b	c	d	e	f	g	h	i	j	k	l	m	n	o
Mean Osteolysis (Osteolytically inactive tumours) mg.Calcium/dl.	-0.15	0.21	-0.04	0.03	0.02	-0.07	-0.10	-0.23	-0.15	-0.14	-0.16	-0.04	-0.07	-0.07	-0.03
S.E.M.	0.12	0.33	0.39	0.39	0.30	0.29	0.41	0.41	0.40	0.44	0.35	0.35	0.35	0.42	0.48

DISCUSSION

The results indicate that the osteolysis produced by human mammary cancer can be significantly inhibited by non-steroidal anti-inflammatory drugs, which also are prostaglandin synthesis inhibitors, and by diphosphonates which probably directly affect bone resorption. The combination of a diphosphonate and non-steroidal anti-inflammatory drug was the most effective agent in our study. Whereas Cl_2MDP produced a significant reduction in tumour osteolysis EHDP had no effect. The effect of the non-steroidal anti-inflammatory agents varied. The most effective drug appeared to be Flurbiprofen since it significantly reduced the osteolysis in the active tumours in all three doses. Ibuprofen in the middle dose was also effective. Although Indomethacin was effective in the osteolytically-active tumours, when all the tumours were considered the reduction statistically was not significant. This is surprising as Indomethacin has been shown to be effective in animal models.

Powles and his colleagues (1976) using a similar culture technique found that 23 (60%) of 38 human mammary carcinomata had significant in vitro osteolytic activity compared with 11 (65%) of our 17 tumours. In our previous study (Galasko et al, 1980)17 (63%)of 27 tumours were osteolytically active. If our two studies are combined 28 (64%) of 44 tumours were active. Powles and colleagues (1976)reported that all their patients presenting with bone metastases or hypercalcaemia had osteolytically active tumours and that over the subsequent three year follow-up period skeletal metastases did not develop in any of their 15 patients with osteolytically inactive tumours.

They also studied 14 tumours, chosen at random for in vitro osteolytic activity in the presence or absence of aspirin which is a prostaglandin inhibitor. The activity of eight of the nine osteolytically active tumours was significantly although not completely inhibited by aspirin. The combination of Cl_2MDP and indomethacin, completely inhibited resorption in nine of the eleven active mammary cancers, in our study.

Our current study confirms the previous in vivo animal experiments(Galasko et al,1979) which showed that the effect of indomethacin in reducing prostaglandin activity in the VX2 carcinoma, osteoclast proliferation in the neighbourhood of the tumour and tumour-mediated osteolysis was dose-dependent. In that study the dose required to affect prostaglandin activity was less than that required to reduce tumour-mediated osteolysis. Reduction in the serum prostaglandin level or those of its metabolites, therefore, **cannot** be used as a guide to the efficacy of treatment.

It is interesting to note that Cl_2MDP was as effective as the prostaglandin synthesis inhibitors. The bone destruction in multiple myeloma is mediated via osteoclasts, the tumour secreting O.A.F. rather than PGE_2. Recent studies have shown that Cl_2MDP reduced bone resorption in patients with myeloma as shown by a decrease in hypercalciuria or urinary hydroxyproline(Siris et al, 1980). Amino hydroxypropylidene diphosphonate (A.P.D.) is another diphosphonate which is a potent inhibitor of bone resorption. It has been shown to reduce serum hypercalcaemia and urinary calcium and hydroxyproline excretion in patients with osteolytic bone lesions due to metastatic mammary cancer or myeloma. (Van Breukelen et al, 1979).

The finding that the combination of diphosphonate and prostaglandin inhibition was the most effective method of reducing tumour induced osteolysis suggests that prostaglandin is not the only osteoclast-stimulating factor secreted by mammary carcinoma and that other forms of bone resorption may be occurring. This confirms the studies of Powles and his colleagues (1976) and our previous in vivo studies (Galasko and Bennett, 1976 and Galasko et al, 1979) which also demonstrated that these agents did not totally eliminate osteoclast proliferation nor the resultant osteolysis.

Our results suggest that these agents may have an important role to play in the management of patients with mammary cancer. The in vivo animal studies (Galasko et al, 1979) indicated that treatment was effective only if started within seven days of inoculation of the tumour, the animals dying with pulmonary metastases 35 days after inoculation of the tumour. Therefore, these drugs need to be tested in a controlled clinical trial in patients with apparently "early" mammary carcinoma as a form of adjuvant therapy following mastectomy.

There have been isolated reports **of** the use of prostaglandin inhibitors in the management of patients with skeletal metastases. The results have been variable but unfortunately biopsies were not taken of the metastases so that it is not possible to determine the osteoclast activity. It may well be that those patients who failed to respond had phase II type skeletal metastases (Galasko, 1976), whereas osteoclast activity may have been prominent in those patients who showed some response. In phase II the osteoclasts disappear although bone destruction continues. Furthermore, in many of the reports the doses used may have been inadequate to significantly affect osteolysis but sufficient to reduce the tumour prostaglandin activity.

ACKNOWLEDGEMENTS

We would like to thank the Medical Research Council and the Boots Company Limited for support. The diphosphonates were donated by the Proctor & Gamble Company, Cincinnati.

REFERENCES

Bennett, A., Charlier, E.M., McDonald, A.M., Simpson, J.S., Stamford, I.F. and Zebro, T. (1977). Prostaglandins and breast cancer. Lancet, 2, 624-626.

Bennett, A., McDonald, A.M., Simpson, J.S. and Stamford, I.F. (1975). Breast cancer, prostaglandins and bone metastases. Lancet, 1, 1218-1220.

Fleisch, H. and Felix, R. (1979). Diphosphonates. Calcified Tissue International, 27, 91-94.

Galasko, C.S.B. (1976). Mechanisms of bone destruction in the development of skeletal metastases. Nature, 263, 507-508.

Galasko, C.S.B. and Bennett, A. (1976). Relationship of bone destruction in skeletal metastases to osteoclast activation and prostaglandins. Nature, 263, 508-510.

Galasko, C.S.B., Rawlins, R. and Bennett, A. (1979). Prostaglandins, osteoclasts and bone destruction produced by VX2 carcinoma in rabbits: effects of administering indomethacin at different doses and times. British Journal of Cancer, 40, 360-364.

Galasko, C.S.B., Samuel, A.W., Rushton, Stella and Lacey, Eve (1980). The effect of prostaglandin synthesis inhibitors and diphosphonates on tumour mediated osteolysis. British Journal of Surgery - in press.

Gindler, E.M. and King, J.D. (1972). Rapid colorimetric determination of calcium in biological fluids with methylthymol blue. American Journal of Clinical Pathology, 58, 376-382.

Powles, T.J., Clark, S.A., Easty, D.M., Easty, G.C. and Neville, A.M. (1973). The inhibition by aspirin and indomethacin of osteolytic tumour deposits and hypercalcaemia in rats with Walker tumour and its possible application to human breast cancer. British Journal of Cancer, 28, 316-321.

Powles, T.J., Dowsett, M., Easty, D.M., Easty, G.C. and Neville, A.M. (1976). Breast cancer osteolysis, bone metastases and anti-osteolytic effect of aspirin. Lancet, 1, 608-610.

Seyberth, H.W., Segre, G.V., Morgan, J.L., Sweetman, B.J., Potts, J. and Oates, J.A. (1975). Prostaglandins as mediators of hypercalcaemia associated with certain types of cancer. New England Journal of Medicine, 293, 1278-1283.

Siris, Ethel, S., Sherman, W.H., Baquiran, D.C., Schlatterer, J.P., Osserman, E.F. and Canfield, R.E. (1980). Effects of dichloromethylene diphosphonate on skeletal mobilization of calcium in multiple myeloma. New England Journal of Medicine, 302, 310-315.

van Breukelen, F.J.M., Bijvoet, O.L.M. and van Oosterom, A.T. (1979). Inhibition of osteolytic bone lesions by (3 - amino - 1 - hydroxypropylidene) - 1, 1 - biphosphonate (A.P.D.) Lancet, 1, 803-805.

Voelkel, E.F., Tashjian, A.H. Jr., Franklin, R.B., Wasserman, E. and Levine, L. (1975) Hypercalcaemia and tumour-prostaglandins: the VX2 carcinoma model in rabbits. Metabolism, 24, 973-986.

POTENTIAL CLINICAL USE OF DIPHOSPHONATES AGAINST BONE METASTASES AND HYPERCALCAEMIA OF MALIGNANCY

D.L. Douglas, J.A. Kanis, F.E. Preston, D.J. Beard,
F.E. Neal and R.G.G. Russell

INTRODUCTION

The diphosphonates are analogues of inorganic pyrophosphate containing P-C-P bonds which are stable towards chemical and enzymatic degradation. Their use as drugs is a relatively recent development, the rationale being that several 1,1-substituted diphosphonates (bisphosphonates) inhibit both the growth and dissolution of hydroxyapatite crystals in vitro and retard bone resorption and bone formation in experimental animals. The pharmacology and experimental background to the use of the diphosphonates is reviewed elsewhere (Russell et al., 1976; Fleisch et al., 1977). Only three diphosphonates have been used in clinical studies, namely EHDP (disodium etidronate, or disodium 1-hydroxy-ethylidene-1, 1-diphosphonate), which has been available the longest, and Cl_2MDP (clodronate disodium, or dichloromethylene diphosphonate) and APD (3-amino, 1-hydroxypropylidene-1, 1-diphosphonate).

All three of these compounds are able to inhibit bone resorption in man, an effect which has been demonstrated most clearly in patients with Paget's disease of bone (Altman et al., 1973; Meunier et al, 1979 Frijlink et al., 1979). Each of these compounds produces a dose-dependent inhibition of excessive bone turnover in Paget's disease, as judged by changes in bone histology and also by the suppression of the elevated serum alkaline phosphatase and urinary peptide-bound hydroxyproline, which are indices of the excessive rates of bone

Patient	Diagnosis	Treatment prior to Cl_2MDP	Patient	Diagnosis	Treatment prior to Cl_2MDP
HD	myeloma	saline	TC	myeloma	pred, cyclo
KH	myeloma	-	JS	myeloma	pred, cyclo
IG	myeloma	pred	FH	myeloma	int. pred, melph
TL	Ca bronchus	pred, saline			
AD	Ca breast	pred,	JW	myeloma	pred, cyclo, saline
JB	Ca larynx	-			
DS	myeloma	pred, cyclo, melph, CCNU, saline	MB	Ca breast	-
			VA	Ca breast	-

TABLE 1 Clinical details of 13 patients with hypercalcaemia of malignancy (pred = prednisolone, melph = melphalan, cyclo = cyclophosphamide, CCNU = chloroethyl cyclohexyl nitrosurea).

formation and destruction respectively.

Although these diphosphonates do inhibit bone resorption in man, there has been remarkably little attention paid to their possible use in preventing the excessive bone resorption that may occur in various cancers, particularly in patients with myeloma or with bone metastases due to carcinoma of the breast or bronchus. Excessive bone resorption due either to myeloma or to osteolytic deposits can cause hypercalcaemia, especially when the disease is progressing rapidly and when there is associated impairment of renal glomerular function. Several studies in the recent past (van Breukelen et al., 1979; Siris et al., 1980; Douglas et al., 1980) have shown that both APD and Cl_2MDP are able to inhibit bone resorption and to reverse hypercalcaemia in such patients.

We have been evaluating Cl_2MDP as an inhibitor of bone resorption in patients with Paget's disease of bone, primary hyperparathyroidism and hypercalcaemia of malignancy and report here our experience in the latter group of patients.

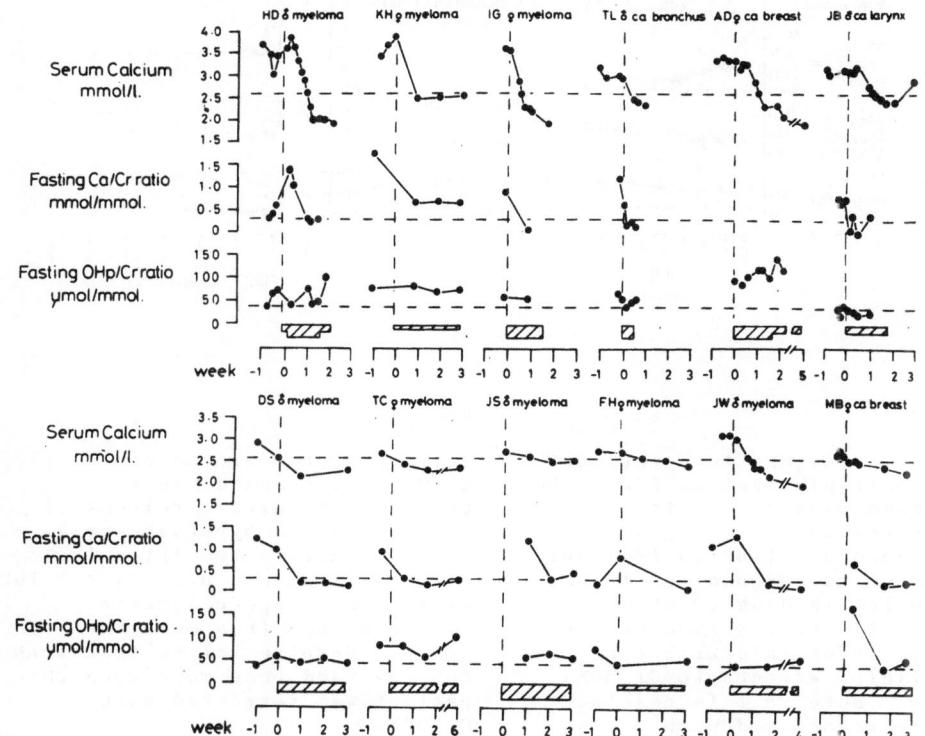

FIG. 1

Changes in serum calcium and fasting urinary calcium and hydroxyproline/creatinine ratios in 12 patients with hypercalcaemia of malignancy treated with Cl_2MDP (0.8-3.2g daily). The hatched bars signify periods of treatment. Data from one patient (VA) with carcinoma of breast who did not respond is not shown.

338

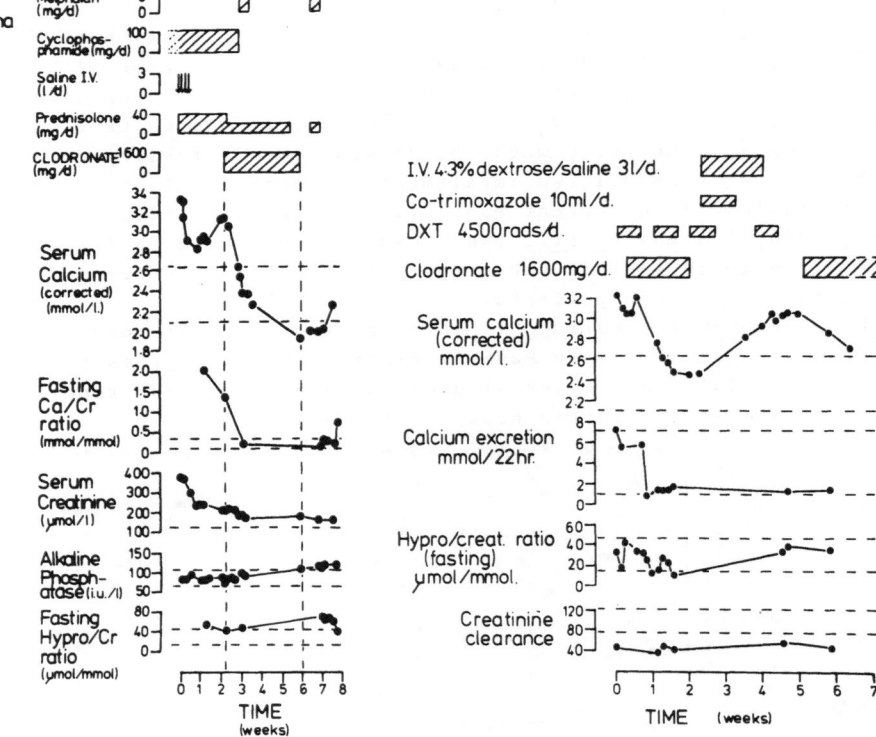

FIG 2

Effect of Cl₂MDP in a patient
with multiple myeloma (JW). He
remained hypercalcaemic despite
prednisolone (40 mg/d) and
intravenous saline (3 l/d) but
appeared to respond to Cl₂MDP.
The multiple drug treatment
given illustrates some of the
difficulties in attributing
beneficial effects to Cl₂MDP
alone. Note fall in calcium
is not associated with a
reduction in hydroxyproline
excretion.

FIG. 3

Effects of two course of
Cl₂MDP (clodronate) in a
patient (JB) with carcinoma of
the larynx and hypercalcaemia.
Note the marked reduction in
serum calcium and urinary calcium
excretion. Hypercalcaemia
recurred when treatment was
stopped despite saline infusions
but reversed once more when the
patient was retreated with
Cl₂MDP.

Each patient received Cl_2MDP usually as a single oral dose of 800-3200 mg daily. The duration of treatment ranged from 4 days to 4 months. All patients had haematological, and serum and urine biochemical measurements before treatment and at frequent intervals (daily or weekly) during treatment. Six of the patients with myeloma were already receiving cytoxic therapy, 8 patients were receiving prednisolone, and 4 patients were receiving intravenous saline as shown in table 1.

RESULTS AND DISCUSSION

Hypercalcaemia was reversed in 12 of the 13 patients (fig. 1) and hypercalciuria in all 13 within days of starting treatment. However, hydroxyproline excretion did not fall consistently as observed previously in patients with hypercalcaemia due to hyperparathyroidism (Douglas et al, 1980) and in those patients with hypercalcaemia of malignancy treated with APD (van Breukelen et al., 1979).

The fall in serum calcium without a simultaneous reduction in urinary excretion of hydroxyproline is difficult to explain, and suggests that Cl_2MDP may not act wholly by inhibiting osteoclastic bone resorption, but may also have other effects, such as by inhibiting osteolytic osteolysis or by decreasing renal tubular reabsorption of calcium. An additional possibility is that the hydroxyprolinuria reflects in part tumour collagen degradation which is unaffected by Cl_2MDP.

In assessing the effects of anti-osteolytic agents it is sometimes difficult to attribute the response to a single drug when patients have received several different treatments including intravenous fluids for acute hypercalcaemia and steroids or cytotoxic agents for their primary disease. A change in concomitant therapy occurred in 3 of the myeloma patients which made it difficult to attribute the fall in serum calcium to Cl_2MDP alone (see fig. 2). However, in the remaining patients Cl_2MDP appeared to be responsible for the fall in serum calcium and urinary calcium excretion (see fig. 3)

These studies suggest that Cl_2MDP is a promising new agent which is capable of reducing the increased bone resorption and hypercalcaemia in many patients with osteolytic deposits in bone. The use of Cl_2MDP and similar compounds as an adjunct to treatment of patients with skeletal neoplasia, with or without hypercalcaemia, is an exciting possibility for future study.

ACKNOWLEDGEMENTS

We thank our colleagues who have contributed to this work and the patients who have taken part. We are most grateful to the Wellcome Trust and to the Procter & Gamble Company, U.S.A., for financial assistance towards these studies.

REFERENCES

Altman, R.D., Johnston, C.C., Khairi, M.R.A., Wellman, H., Serafini, A.N. and Sankey, R.R., 1973. Influence of disodium etidronate on clinical and laboratory manifestations of Paget's disease of bone (Osteitis Deformans). N. Eng. J. Med., 289: 1379-1384.

van Breukelen, F.J.M., Bijvoet, O.L.M., van Oosterom, A.T., 1979. Inhibition of osteolytic bone lesions by 3-amino-1-hydroxypropylidene-1, 1-bisphosphonate (APD). Lancet, i: 803-805.

Canfield, R., Rosner, W., Skinner, J., McWhorter, J., Resnick, L., Feldman, F., Kammerman, S., Ryan, K., Kunigonis, M. and Bohne, W., 1977. Diphosphonate therapy of Paget's disease of bone. J. Clin. Endocr. Metab., 44: 96-106.

Douglas, D.L., Duckworth, T., Russell, R.G.G., Kanis, J.A., Preston, F.E., Prenton, M.A. and Woodhead, J.S., 1980. Effect of dichloromethylene diphosphonate in Paget's disease of bone and in hypercalcaemia due to primary hyperparathyroidism or malignant disease. Lancet, in press.

Fleisch, H. and Russell, R.G.G., 1977. Experimental and clinical studies with pyrophosphate and diphosphonates. In: D.S. David (Editor), Calcium metabolism in renal failure and nephrolithiasis, Wiley, N.Y. pp. 293-336.

Frijlink, W.B., Bijvoet, O.L.M., Velde, J. and Heynen, G., 1979. Treatment of Paget's disease with (3-amino-1-hydroxypropylidene)-1, 1-bisphosphonate (APD). Lancet, i: 799-802.

Khairi, M.R.A., Altman, R.D., DeRosa, G.P., Zimmerman, J., Schenk, R.K. and Johnston, C.C., 1977. Sodium etidronate in the treatment of Paget's disease of bone. Ann. Int. Med., 87: 656-663.

Meunier, P., Chapuy, M.C., Courpron, P., Vignon, E., Edouard, C. and Bernard, J., 1975. Effets cliniques, biologiques et histologiques de l'ethane-1-hydroxy 1, 1-diphosphonate (EHDP) dans la maladie de Paget. Revue du Rhumatisme, 42: 699-705.

Meunier, P.J., Chapuy, M.C., Alexandre, C., Bressot, C., Edouard, C., Vignon, E., Mathien, L. and Trechsel, U. 1979. Effects of disodium dichloromethylene diphosphonate on Paget's disease of bone. Lancet, ii: 489-492.

Russell, R.G.G. and Fleisch, H., 1976. Pyrophosphate and diphosphonates. In: G.H. Bourne (Editor), The biochemistry and physiology of bone: calcification and physiology, Academic Press, N.Y. 61-104.

Russell, R.G.G., Smith, R., Preston, C.J., Walton, R.J. and Woods, C.G., 1974. Diphosphonates in Paget's disease. Lancet, i: 894-898.

Siris, E.S., Sherman, W.M., Baquiran, D.C., Schlatterer, J.P., Osserman, E.F. and Canfield, R.E., 1980. Effects of dichloromethylene diphosphonate on skeletal mobilisation of calcium in multiple myeloma. New Eng. J. Med., 302: 310-315.

MULTIPARAMETRIC BIOCHEMICAL STUDY IN THE DIAGNOSIS OF BONE METASTASIS OF BREAST CANCER

J.L. Boublil, G. Milano, M. Namer, M. Viot, A. Ramaioli, M. Schneider, C.M. Lalanne

INTRODUCTION

Breast cancer is the most common malignant tumor affecting women, and the most frequent site of distant metastases in this localization is bone. Indeed, 85% of patients who die from breast cancer have bone metastasis (Haagensen, 1956; Ackerman, 1970) and early bone metastasis detection is thus extremely important. While conventional X-ray skeletal surveys are not sensitive enough to detect early bone metastasis, radioisotopic bone scanning has been reported highly sensitive in localizing skeletal metastasis; metastases show up on scans earlier than on X-rays by an average of 4 months (Charkes, 1975; Hoffman, 1972). However, these physical methods only reveal patent lesions.

PURPOSE OF THE STUDY

Our goal was to detect subclinical bone metastasis at the moment of early modification of bone structure, as suggested by other authors (Prockop and Sjoerdsma, 1961; Platt et al. 1964; Bonadonna et al., 1966; Powles et al. 1975; Gielen et al., 1976). This search for sensitivity led us to consider biological parameters reflecting bone metabolism, and the principle of a multifactorial biochemical study was adopted. After selection, the most discriminant biological parameters in the diagnosis of bone metastasis were grouped together to obtain a discriminant index. Next, in a prospective study, we evaluated whether this index had a predictive value for bone metastasis during follow-up and could thus be used to monitor treatment.

MATERIALS AND METHODS

Materials

In a retrospective study, 95 patients with breast cancer, aged 30 to 88, were treated and followed up at our Center over a two year period. Each patient underwent clinical examination, a radiological skeletal survey, bone scintigraphy (Te 99) and bone biopsy. Using these findings, the patients were then classified in two groups according to the presence or absence of bone metastasis. The group Mo (n = 50) showed no radiologic or scintigraphic abnormality; both X-rays and scans were negative. The group M+ (n = 45) had definite

radiologic and scintigraphic lesions; X-rays and scans were positive
and there was biopsy-confirmed metastasis. Patients in group Mo
were followed over an additional year to make sure they were not
developing bone metastasis at the time of the multiparametric biochemical evaluation.

Methods

The biochemical evaluation of bone metabolism was assayed every
two months by the following tests: (a) in serum: calcium (Ca), phosphorus (P) and bone isoenzyme of alkaline phosphatase (bone isoE ALP);
(b) in urine: calcium, phosphorus and the hydroxyproline/creatinine
ratio (HP/creat.). We preferred this ratio instead of total urinary
hydroxyproline in order to allow for errors related to urine collection (Powles et al., 1975). A low gelatin diet was necessary 24 hr
before urine collection to avoid false positive hydroxyproline measurements. Calcium was measured by a semi-automated method of CORNING
France, and phosphorus with a commercial kit from HARLECO (Coopérative
Pharmaceutique Française). Hydroxyproline was measured with the
commercial HYDROPRONOSTICON kit (ORGANON TEKNIKA France), creatinine
by the CENTRIFICHEM from UNION CARBIDE and the bone isoenzyme of
alkaline phosphatase with the commercial kit from HELENA France.

RESULTS
Retrospective study

Potential biological discriminators were evaluated one at a time
by computer analysis for their ability to differentiate the two groups
Mo and M+. The hydroxyproline/creatinine ratio was the factor which
best separated the two groups; it correctly classified 90% of all
patients in their respective group. In a second computer analysis,
the other biological parameters were also assayed one at a time to
determine which ones best aided the HP/creat. ratio in differentiation. The only significant factor was the bone isoenzyme of alkaline
phosphatase. Under these conditions, the other biological tests -
calcium and phosphorus in blood and urine - were not statistically
significant in discrimination.

Using a mathematical method, the following equation was then
established for the discriminant index:
I = 0.08254 (HP/creat.) + 0.0131 (bone isoE ALP) - 3.22957

Figure 1 gives the individual values of this index. All patients
without bone metastasis show a negative index. In contrast, of 45
patients with proven bone metastases, 38 have a positive index.

False negatives thus represented 15%.

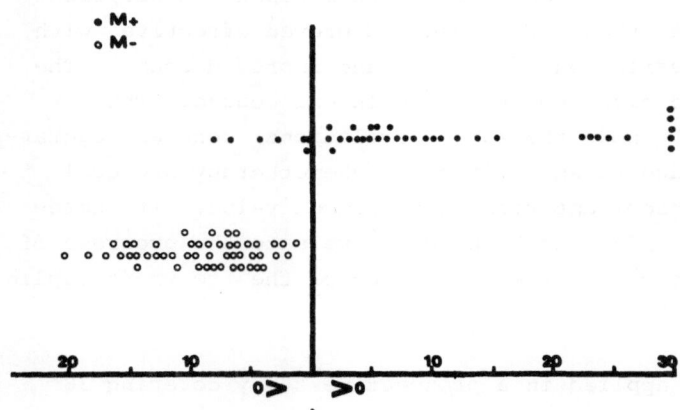

Fig. 1. Individual distributions of the index values for patients in groups Mo and M+

Once established, this index was evaluated for its practical value during patient follow-up. Figure 2 illustrates index evolution during the clinical course of the disease for two group M+ patients, who had bone metastasis and a concomitant positive index at the beginning of their survey.

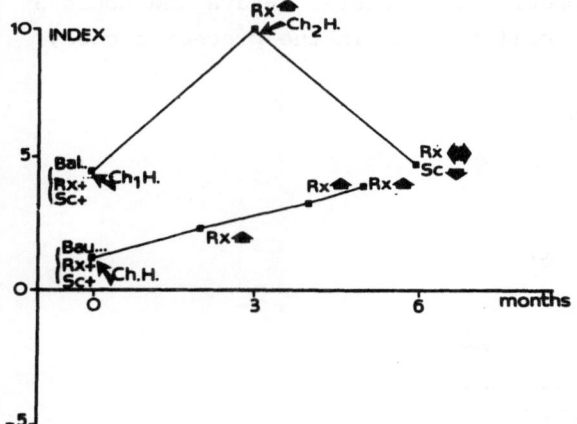

Fig. 2. Index value variation during disease evolution for two breast cancer patients with bone metastases undergoing treatment

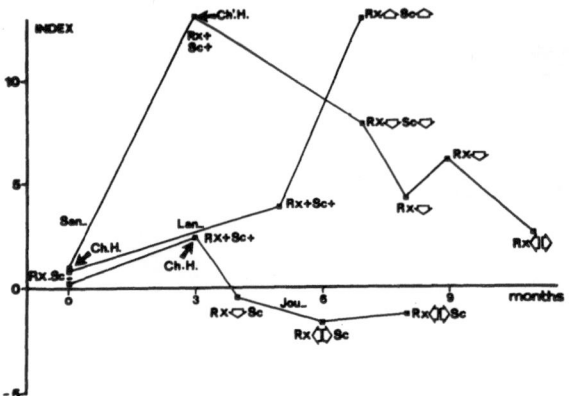

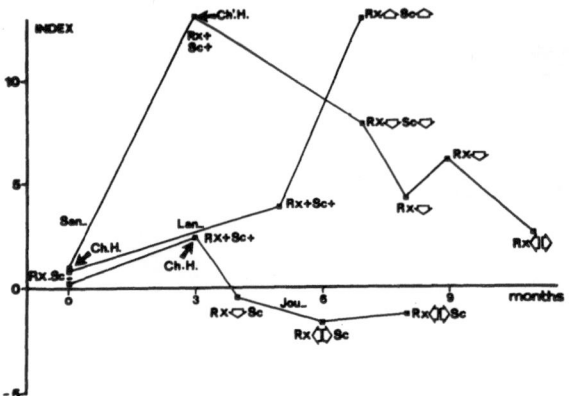

344

The upper curve (Patient 1) reveals that an initial chemotherapy regimen was ineffective in stabilizing the bone lesions; indeed, the lesions were aggravated, as shown by the X-rays taken. A different chemotherapy regimen was then introduced and proved effective, with stabilization of the lesions on the X-rays and improved scans. The index values correlated closely with the clinical course. The lower curve (Patient 2) shows the same correlations: constant aggravation of bone lesions due to an inefficient chemotherapy protocol closely parallels a concomitant rise in the index value. It therefore appears that this index can be used to evaluate the progress of bone lesions, and subsequently the efficiency of the treatment applie

Prospective study

This index was then applied in a prospective study covering 38 patients who all presented a negative index at the outset. After a certain time, 5 of these patients developed a positive index when both radiographic and scintigraphic findings remained normal. One patient, followed for a year, has shown no radiologic or scintigraphi signs of metastases up until now. Another patient, followed up for only 4 months, is in the same situation. These cases could be false positives, but more time is required before a final appraisal.

Figure 3, concerning the remaining 3 patients who developed a positive index, shows the most interesting feature of this index: the fact that, at least in some cases, it has a predictive value. For thei 3 patients, bone metastases appeared on skeletal X-rays and scans 3 months after the index became positive. As in the preceding case,

Fig. 3. Positive index values for three patients with breast cancer before evidence of bone metastases

modification of the chemotherapy regimen once bone metastases were confirmed led to constant improvement of the index, X-rays and scans. Attention should be paid to the "rebound" which occurred at 9 months (descending part of the curve): it can be explained, in view of the constantly improving radiologic images, by analysis of the two parameters composing the index. At the time of the rebound, the HP/creat. ratio had returned to normal due to the stopping of bone lysis. In contrast, a significant rise occurred in bone isoE ALP due to osteoblastic activity (which showed up on X-rays as progressively increasing osteocondensation).

CONCLUSION

The usefulness of urinary HP in the follow-up of breast cancer bone metastases no longer needs be proven, and the bone fraction of ALP can now be evaluated. The association of these 2 parameters, each reflecting different aspects of bone metabolism, is more effective than each one taken alone for diagnosing bone metastases in breast cancer. As well as its diagnostic value, this index evaluates treatment efficiency and constitutes an inexpensive, easy-to-use method for following patients needing constant treatment monitoring. Furthermore, this index had a possible bone metastasis predictive value in a certain number of cases. Of course, its real value in this respect will become evident once a much longer study covering many more cases is completed. Such a study has been in progress at our Center for over 3 years and covers over 200 cases. Finally, since certain conditions such as acute arthritis and Paget's disease may result in false positives, care must be taken to eliminate such cases.

REFERENCES

Ackerman, L.V., Del Regato, J.A., 1970. Cancer diagnosis, treatment and prognosis. Mosby, St. Louis, 830 pp.
Bonadonna, G., Merlino, M.J., Myers, L.W.P., Sonenberg, M., 1966. Urinary hydroxyproline and calcium metabolism in patients with cancer. New Engl J Med, 275: 298-305.
Charkes, N.D., Malmud, L.S., Caswell, T. et al., 1975. Preoperative bone scan use in women with early breast cancer. JAMA, 233: 516-518.
Gielen, F., Dequeker, J., Drochmans, A., Wildiers, J., Merlevede, M., 1976. Relevance of hydroxyproline excretion to bone metastasis in breast cancer. Br J Cancer, 34: 279-285.
Haagensen, C.D., 1956. Diseases of the breast. Saunders, Philadelphia, p. 534.
Hoffman, H.C., Marty, R., 1972. Bone scanning: its value in the preoperative evaluation of patients with suspicious breast masses. Am J Surg, 124: 194-199.
Platt, W.D., Doolittle, L.M., Hartshorn, J.W., 1964. Urinary hydroxyproline excretion in metastatic cancer of the breast. New Engl J Med, 287-290.
Powles, T.J., Leese, C.L., Bondy, P.K., 1975. Hydroxyproline excretion in patients with breast cancer and response to treatment. Br Med J, 2: 164-166.
Prockop, D.J., Sjoerdsma, A., 1961. Significance of urinary hydroxyproline in man. J Clin Invest, 40: 843-849.

ACUTE CHANGES IN CALCITONIN LEVELS IN LUNG CANCER PATIENTS TREATED WITH C. PARVUM: DO THESE REFLECT IN VIVO KILLING OF TUMOUR CELLS?

H.D. Mitcheson, C.J. Hillyard, I. MacIntyre and J.E. Castro

INTRODUCTION

Calcitonin (CT) is a useful biochemical marker for monitoring progress of patients with bronchial carcinoma (McKenzie et al, 1977; Silva et al, 1979). There is considerable evidence that such calcitonin is produced in most cases by the malignant tissues and is not of thyroid origin (Silva et al, 1974; Ellison et al, 1975; Hillyard et al, 1976; Schwartz et al, 1979). We have measured immunoreactive CT in the plasma of patients entered in a prospective randomised study of C.parvum treatment for inoperable bronchial carcinoma.

PATIENTS AND METHODS

Patients: 51 patients with inoperable bronchial carcinoma were studied. 30 had squamous cell, 8 oat cell and 13 carcinomas of other types. All 51 patients received radiotherapy. 25 had no other treatment and acted as controls; 26 were additionally treated with Corynebacterium parvum (Cp) (Wellcome strain CN 6134, 7 mg dry wt/ml) given at a dose of 10 mg/m^2 surface area by intravenous infusion at monthly intervals to a planned total of 4 infusions for each patient. Venous blood samples were taken immediately before, 1 h., 24 h., 48 h. and 5 days after each Cp infusion. After completion of treatment, blood was sampled every 3 months. Control patients also had blood sampled every 3 months.

Plasma calcitonin assay: Peripheral blood samples were collected into cold heparinised tubes, centrifuged and separated immediately. Plasma was frozen and stored at -20°C until assay. Calcitonin was measured by an overnight radioimmunoassay similar to that described by Coombes et al (1974). The antiserum used was raised in rabbits and is directed against the central and C. terminal parts of the calcitonin molecule. Normal calcitonin concentrations (< 0.08 μg/ℓ) are undetectable using this assay.

Whisky test: 6 patients had CT release measured after stimulation with oral whisky, a potent CT secretogogue (Dymling et al, 1976). Whisky given to normal healthy volunteers increases CT but not above the detection limits of this assay (Hillyard et al, 1977).

Surgery: As a control for non-specific stress causing CT release, 2 patients had CT levels compared after oral whisky and major surgery not related to their tumours (one had urethroplasty, the other transurethral resection of prostate).

Statistics: Non-parametric data were ranked using the Wilcoxon test for paired data.

RESULTS

Elevated plasma CT was found in 39 of the 51 patients (76%) before treatment. The highest level was in a patient with a squamous cell carcinoma. 32 patients had sequential CT measurements and in 27 these related accurately to clinical progress (e.g. Fig. 1). In 2 the CT levels did not correlate with clinical progress and in 3 others CT was undetectable.

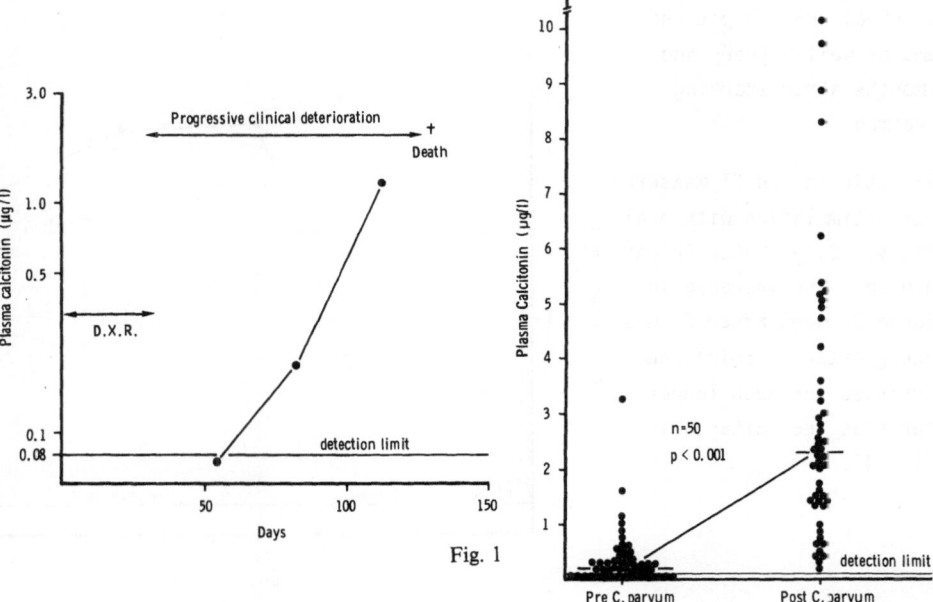

Fig. 1

Fig. 2

Cp caused a massive acute increase in plasma calcitonin in all patients (Fig. 2). This developed several hours after infusion, was maximal at 48 h. and returned to basal after 5 days. For 23 patients receiving a total of 50 infusions the median CT concentration before infusion was 0.18 µg/ℓ (range < 0.08 - 3.3) and the median after 48 h. was 2.32 µg/ℓ (range 0.19 - 25.88). This increase was statistically highly significant (p < 0.001).

Patients who responded to treatment with radiotherapy and Cp showed
reduction in tumour size and became well.   Fig. 3 shows sequential CT
levels in one such patient
who had a squamous cell
bronchial carcinoma. His
CT level was elevated
before treatment, increased
acutely with each Cp infusion
and fell progressively after
each infusion. After the
fourth infusion CT was no
longer detectable. 14
months later the CT level
increased on one occasion
but subsequently returned
to normal and the patient
remains well 2 years and
6 months -after starting
treatment.

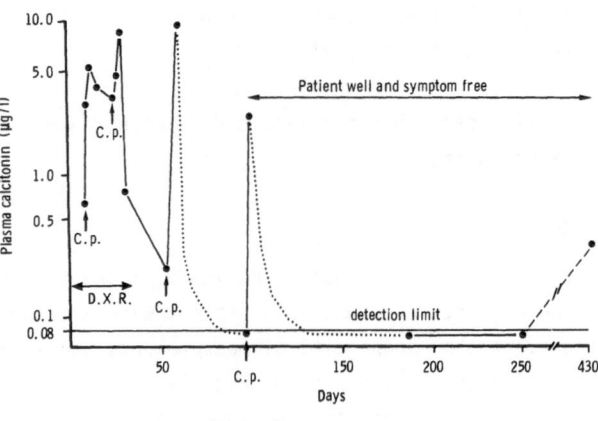

Fig. 3

Six patients had CT measured
after stimulation with oral
whisky. 24 h. later Cp was
infused. The increase in
plasma CT seen after Cp was
much greater (5-fold) and
persisted for much longer
than that seen after whisky
(Fig. 4).

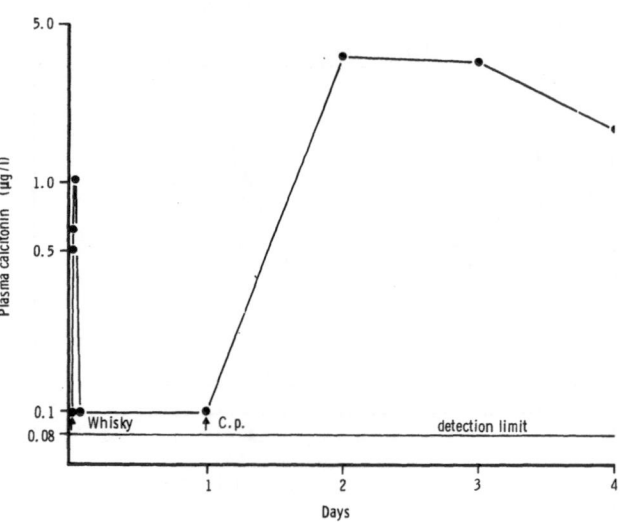

Fig. 4

Two other patients had CT
release measured after
stimulation with oral
whisky. 24 hours later
they underwent surgery
not related to their
bronchial neoplasms. Both
patients had an acute
increase in CT after whisky
but surgery did not
provoke CT release (Fig. 5)

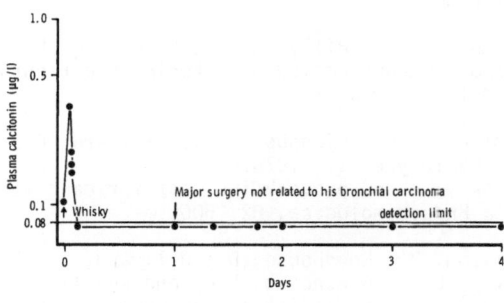

Fig. 5

DISCUSSION

39 of the 51 patients (76% with bronchogenic carcinoma had abnormal CT
levels. This is greater than the 59% reported by McKenzie et al (1977),
52% by Silva et al (1979) and 38% by Schwartz et al (1979) and may be due
to our patients all having advanced inoperable tumours. We confirmed that
calcitonin is a useful biochemical marker for monitoring the progress of
patients with bronchial carcinoma. Calcitonin is produced in most cases
by the malignant tissue and is not of thyroid origin (Silva et al, 1974;
Ellison et al, 1975; Hillyard et al, 1976; Schwartz et al, 1979), however
one patient with adenocarcinoma of the lung has been reported (Silva et al,
1975) where the hypercalcitoninaemia was due to thyroid secretion.

Cp caused a massive acute increase in plasma CT in all patients. This can
not be attributed solely to simple release of available CT from thyroid
and malignant tissue since the increase was 5-fold and persisted for much
longer than that caused by oral whisky.

Patients treated with Cp were very ill for several days. We reasoned that
the stress of treatment stimulating the adreno-pituitary axis might cause
increased synthesis and increased secretion of CT. However patients who
underwent the stress of major surgery did not develop hypercalcitoninaemia
despite having abnormally increased CT levels after oral whisky. Those
who responded well to treatment with radiotherapy and Cp had a dramatic
acute rise in CT with Cp and a subsequent lower basal level of CT. We
suggest that Cp may cause tumour cell death, cell lysis and liberation of
stored ectopic CT into the circulation causing the acute hypercalcitoninaemia,
followed by a lower basal CT level produced by the reduced tumour cell burden.

References

Coombes, R.C., Hillyard, C., Greenberg, P.B. and MacIntyre, I. 1974.
Plasma immunoreactive calcitonin in patients with non-thyroid tumours.
Lancet, i, 1080.

Dymling, J.F., Ljungberg, O., Hillyard, C.J., Greenberg, P.B., Evans, I.M.A.
and MacIntyre, I. 1976.
Whisky: A new provocative test for calcitonin secretion.
Acta Endocrinologica, 82, 500.

Ellison, M., Woodhouse, D., Hillyard, C., Dowsett, M., Coombes, R.C.,
Gilby, E.D., Greenberg, P.B. and Neville, A.M. 1975.
Immunoreactive calcitonin production by human lung carcinoma cells in
culture.
Br. J. Cancer, 32, 373.

Hillyard, C.J., Coombes, R.C., Greenberg, P.B., Galante, L.S. and
MacIntyre, I. 1976.
Calcitonin in breast and lung cancer.
Clin. Endocrinol. 5, 1.

Hillyard, C.J., Cooke, T.J.C., Coombes, R.C., Evans, I.M.A. and MacIntyre, I
1977
Normal plasma calcitonin: circadian variation and response to stimuli.
Clin. Endocrinol., 6, 291.

McKenzie, C.G., Evans, I.M.A., Hillyard, C.J., Hill, P., Carter, S.,
Tan, M.K. and MacIntyre, I. 1977.
Biochemical markers in bronchial carcinoma.
Br. J. Cancer, 36, 700.

Schwartz, K.E., Wolfsen, A.R., Forster, B. and Odell, W.D., 1979.
Calcitonin in non-thyroidal cancer.
J. Clin. Endocrinol. Metab. 49, 438.

Silva, O.L., Becker, K.L., Primack, A., Doppman, J. and Snider, R.H. 1974.
Ectopic secretion of calcitonin by oat-cell carcinoma.
New Eng. J. Med. 1122.

Silva, O.L., Becker, K.L., Primack, A., Doppman, J.L. and Snider, R.H. 1975.
Hypercalcaemia in bronchogenic cancer. Evidence for thyroid origin of the
hormone.
J.A.M.A. 234, 183.

Silva, O.L., Broder, L.E., Doppman, J.L., Snider, R.H., Moore, C.F.,
Cohen, M.H. and Becker, K.L. 1979.
Calcitonin as a marker for bronchogenic cancer.
Cancer, 44, 680.

SERIAL QUANTITATIVE BONE SCANNING OF METASTATIC TUMOUR IN RATS

D.G. Williams, S.P. Parbhoo, J.E. Agnew and B.A. Stoll

INTRODUCTION

Skeletal scintigraphy is claimed to be a sensitive method of detecting bone metastases, particularly since the introduction of the Technetium-99M radionuclides linked to bone-seeking diphosphonate compounds, such as methylene diphosphonic acid (MDP) (Büll et al, 1977a). Quantitative estimation of the uptake of these compounds has been advocated as a means of assessing the progress of bone metastases and of their response to treatment (Büll et al, 1977b). It requires the use of a gamma camera attached to a computer system.

Serial quantitative scanning has been reported in an attempt to follow the effect of chemotherapy in patients with advanced breast cancer. (Alexander et al 1976). The rate of uptake of Technetium MDP is thought to be related to osteoblastic activity but there is a paucity of investigations on the relationship between quantitative change in the scan and serial change in tumour size.

The aim of this investigation is to follow the natural course of a metastasis in rat bone of Walker 256 carcinosarcoma, using serial quantitative 99m Tc-MDP scanning. An attempt is made to correlate the findings with histological and radiographic changes in the tumour.

MATERIALS AND METHODS

Animal Tumour System

Injection of Walker 256 carcinosarcoma cells into the aorta of a rat will cause osteolytic bone tumour deposits in the legs and also hypercalcemia (Powles et al 1972) For the purposes of the experiments, suspensions of Walker 256 cells (Chester Beatty Research Institute, Strain P385) were obtained by aspirating ascites from host animals in which tumour cells had been passaged. Suspensions containing 10^3 viable tumour cells in 0.2 ml of saline were prepared for injection.

The abdominal aortas of male Wistar rats weighing 80-120 gm were exposed under ether anaesthesia and the common iliac vessels supplying the left leg were temporarily clamped. The cell suspension was injected into the aorta in a caudal direction, using a specially-angled 30 FG hypodermic needle, such that the cells injected were directed into the right common iliac vessels of the right leg. Control animals matched for weight and age were injected with 0.2 ml saline containing no cells.

This technique produced osteolytic bone lesions in the right legs of the rats, predominantly around the knee joints. The bone deposits increase uniformly in size over a period of 16-18 days until the death or sacrifice of the rat. There were 15 rats in each of the control non-injected and saline-injected groups and 14 animals in the experimental group.

MONITORING OF TUMOUR 1. Bone Scanning

Commercially obtained 99m Tc-MDP (The Radiochemical Centre, Amersham, England) was prepared in conventional manner. A dose of 0.8 mCi. in a volume of 0.2 ml was injected each time into a tail vein of each rat $1\frac{1}{2}$-2 hours prior to scanning. Under ether anaesthesia, the animals were each placed prone with limbs outstretched and fixed in a standard position on the surface of a high-resolution gamma camera interfaced with a 32K mini computer. Counting commenced and continued until a total of 150,000 counts was obtained, producing a total body skeletal scan. This involved a scanning time of 3 - 4 minutes. The data were digitally recorded on a 64 x 64 grid and stored on a magnetic tape.

2. Serial Quantitative Analysis of Scan

The scan data for each animal were processed to produce a numerical whole skeleton 'print-out'. The uptake of radionuclide in the tumour-bearing area of each leg was determined by summating the number of counts contained in a specified 'region of interest' (ROI) on the print out encompassing a matrix of 9 cells at the maximum resolution of the camera. This represented an area which was known to include both femoral and tibial epiphyses and adjacent metaphyses and each ROI represented an anatomical area of 1.32 cm square.

The ratio of counts in this area to the whole body count was calculated and expressed as a percentage (percentage uptake) for each limb in each animal. The ratio of counts in the ROI in the right leg to the counts in the ROI in the left leg (CR/CL) was also estimated for each animal and expressed as the 'inter-limb' ratio. The values for percentage uptake in controls and experimental animals were recorded and the change in inter-limb ratios on serial scanning were noted.

Statistical analyses of the data were performed using the student's "t" test for determining the level of significance of the differences between the values of control and experimental groups and between the values obtained for changes in the inter-limb ratios in the experimental group.

3.   Radiography

Fine detail skeletal radiography was carried out on all animals on alternate days from the time of tumour induction, corresponding with the time of bone scanning, using fine grain (Kodak-type M) film. The time of first appearance of a lytic lesion was noted and an estimate of its size and rate of growth was made.

4.   Histology

Histological sections were examined from all tumour-bearing and normal hind legs. Longitudinal sections in the sagittal plane through the knee joints were cut, fixed, decalcified and stained with haematoxylin and eosin and examined microscopically. Six animals were killed following tumour induction at differing time intervals during the course of the scanning programme in order to determine the natural history of the tumour. Histological material was obtained from all other animals at the end of the scanning programme to confirm the presence of tumour.

RESULTS

The percentage uptake of 99m TcMDP in the knees of the control rats showed no significant difference in the mean uptake between normal non-injected animals and saline-injected animals, nor between injected and non-injected legs in the same rat, nor was there any difference between the mean uptake in single scans and the mean in those animals subjected to sequential scanning. The overall mean value of 4.01% + 0.23 (n=50) corresponds well with the percentage uptake found by other workers for different radionuclides (Genant, et al 1974). The co-efficient of variation indicates a predictable uptake for normals and allows of ready recognition when differencs exist between control and experimental animals. The mean value of inter-limb ratios, i.e. right-left knee counts (CR/CL) was close to unity in all controls (0.99 + 0.01) again permitting ready recognition of inter-limb differences related to experimental manipulation.

The results of serial bone scanning in the tumour-bearing rats are shown in the graph.

354

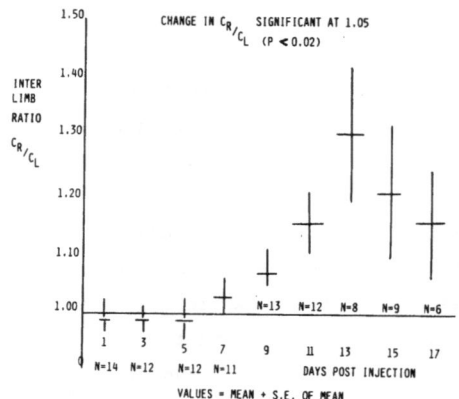

CHANGE IN c_{R/C_L} SIGNIFICANT AT 1.05 (P < 0.02)

VALUES = MEAN ± S.E. OF MEAN

99m Technetium MDP Bone Scanning in Rats.

Graph showing mean values of inter limb ratios of all animals on each day of sequential bone scanning plotted against the number of days following tumour injection in experimental rats.

An inter-limb ratio greater than 1.05 has been taken to indicate significant increase in radionuclide uptake in the tumour-injected limb. There was no increase in the uptake of radionuclide in the tumour-injected limbs for the first 5 days. A significant difference was, however, present by the 9th day after tumour-implantation and the uptake subsequently increased until a peak was reached by Day 13. Diminution in uptake began after Day 15.

Study of fine resolution radiographs taken in conjunction with the bone scans showed the first appearance of recognisable lytic lesions to be after Day 10.

These lytic areas increased in size until destruction of the bony metaphysis and epiphysis had occurred. Measurement of these lesions indicated that the earliest recognizable area of lysis measured 0.2 cm diameter and that the lytic area doubled in size in 48 hours.

The earliest appearance of tumour cells in the histological study of the tumour's natural history was at 5-6 days after injection. Their appearance in the bone marrow at the metaphysis was followed by the proliferation of new bone on existing bony trabeculae. As the tumour cells increased in numbers, bone destruction and replacement of marrow and of cortical bone by tumour cells was noted.

DISCUSSION

The results of isotope studies in the control animals confirm the reproducibility of the counting technique and suggest that any observation of deviation from unity in the inter-limb ratio is of significance.

The increased sensitivity of the computerized scan readings over conventional x-ray examination is shown by the observation that the first radiographic evidence of the tumour was preceded up to 48 hours earlier by a significant change in the quantitative scan. Since the minimum size of lytic lesions detectable in the x-ray was 0.2 cm diameter, the scan was recording activity in a lesion smaller than this.

A major histological change found associated with tumour growth was new bone formation and evidence of simultaneous bone destruction as suggested by the present of osteoclasts. In our experiments, progression in the level of uptake in the quantitative scan mirrored the histological appearance of new bone formation. However, as tumour bulk increased and bone destruction predominated, new bone formation ceased. This change was reflected in the later fall seen in the uptake as the avidity for radionuclide diminsihed.

Clinically, quantitative bone scanning has been advocated for monitoring response of bone metastases to treatment, particularly in the scan-positive, x-ray-negative asymptomatic patient undergoing systemic chemotherapy. The technique is equally of value in the patient with radiographically-demonstrable metastases, if scanning techniques permit evidence of response before x-ray techniques. Radiographic evidence of healing is rarely established until 4-6 months after systemic treatment is started and even then is subject to considerable observer-bias. We are currently assessing the role of this technique in patients with metastatic breast cancer undergoing systemic therapy (Parbhoo, et al 1980).

REFERENCES

ALEXANDER J.L., GILLESPIE P.J., EDELSTEYN G.A., Serial Bone scanning using Technetium 99M Diphosphonate in patients undergoing cyclical combination chemotherapy for advanced breast cancer. Clinical Nuclear Medicine 1976 1 13-17.
BULL U., PFIEFFE R J.P., NIENDORF H.P., TONGENDORFF J. A computer assisted comparison of 99m Tc-Methylene Diphosphonate and 99m Tc-polyphosphonate bone imaging. British Journal of Radiology 1977 629-636.
BULL U., SCHUSTER H., PFIEFFER J.P., TONGENDORFF J., NIENDORF H.P. Bone to bone and joint to joint ratios in normal and diseased skeletal states using region of interest technique and bone seeking radio-pharmaceuticals. Nuklearmedizin 1977 16 104-112.
GENANT H.K., BAUTOVICH G.J., SINGH M., LATHROP K.A., HARPER P.V. Bone seeking radionuclides: an in vivo study of factors affecting skeletal uptake. Radiology 1974 113 373-383.
PARBHOO S.P. ALANI H., STOLL B.A., AGNEW J.E. Proceedings of E.O.R.T.C. 1980
POWLES T.J., CLARK S.A., EASTY D.M., EASTY G.G., MUNRO-NEVILLE A. The inhibition by aspirin and indomethacin of osteolytic tumour deposits and hypercalcemia in rats with Walker tumour, and its possible application to human breast cancer. British Journal of Cancer 1973 28 316-321.

EXPERIMENTAL STUDY ON CHARACTERISTICS OF MICROCIRCULATION IN TUMOR TISSUE, WITH REFERENCE TO CANCER CHEMOTHERAPY

M. Suzuki, K. Hori, I. Abe, S. Saito and H. Sato

INTRODUCTION

Selective increase of tumor blood flow, together with drug sensitivity of tumor cells, is important in cancer chemotherapy with reference to enhancement of the delivery of anticancer drugs selectively to tumor tissue.

Several authors (Kligerman and Hensel, 1961, Gullino and Grantham, 1962, Cater et al., 1966, Edlich et al., 1966, Rankin et al., 1977, Mattson et al., 1978) have reported that tumor vessels might be sensitive to some vasoactive drugs; however, there are few research reports about selective increase of blood flow in tumor tissue.

This report deals with some results obtained in a series of experiments on the functional characteristics of tumor tissue in which blood flow was increased markedly by angiotensin-induced hypertension, enhancing the chemotherapeutic effect due to in-creased drug delivery selectively into tumor tissue. A part of this investigation has been reported elsewhere (Suzuki et al.,1977, 1978, 1979a,b).

MATERIALS AND METHODS

Animals and tumors

Male Donryu rats (Nippon Rat Co., Urawa, Japan), weighing 110 to 130g, were used. Tumor cells of Yoshida rat ascites hepatoma AH109A and AH272 maintained in this laboratory were employed in this series of experiments.

Measurement of blood pressure

The mean arterial blood pressure was monitored electrically through a poly-ethylene catheter inserted into the left femoral artery or the left common carotid artery.

Elevation of blood pressure

The blood pressure was elevated gradually by the infusion of angiotensin II (Hypertensin, CIBA, Basel, Switzerland) into the tail vein, under operation of an infusion pump. The dose of angiotensin II infused was at a rate of 1-2 μg/kg/min.

Analysis of pressure-flow relationship

Local tissue blood flow was determined by a thermoelectrical method with a crossed thermocouple flow meter (Unique Medical Co., Tokyo, Japan) as modified by Takahashi (1964) and hydrogen clearance technique (Aukland et al., 1964). Changes in blood flow by thermoelectrical method were examined as follows: Blood flow at normal pressure was designated as 100% and the one at the moment of sacrificing the animal was designated as 0%.

In order to determine the pressure-flow relation by hydrogen clearance technique, the method described by Pasztor et al (1973) was employed. The correlation between pressure and flow was analyzed by examining either normal tissues (the liver, brain, bone marrow of the femur and subcutis) or tumor tissue. The details of the method have been given elsewhere (Suzuki et al., 1978, 1979).

Chemotherapeutic effect

Tumor cells of AH272(2×10^6) were inoculated subcutaneously to the back of each rat. The animals were divided into following 3 groups. Group 1 (8 rats) served as the control. Group 2 (8 rats) was given mitomycin-C alone. Group 3 (14 rats) was treated with mitomycin-C in combination with angiotensin II. The treatments started on day 17 after transplantation and once a day for the following 5 days, giving a daily dose of 0.5mg/kg of mitomycin-C. The process of treatment in Group 3 was as follows: (1) The blood pressure was elevated gradually. (2) When the mean arterial blood pressure rose to 140 mmHg, anticancer drug was injected in one shot into the tail vein. (3) This pressure was kept for 10 minutes following administration of the drug. The pressure was monitored by using monitor rats instead of Group 3.

In vivo analysis of blood flow in tumor vessel

In vivo observation of tumor blood flow was studied micro-scopically in an early stage of tumor (AH109A) growth in a trans-parent chamber modified by Yamaura et al., (1971) set up in the back of rat. Microcinematograph was taken with a 16mm high spead camera (500 fr/sec), being analyzed with the use of film motion analyzer.

RESULTS

Pressure-flow relationship in tumor tissues and normal tissues

The results obtained from 12 cases of subcutaneously trans-planted AH109A tumor by means of thermoelectrical method were summarized as follows: With elevation of the mean arterial blood pressure from normotension up to approximately 150 mmHg by infusion of angiotensin II, tissue blood flow in tumor was increased to $480.3 \pm 255.1\%$ (mean $\pm$ SD) (P<0.01).

The pressure-flow relationship obtained by hydrogen clearance technique for intramuscular tumor of the thigh produced by trans-plantation of AH109A cells was as follows: When the pressure was elevated from 101.1 ± 3.3 to 147.8 ± 3.6 mmHg by angiotensin II, tumor blood flow rose from 10.0 ± 5.6 to 36.7 ± 22.6 ml/min/100g (P<0.01), i.e. the flow was increased to $390.0 \pm 120.9\%$ by angio-tensin-induced hypertension. Similar results were obtained for intrahepatically transplanted AH109A tumor and subcutaneously transplanted one.

Almost unchanged or rather decreased blood flow was observed in normal tissues such as the liver, brain, bone marrow and subcutis either by thermoelectrical method or hydrogen clearance technique when the mean arterial pressure was elevated up to approximately 160 mmHg.

Enhancement of chemotherapeutic effect

Although moderate effect was observed in group 2 given mito-mycin-C alone as compared to the growth in group 1 as the control, the regrowth of tumor was recognized in all animals of group 2 about one week after ending the treatment.

In group 3, however, marked enhancement of the chemotherapeutic effect was noted in combination with angiotensin II. The regrowth of tumor occurred in nine out of 14 animals, being delayed about 4 days, compared with group 2. In the remaining 5 rats, the tumors disappeared completely and the animals became free of tumor. On the effect for tumor growth, the difference between group 2 and group 3 was highly significant ($P < 0.01$). Besides the effects on the main tumors in group 3, moderate to marked decrease of lymph-node metastasis was noted in size and incidence, unlike other groups.

In vivo analysis of blood flow in tumor vessels

Marked increase of blood flow was also observed in an early stage of tumor growth in a transparent chamber during angiotensin-induced hypertension. In the analysis of microcinematograph taken with a high speed camera, some 2 fold dilated vessels were noticed, during a period when the pressure was elevated to 140 mmHg. Furthermore, the velocity of blood flow became evidently much faster.

DISCUSSION

There is no autoregulation of blood flow in tumor vessels. They are passive and the vascular bed is unaffected directly by angiotensin II. As a result, tumor blood flow was increased by several fold during the period when the mean arterial blood pressure was elevated to approximately 150 mmHg, while it was almost unchanged or decreased in normal tissues. Selective increase of blood flow by angiotensin-induced hypertension is a unique functional characteristic in tumor tissue, and it is inferred that it would give selective enhancement of the delivery of anticancer drugs, administered systemically, into malignant tissues. Enhanced chemotherapeutic effect clearly resulted because of increased drug delivery based on the characteristics of tumor tissue.

Since the first attempt to quantitate blood flow of tumors by Gullino and Grantham (1961), the number of related reports has increased. The results obtained demonstrate that tumor blood flow was rather small at normotension, suggesting that drug delivery is a bottleneck in the way of cancer chemotherapy, quite apart from the problem of drug sensitivity of tumor cells.

A possible enhancement of chemotherapeutic effects could be estimated even in micrometastatic foci, considering the character- istics of microcirculation in the early stages of a tumor focus growing in a transparent chamber as a model of micrometastasis in cancer.

REFERENCES

Aukland, K., Bower, B.F. and Berliner, R.W., 1964. Measurement of local blood flow with hydrogen gas. Circulation Res., 14: 164-187.

Cater, D.B., Adair, H.M. and Grove, C.A., 1966. Effects of vasomotor drugs and "mediators" of the inflammatory reaction upon the oxygen tension of tumours and tumour blood-flow. British J. Cancer, 20: 504-516.

Edlich, R.F., Rogers, W., DeShazo, C.V., Jr. and Aust, J.B., 1966. Effect of vasoactive drugs on tissue blood flow in the hamster melanoma. Cancer Res., 26: 1420-1424.

Gullino, P.M. and Grantham, F.H., 1961. Studies on the exchange of fluids between host and tumor. II. The blood flow of hepatomas and other tumors in rats and mice. J. Natl. Cancer Inst., 27: 1465-1491.

Gullino, P.M. and Grantham, F.H., 1962. Studies on the exchange of fluids between host and tumor. III. Regulation of blood flow in hepatomas and other rat tumors. J. Natl. Cancer Inst., 28: 211-229.

Kligerman, M.M. and Henel, D.K., 1961. Some aspects of the microcirculation of a transplantable experimental tumor. Radiology, 76: 810-817.

Mattson, J., Appelgen, L., Karlsson, L. and Peterson, H. -I., 1978. Influence o vasoactive drugs and ishaemia on intra-tumour blood flow. Europ. J. Cancer, 14: 761-764.

Pasztor, E., Symon, L., Dorsch, N.W.C. and Branston, N.M., 1973. The hydrogen clearance method in assessment of blood flow in cortex, white matter and deep nuclei of baboons. Stroke, 4: 556-567.

Rankin, J.H.G., Jirtle, R. and Phernetton, T.M., 1977. Anomalous responses of tumor vasculature to norepinephrine and prostagrandin E_2 in the rabbit. Circ. Res., 41: 496-502.

Suzuki, M., Hori, K., Abe, I., Saito, S. and Sato, H., 1977. Characteristic blood circulation in tumor tissue, with reference to local permeation of drug in cancer chemotherapy. Proc. Jap. Cancer Assoc., The 36th Annual Meeting. P.149.

Suzuki, M., Hori, K., Abe, I., Saito, S. and Sato, H., 1978. Characteristic blood circulation in tumor tissue, with reference to cancer chemotherapy. Cancer and Chemotherapy, 5(Suppl. 1): 77-80.

Suzuki, M., Hori, K., Abe, I., Saito, S. and Sato, H., 1979. Characteristic of microcirculation in tumor. Cancer and Chemotherapy, 6(Suppl. II): 287-291.

Suzuki, M., Hori, K., Abe, I., Saito, S. and Sato, H., 1979. Characteristic microcirculation of tumor. J. Jap. Coll. Angiol., 19: 233-236.

Takahashi, T., 1964. Studies on hepatic circulation by crosed double thermocouple. Folia Pharmacol. Jap., 60; 308-325.

Yamaura, H., Suzuki, M. and Sato, H., 1971. Transparent chamber in the rat skin for studies on microcirculation on cancer tissue. Gann. 62: 177-185.

DEVELOPMENT OF SEVERE RADIATION PHEUMONITIS IN PATIENTS WITH OAT CELL CARCINOMA DURING COMBINED MODALITY THERAPY

J.H. Karstens, J. Ammon and W. Frik

INTRODUCTION

The concomitant use of various cancer chemotherapeutic agents in combination with radiotherapy and corticosteroids is included in the treatment scheme for several malignancies. Especially in patients with small cell carcinoma of the lung the initial treatment is combination chemotherapy with chest and skull irradiation. In these patients the lung radiation therapy is capable of rapid tumor shrinkage. The addition of chemotherapy to chest irradiation has furthermore allowed effective control of distant metastases. The combination of these two regimen (combined modality therapy) is now the treatment of choice for patients with small cell carcinoma of the lung (Makoski et al., 1977).

Among the side effects of this therapy drug-induced lung disease is a well know complication in the monotherapy with several antineoplastic drugs (Morrison et al, 1979). Recently diffuse interstitial changes in the lung have also been described in patients treated by a polychemotherapy regimen without previous radiotherapy (Bargon et al., 1978). In patients with bronchial neoplasm the addition of radiotherapy to chemotherapy appears to induce diffuse pulmonary interstitial changes (Bleher et al., 1979).

We studied the radiographic effects on lung tissue in a group of patients with small cell carcinoma (extensive disease). The patients were treated by a combination of radiotherapy and polychemotherapy (Ammon et al., 1979). Some of these patients developed a radiation pneumonitis with severe dyspnoe, fever and non-productive cough. These cases are notable in view of the severity of the radiation pneumonitis which occurred after the abrupt or rapidly tapered cessation of corticosteroids. To our knowledge severe radiation pneumonitis precipitated by withdrawal of corticosteroids has only been reported in patients with malignant lymphoma (Kaplan, 1972; Parris et al., 1979).

METHODS, MATERIALS AND FINDINGS

From 1976 until 1979, 52 patients with a histological confirmed diagnosis of small cell carcinoma (extensive disease) of the lung received radiation therapy and combined chemotherapy. The pre-therapeutic evaluation of these patients usually included CT of the skull, liver- and bone-scanning and chest radiography. As for the radiotherapy a median dose of 40 Gy was delivered through an anterio: field which included the apparent tumor mass and the mediastinum. The medium field size was 8 x 12cm. Treatment was administered continuously with 20 fractions by a 42-MeV-Betatron, using photons, without a split course. A chemotherapeutic regimen, based on the publication of Hornback et al. (1976) preceeded the radiotherapy. The addition of corticosteroids apparently gives better results (Senn, Jungi, 1976). Table 1 briefly summarizes our regimen. Radiotherapy was in the majority of cases started after the sixth course of chemotherapy.

Week	Mo	Tu	We	Th	Fr	Sa	So
1	A	V	C	C	-	-	-
2	-	-	-	-	-	-	-
3	A	V	C	C	-	-	-
4	-	-	-	-	-	-	-
5	A	V	C	C	-	-	-
6	-	-	-	-	-	-	-
7	A	V	C	C	-	-	-

A - 40 mg Adriamycin/m^2
V - 1 mg Vincristine
C - 500 mg Cyclophosphamide

Table 1: Scheme of cytostatic therapy for patients with small cell carcinoma.

Four patients (8%) developed radiation pneumonitis with severe symptoms. The data of these four patients are given in Table 2. This table shows the temporal relationship between corticosteroid withdrawal and the onset of symptoms.

Patient	age	radiation dose	No. of cytost. cycle	onset of symptoms after prednisone withdrawal	survival time
P. Ma.	77	42 Gy	V	9 days	4 years (alive)
F. Kl.	55	40 Gy	IV	8 days	11 month
M. Li.	68	31 Gy	VIII	5 days	12 month (alive)
R. Kr.	40	27 Gy	V	3 days	7 month

Table 2: Temporal relationship between corticosteroid withdrawal and onset of symptoms.

REPRESENTATIVE CASE REPORT

A 55-year old man came to treatment with a massive lesion of the left lung. Excision of a supraclavicular lymphnode revealed small cell carcinoma. Because of severe dyspnea he underwent radiotherapy as an initial treatment. The patient remained free of symptoms for three months when a recurrence made chemotherapy necessary. Eight days after the 4th course the patient was readmitted with severe dyspnea, fever, malaise and cough. Chest radiography revealed mixed interstitial and alveolar infiltrates with a distribution corresponding to the radiation field previously used (Fig.1a). Because of the probable diagnosis of radiation pneumonitis secondary to steroid withdrawal prednisone (40 mg daily) and additional antibiotics and gammaglobulin were administered. Repeated chest radiography 14 days later showed almost complete regression of the infiltrates (Fig.1b). The prednisone dose was slowly tapered over a period of 6 weeks. The patient received the additional courses. Prednisone was eliminated in the further courses.

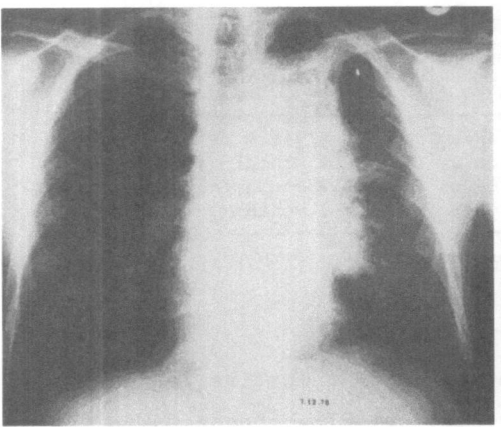 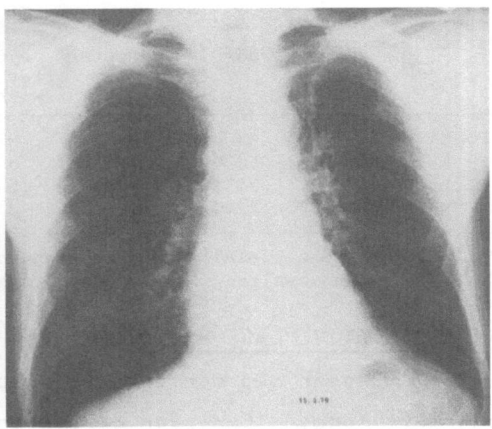

Fig. 1a: The distribution of
infiltrates corresponds to
the radiation field previously
used.(7.12.78)

Fig. 1b: Chest radiography
3 months later shows almost
complete regression of the
infiltrates.(15.3.79)

DISCUSSION

Patients who receive radiation to lungs in the course of
radiotherapy develop radiation pneumonitis two to four months after
onset of treatment, and a number of these develop fibrosis 8-12
months later. The actual incidence of the pulmonary complication
is difficult to determine. In patients with bronchial neoplasms
13% of the patients may show radiographic changes (Hellman et al.,
1964). Both the occurrence and severity of radiation pneumonitis
depend on several factors, the concomitant use of antineoplastic
drugs and radiotherapy in patients with lung cancer is reported
to give a rather high incidence of late changes in lung tissue
(Bleher et al., 1979).

There are no reports about the possible role of steroid withdrawal causing severe radiation pneumonitis in patients with small
cell carcinoma of the lung. Our findings are based on a group of
52 patients treated by a combined modality therapy (Table 1).
Four patients (8%) developed a severe increasing dyspnea. Chest
X-ray findings in these four cases revealed infiltration corresponding to the portals of the previous radiotherapy.

Table 2 shows the temporal relationship between steroid
withdrawal and the dramatic onset of symptoms. In these patients

radiation pneumonitis occurred after after the corticosteroids were abruptly discontinued or tapered off rapidly. The complete regression after the reinstitution of prednisone established the diagnosis of steroid withdrawal caused pneumonitis.

Differential diagnoses of pulmonary infiltrates in patients with disseminated malignant disease receiving combined radiotherapy and chemotherapy can be numerous. Several interstitial lung diseases including lymphangiosis carcinomatosa have to be included (Stender, 1977; 1978). Interstitial pneumonia may be caused by a variety of organisms, including pneumocystis carinii (Dee et al., 1979). A definitive diagnosis is needed and often a lung biopsy is necessary in patients with diffuse pulmonary opacities, who are immuno-insufficient from an underlying metastatic malignant disease (Jahn, 1977).

In our patients the distribution of pulmonary infiltrates corresponding to the radiation field strongly supported the diagnosis of radiation pneumonitis. This fact and the preceeding abrupt cessation of corticosteroids proved helpful in finding a decision to give a trial of prednisone. The prompt symptomatic improvement in the first 24 hours and the resolution of pneumonitis on chest X-ray film confirmed the diagnosis in all four cases. The additional therapy with antibiotics (Gross, 1977) did certainly not contribute to this improvement.

CONCLUSIONS

(a) Among the several causes of radiation pneumonitis with severe symptoms withdrawal of corticosteroids should be considered as a possible cause.

(b) This is especially important in patients receiving combined chemotherapy and radiotherapy for malignant lymphoma or small cell carcinoma of the lung.

(c) In these patients a trial of prednisone therapy should be given, when there is a temporal relationship between steroid withdrawal and the onset of symptoms. The rapid symptomatic and radiographic improvement establishes diagnosis.

(d) If concomitant steroid therapy is considered necessary in patients receiving radiotherapy and chemotherapy, it should be very slowly tapered.

REFERENCES:

Ammon, J., J. Kreidler, J. Goronzy:
Ergebnisse einer zytostatischen Kombinationsbehandlung der metastasierten Mamma- und kleinzelligen Bronchialkarzinome unter teilweiser Blockade des Zellzyklus.
In: Kombinierte Strahlen- und Chemotherapie.
Hrsg.: Wannenmacher, M.
Verlag Urban & Schwarzenberg, München - Wien - Baltimore (1979)

Bargon, G., B. Anger, W. Schreml, W. Kubanek, H. Heimpel:
Progrediente Lungenfibrose unter der Kombinationstherapie mit BCNU,
Cyclophosphamid und Cytosin-Arabinosid.
Fortschr. Röntgenstr. 129 (1978) 312

Bleher, E. A., K. Salonen, U. Tillmann:
Pneumonitis und Fibrose nach alleiniger Strahlentherapie und nach kombinierter
Behandlung mit Chemotherapie beim Bronchuskarzinom.
Schweiz. med. Wschr. 109 (1979) 857

Dee, P., W. Winn, K. Mc Kee:
Pneumocystis carinii Infection of the Lung:
Radiologic and Pathologic Correlation.
Am. J. Roentgenol. 132 (1979) 741

Gross, N. J.:
Pulmonary effects of radiation therapy.
Ann. Int. Med. 86 (1977) 81

Hellman, S., M. M. Kligerman, C. F. von Essen et al.:
Sequelae of radical radiotherapy of carcinoma of the lung.
Radiology 82 (1964) 1055

Hornback, N. B., L. Einhorn, H. Shidnia, B. T. Joe, M. Krause, B. Furnas:
Oat cell carcinoma of the lung. Early treatment results of combination radia-
tion therapy and chemotherapy.
Cancer 37 (1976) 2658

Jehn, U.:
Die Diagnostik der Pneumocystis carinii-Pneumonie des Erwachsenen.
Dtsch. med. Wschr. 102 (1977) 486

Kaplan, H. S.:
Hodgkin's Disease.
Harvard Univ. Press, Cambridge, Massachusetts (1972)

Makoski, H.-Br., G. Schmitt, R. Osieka, C. G. Schmidt:
Integrierte Behandlung des inoperablen kleinzelligen Bronchialkarzinoms.
Strahlentherapie 153 (1977) 649

Morrison, D. A., A. L. Goldman:
Radiographic Patterns of Drug-Induced Lung Disease.
Radiology 131 (1979) 299

Parris, T. M., J. G. Knight, Ch. E. Hess, W. C. Constable:
Severe Radiation pneumonitis precipitated by withdrawal of corticosteroids:
A diagnostic and therapeutic dilemma.
Am. J. R. 132 (1979) 284

Senn, H. J., W. F. Jungi und Schweizerische Arbeitsgruppe für klinische Krebs-
forschung (SAKK):
Adriamycin versus Adriamycin + Vincristin + Corticosteroide bei disseminierten
und/oder inoperablen Weichteilsarkomen.
In: M. Ghione, J. Fetzer, H. Maier (Hrsg.), Ergebnisse der Adriamycin-Therapie.
Springer-Verlag, Berlin - Heidelberg - New York, (1975)

Stender, H. St.:
Das Röntgenbild der interstitiellen Pneumonie und allergischen Alveolitis.
Radiologe 17 (1977) 21

Stender, H. St.:
Röntgendiagnostik der Lungengerüsterkrankungen.
In: Erkrankungen des Lungenparenchyms.
Klinisch radiologisches Seminar Band VIII.
Hrsg. Frommhold, W., P. Gerhardt.
Georg-Thieme-Verlag, Stuttgart (1978)

EFFECT OF HEMITHORAX IRRADIATION OF YOUNG MICE ON PULMONARY METASTATIC DEPOSITS FROM SUBSEQUENTLY DEVELOPING SPONTANEOUS MAMMARY TUMOURS

J. Shewell

There is considerable experimental evidence that local lung irradiation increases successful metastatic deposition of tumour cells, in both spontaneous and artificial (tumour cell inoculation) model systems. This experiment demonstrates increased pulmonary metastasis in the lungs of mice given hemithorax irradiation one week after weaning, before spontaneous tumours developed, and followed through their lifespan. 120 C_3H/Bts female mice were irradiated with 500R 220 kVp X-rays to the right or left hemithorax at 4 weeks old. 120 paired litter-mate controls were sham-irradiated. The mice were mated at 8 weeks old, and pairs of irradiated/control mice killed at selected intervals up to 15 months after irradiation to follow long term changes. Half the remaining (190) mice developed mammary tumours (51% non-irradiated, 43% irradiated). Tumour diameters were measured, and volume doubling times calculated. Mice were killed before the tumour ulcerated. At post-mortem examination gross lung colonies were scored, and confirmed by histological examination. Lung lobes with no gross colonies were examined histologically for tumour cell emboli and microscopic invasive metastases. There was a significantly increased incidence of gross metastases in irradiated mice compared with controls (52.2% $\pm$ 10.4 to 23.5% $\pm$ 7.3, χ^2 5%), and also of microscopic metastases (60.9% $\pm$ 10.2 to 35.3% $\pm$ 8.2). The number of metastatic colonies in the irradiated lung (either R or L) was greater than that in the shielded lung (non-irradiated control R/L 2.6 $\pm$ 0.2, irradiated R/non-irradiated L 4.3 $\pm$ 0.5, irradiated L/non-irradiated R 2.6 $\pm$ 0.7).

This work was supported by a grant from the Cancer Research Campaign, which is gratefully acknowledged.

THE CHEMOTHERAPY OF MICROMETASTASES - AN OVERVIEW OF CURRENT STATUS

S.K. Carter

INTRODUCTION

Adjuvant chemotherapy of adult solid tumors has been a major recent thrust of clinical research. It has received a great deal of publicity and at times has appeared to be a major therapeutic breakthrough. As with many other therapeutic excitements adjuvant chemotherapy has gone through a variable course. There was the slow beginning involving experimental studies and early tentative clinical studies. This built up to a crescendo of excitement with the early results of trials in breast cancer and osteosarcoma. A mass of clinical studies began as a result of the excitement. As the breast and osteosarcoma studies become less positive with longer follow-up wild enthusiasm has been replaced by sober reevaluation. Where the curve goes in the future is unknown but hopefully it will move steadily upward until the original positive expectations are fulfilled.

Adjuvant chemotherapy in adult solid tumors can be defined as cytotoxic drug treatment given in the following situations:

1) Immediately after the primary tumor and regional lymph nodes have been removed or ablated by surgery and/or irradiation

2) Where clinical, laboratory and radiologic investigation are negative for metastatic disease

3) Where historical experience indicates a high probability of ultimate metastatic failure.

Unfortunately, at the time of initial diagnosis a significant number of patients already have microscopic foci of metastatic disease, which is undectable by present diagnostic means, and it erroneously appears that the tumor is localized. In localized solid tumors the traditional choice of initial treatment is surgery and/or radiotherapy but neither of these modalities can be considered curative when the disease has metastasized beyond the primary site and nearby lymph nodes or extensively involves a vital organ. Relapses following surgery and/or radiotherapy are largely due to metastases existing before treatment.

The translation from advanced disease activity to adjuvant usage has several built-in assumptions derived mainly from the cell kill hypothesis (Skipper et al., 1964) (Schabel, 1975):

1) The kinetics of microscopic residual disease will be more favorable for cytotoxic kill than in the advanced state. Since the tumor growth in micrometastases will be at an earlier point in the Gompertzian growth curve the doubling time of the tumor will be shorter and the growth fraction higher.

2) Because of the above, chemotherapy can be given at slightly reduced dose levels as compared to the metastatic disease situation. This concept is an empiric

necessity since severe toxicity is much less acceptable in the symptom-free post surgical patient. In addition drug related mortality in patients possibly already cured by their local and regional therapy would be a severe negative factor in acceptance of the treatment in the future.

3) Drug treatment should be prolonged since it is highly unlikely that a single course of drug would achieve total initial cell kill.

BREAST CANCER

Breast cancer is in the forefront of the combined modality strategy involving the use of chemotherapy. No matter what effective local control therapy is utilized metastatic relapse remains the major cause of treatment failure and ultimate demise. The histologic status of axillary lymph nodes is the most potent prognostic variable for this metastatic failure. In women with positive axillary nodes the median time to relapse is 3 years and slightly less than 25% will be disease free at 10 years. This compares to an approximate 75% relapse free rate for women with negative nodes at 10 years. Where four or more nodes are found to be positive the ten year relapse rate ranges from 83.6 to 86.2% with total survival being 13.4 to 25.6% (Fisher, Slac et al., 1975) (Valagussa et al., 1978).

In 1972 a large scale controlled trial of the use of chemotherapy as an adjuvant to surgical operation in women in whom cancer had already spread was initiated by the National Surgical Breast Project (NSABP), headed by Dr. Bernard Fisher. Half of the women were given L-phenylalanine mustard (L-PAM) after radical mastectomy and half were given a placebo (Fisher, Carbone et al., 1975). Treatment failures had occurred in 22 percent of 108 patients receiving placebo and 9.3 percent of 103 women given L-phenylalanine mustard at the time of first literature report. This difference was only statistically significant for premenopausal women and continued follow-up has shown no meaningful difference for women who are postmenopausal.

A follow-up of the NSABP data (Fisher, 1979) has shown that at 48 months of follow-up the percentage of treatment failures overall is 48% in 169 placebo and 40% in 179 L-PAM patients with the P-value being 0.02. When the data are looked at broken down by menopausal status the data are as follows:

AGE		NUMBER OF PATIENTS	% TREATMENT FAILURE	P-VALUE
≤ 49				
	Placebo:	60	55.0	0.005
	L-PAM	59	34.0	
≥ 50				
	Placebo:	109	45.0	0.29
	L-PAM	120	43.0	

The only situation in which the L-PAM is statistically significantly superior to placebo is with premenopausal patients with 1-3 positive nodes where the failure rate is 44% with placebo in 31 patients as against 13% with L-Pam in 32 patients at

4 years. The P-value is 0.005.

The first CMF adjuvant study was initiated on June 1, 1973 (Bonadonna et al, 1978) (Bonadonna et al, 1976) (Bonadonna et al, 1977). Patients with primary tumors staged T_{1b}-T_{2b}-T_{3b} or T_4 by the UICC TNM international classification were not considered eligible for inclusion in the protocol. Also excluded were those with N_2 or N_3 lesions which meant either nodes fixed to one another or to other structures or supraclavicular; infraclavicular nodes or edema of the arm. After mastectomy randomization was to CMF begun within four weeks of surgery or to no further treatment.

As of February 1, 1979, (Bonadonna et al, 1979) the clinical benefit in terms of relapse free survival of adjuvant CMF overall in 207 CMF treated women as compared to the 179 controls remains highly significant (P=0.0001). This benefit is seen exclusively in premenopausal women.

The CMF data are clearly positive in premopausal women but not of much benefit in postmenopausal patients. When the L-PAM data and the CMF data are put together with earlier single course thio-tepa data of the NSABP (Fisher, Slack et al, 1975) an enigma is seen. All are negative in postmenopausal women and a dichotomy exists in premenopausal women. A single course of thio-tepa is of value for the subset of $\geq$ 4+ nodes but not for the better risk group of 1-3+ nodes. The more aggressive 18 months of L-PAM is of value for the 1-3+ nodes but not for the $\geq$ 4+ nodes. CMF is effective for both subsets. Since CMF is more effective in advanced disease this is encouraging for advanced disease activity being predictive for adjuvant effect.

Current controlled protocols are ongoing in the United States cooperative groups and in several cancer centers. In addition some cancer centers are undertaking single arm studies relating to historical controls. While some preliminary reports are available (Tancini, 1979) (Budzar, 1979) (Wendt, 1979)(Glucksberg, 1979) and (Meakin, 1977) it is still too early to make any meaningful interpretation especially since none, with any data to report, have a surgery only control. With longer analysis it is now obvious the L-PAM alone is a poor control for postmenopausal women and studies which use this as a control will be particularly difficult to interpret.

OSTEOGENIC SARCOMA

Osteogenic sarcoma is a tumor that has been at the cutting edge of the combined modality approach to cancer treatment. Along with breast cancer it is a solid tumor which has been viewed as proving the value of adjuvant chemotherapy. For nearly a decade the concept of adjuvant drug treatment has been applied to most patients with this tumor. After initial claims of dramatic efficacy controversy has arisen and the true value of the approach still remains to be totally established.

In this tumor reports with high dose methotrexate by the Sidney Farber Institute (Jaffe et al, 1974) and with adriamycin by Cancer and Leukemia Group B (Cortes et al 1974) indicated relapse free survival advantages over earlier historical controls. In the Sidney Farber series the results are compared to a historical control of 71 patients with local control who were treated between 1950 and 1972. These two groups were comparable in age distribution and sex but were not matched for any other prognostic variable, such as methodology of local control, histology, tumor location, tumor size, or pretreatment work-up for evidence of metastatic disease.

In the CALGB study the data of Marcove et al (1971) was utilized as a historical control. Five of the 21 study patients had relapsed at the time of the initial report (subsequent reports have about half free of disease at two years). Of the 21 study cases, only 15 had radical amputation. Of the 6 who had "subradical" amputation, 4 had recurred at the time of the report.

The Mayo Clinic (Ritts et al, 1978) has compared transfer factor prepared from long-term survivors with a combination chemotherapy regimen of high-dose methotrexat adriamycin and vincristine (MAO). If transfer of delayed hypersensitivity did not occur, those patients were crossed over to MAO immediately. Eighteen patients were entered on each arm of the study. Five patients did not demonstrate systemic reactivity after the third dose of transfer factor and were crossed over to drugs. Another 4 also failed to demonstrate transfer but refused to take chemotherapy. At 18 months the 9 patients on transfer factor had a disease free percentage of 55% compared to 32% in the 18 patients on MAO. Neither of these were superior to the contemporary historical control at the Mayo Clinic with amputation only.

An extensive literature now exists with a variety of adjuvant regimens utilizing either high dose methotrexate (HDMTX) or adriamycin, alone or together in combination with other drugs. When two year relapse free survival is analysed the results vary widely with a range of 26 to 65% which is clearly overlapping with the range of historical controls. It is also obvious that no combination of HDMTX plus adriamyci with or without other drugs can be shown to be clearly superior to HDMTX alone in the Sidney Farber Cancer Center initial series (Jaffe et al, 1972) or adriamycin alone.

There now exists a significant differential between two year relapse free survival and two year overall survival. This is most likely due to the impact of secondary therapy applied at the time of recurrent manifestations of disease. These now include resection of pulmonary metastases, secondary chemotherapy, irradiation or some combination of the modalities. Two year survivals range from 30 to 61% after resection of pulmonary metastases in association with a wide range of therapie. This ability to prolong survival significantly, after relapse, invalidates the utilization of overall survival as an evaluation of adjuvant chemotherapy in comparison to early historical control series.

Osteogenic sarcoma has seemed to many to be an optimal tumor to test the concepts of adjuvant chemotherapy for the treatment of micrometastases. This has been because of its high risk-to-recurrence population and because it was felt that a valid historical control existed. What has been demonstrated however is that osteosarcoma is a tumor with many prognostic variables which combined with its rarity make selection biases in clinical trials difficult to exclude. Most of the reported trials have involved small numbers of patients and have been initially reported with short follow-up times in comparison to their historical controls. This has lead to actuarial projections of NED survival which have been more optimistic than the reality of long-term follow-up.

DISCUSSION

Preliminary results in breast cancer and osteogenic sarcoma have stimulated a great deal of enthusiasm that this approach would have a great impact on end-results in these tumors. As further analysis of these studies has taken place, the positivity has diminished and the cautions of the authors in their original papers as to the preliminary nature of their data have been shown to be valid. Unfortunately the cautions were not always heeded, and so there is a sense of disappointment in some quarters, although the studies still remain positive and clearly established that we are on the right track. It is clear however that the immediate impact will not be as great as once had been hoped. It appears that we will need a greater degree of activity for our drugs in advanced disease than was previously thought, to achieve the desired cell kill in the adjuvant situation. The possibility also exists that the exponentially growing rodent transplant models are not predicting accurately and that the kinetics of the residual tumor cell burden after surgery may not be as favorable as had been thought.

REFERENCES

Bonadonna, G., Erusamolino, E., Valagussa, P., Rossi, Al, Brugnatelli, L., Brambilla, C., DeLena, A., Tancini, G., Bajetta, E., Musumeci, R., Veronesi, U., 1976. Combination chemotherapy as an adjuvant treatment in operable breast cancer. N.Eng. J. Med. 294: 405.

Bonadonna, G., Fossi, A., Valagussa, P., Banfi, A, and Veronesi, U., 1977. The CMF program for operable breast cancer with positive axillary nodes. Updated analysis on the disease-free interval site of relapse and drug tolerance. Cancer 39: 2904.

Bonadonna, G., Valagussa, P., Rossi, A., Zucali, R., Tancini, G., Bajetta, E., Brambilla, C., DeLena, M., DiFronzo, G., Banfi, A., Rilke, F., and Veronesi, U., 1978. Are surgical adjuvant trials altering the course of breast cancer. Seminars Oncol. 5: 450.

Bonadonna, G., Valagussa, P., Rossi, A., Tancini, G., Bajetta, E., Marchini, S., and Varonesi, U., 1979. CMF adjuvant chemotherapy in operable breast cancer. In: S. Salmon and S. Jones (editors) Adjuvant Therapy of Cancer II. Grune & Stratton, New York.

Budzar, A., Blumenschein, G., Gutterman, J., Tashima, C., Hortobagyi, G., Smith, T., Campos, L., Wheeler, W., Hersch, E., Freireich, E., and Gehan, E., 1979. Postoperative adjuvant chemotherapy with 5-fluorouracil, adriamycin, cyclophosphamide and BCG. A follow-up report. JAMA

374

Cortes, E., Holland, J., Wang, J., et al, 1974. Amputation and adriamycin in primary osteogenic sarcoma. N. Eng. J. Med. 291-298.

Fisher, B., 1979. Breast Cancer: Studies of the National Surgical Adjuvant Primary Breast Cancer Project (NSABP). In: S. Salmon and S. Jones (editors) Adjuvant Therapy of Cancer II. Grune & Stratton, New York.

Fisher, B., Carbone, P., Economou, S., et al, 1975. L-phenylalanine mustard (L-PAM) in the management of primary breast cancer. N. Eng. J. Med. 292: 117.

Fisher, B., Slack, N.H., Katrych, D., Wolmark, N., 1975. Ten year follow-up results of patients with carcinoma of the breast in a cooperative clinical trial evaluating surgical adjuvant chemotherapy. Surg. Gynecol. Obstet. 140: 52

Glucksberg, H., Rivkin, S., Rasmussen, S., 1979. Adjuvant chemotherapy for stage II breast cancer: A comparison of CMFVP versus L-PAM. In: S. Salmon and S. Jones (editors) Adjuvant Therapy of Cancer II. Grune & Stratton, New York.

Jaffe, N., 1972. Recent advances in the chemotherapy of metastatic osteogenic sarcoma. Cancer 30: 1627.

Jaffe, N., Frei, E., Traggis, D., et al, 1974. Adjuvant methotrexate and citrovorum factor treatment of osteogenic sarcoma. N. Eng. J. Med. 291.

Marcove, R., Mike, V., Hajek, J., Levin, A., Hutter, R., 1971. N. Y. State J. Med. 71: 855.

Meakin, J., Allt, W., Beale, F, et al, 1977. Ovarian irradiation and prednisone following surgery for carcinoma of the breast. S. Salmon and S. Jones (editors) Adjuvant Therapy of Cancer II. Grune & Stratton, New York.

Ritts, R., Pritchard, D., Gilchristo, G., et al, 1978. Transfer factor versus combination chemotherapy: An interum reprot of a randomized post-surgical adjuvant study in osteogenic sarcoma. In: W. Terry, D. Windhorst (editors) Immunotherapy of Cancer: Present Status of Trials in Man. Raven Press, New York.

Schabel, F., 1975. Concepts for systemic treatment of micrometastases. Cancer, 35: 15.

Skipper, H., Schabel, F., Wilcox, W., 1964. Experimental evaluation of potential anticancer agents. XIII. On the criteria and kinetics associated with "curability" of experimental leukemia. Cancer Chemother. Rep., 35: 1.

Tancini, G., Bajetta, E., Marchini, S., Valagussa, P., Bonadonna, G., Veronesi, U., 1979). Operable breast cancer with positive axillary nodes (N+): Results of 6 versus 12 cycles of adjuvant CMF in premenopausal women. Proc. Am. Assoc. Cancer Res. 20: 172.

Valagussa, P., Bonadonna, G., Veronesi, U., 1978. Patterns of relapse and survival following radical mastectomy: Analysis of 716 consecutive patients. Cancer 41: 1170.

Wendt, A., Jones, S., Salmon, S., Giordano, G., Jackson, R., Miller, R., Heusinkveli R., Moon, T., 1979. Adjuvant treatment of breast cancer with adriamycin-cyclophosphamide with or without radiation therapy. In: S. Salmon and S. Jones (editors) Adjuvant Therapy of Cancer II. Grune & Stratton, New York.

ADJUVANT RAZOXANE IN RESECTABLE COLORECTAL CANCER

J. Gilbert, P. Cassell, K. Hellmann, M. Evans and J. Peto

INTRODUCTION

Survival of patients with resectable colorectal cancer (CRC) has not been materially influenced during the last 20 years by either adjuvant chemotherapy or any new surgical development. Attempts to influence survival in CRC by adjuvant chemotherapy are limited by the fact that of the few drugs that have shown activity in the advanced form of this disease only 5-fluorouracil (5-FU) and razoxane are suitable for long term administration. 5-FU as adjuvant chemotherapy for CRC has been widely and intensively studied over many years, but the results leave doubt as to whether there is a significant statistical or clinical benefit (1-3).

Adjuvant razoxane was therefore examined in a three-year multicentre trial. The drug has the advantage that it can be taken by mouth and that it has only a very low degree of toxicity, with neutropenia as the dose limiting side effect. The trial was prospective and all patients with resectable CRC who presented to the participating surgeons were considered for inclusion in it.

PATIENTS AND METHODS

One hundred and sixty-two patients from four centres were randomized into control and treatment groups and 134 are evaluable. Thirteen patients have been excluded for a variety of reasons (died before 1st follow-up appointment 7; Ca. not confirmed 3; not resected 1, second operation before treatment 2)* The control patients were managed according to the usual practice of the participating centre. One control patient received other chemotherapy (5-FU, vincristine, MeCCNU). Palliative local radiotherapy was used for pain in some cases. The treatment group received razoxane 125mg twice daily by mouth for five days per week (Monday to Friday) indefinitely. The drug was started at the first follow-up appointment, usually between 3 and 6 weeks after operation.
*plus a further 15 withdrawals.

The dose of razoxane was reduced or stopped if the white cell count fell below 3,000/cmm. The drug was restarted as soon as the white cell count began to rise above 3,000/cmm. All patients had a clinical examination at regular intervals and all patients on razoxane had a full blood count weekly for the first four weeks and then monthly.

RESULTS

One hundred and thirty-four patients are evaluable and the results are analysed by the Peto log-rank test. There are no significant differences between controls and razoxane treated Duke's A or D patients, but numbers were small. Detailed analysis is confined to the 96 patients in Duke's groups B and C.

Duke's Groups B and C

In this combined minimal residual disease group there were 49 control and 47 treated patients (table 1). Matching was satisfactory for Duke's staging, sex, age and site of tumour, but there was an excess of poorly differentiated tumours in the control group (table 2).

Sixteen control patients have died compared to twelve in the treatment group. All 16 control patients died of cancer, but 3 patients in the treatment group died of intercurrent disease. For the purposes of survival analysis intercurrent deaths are considered as 'lost to follow-up' at the time of death.

Comparison of cancer mortality of all evaluable
B & C patients

Analysis shows that the difference between control and treatment group approaches statistical significance (p = 0.07). When patients who were originally randomized to the treatment group, but who never receive any razoxane are analysed with the controls, but patients who received razoxane for less than one month continue to be included in the treatment group, the difference between contro. and treated groups increases to p < 0.05 (Fig.1).

TOXICITY

The doses of razoxane used in this trial were exceptionally wel. tolerated and gave few side effects (table3).

FIGURE 1

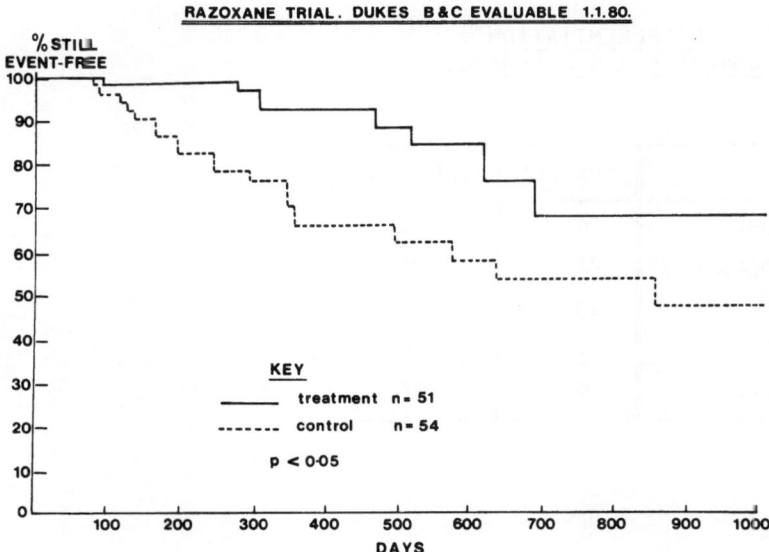

RAZOXANE TRIAL. DUKES B & C EVALUABLE 1.1.80.

TABLE 1

RAZOXANE COLORECTAL TRIAL
1.1.80

EVALUABLE PATIENTS
DUKE'S GROUPS B & C

DUKE'S GROUP	CONTROL	TREATMENT
B	20	23
C	29	24
TOTAL	49	47

TABLE 2

RAZOXANE COLORECTAL TRIAL
1.1.80

DIFFERENTIATION
DUKE'S B & C EVALUABLE

	CONTROL	TREATMENT
POORLY	6	2
MODERATELY	22	19
WELL	20	25
MUCOUS	1	1
TOTAL	49	47

TABLE 3

RAZOXANE COLORECTAL TRIAL
1.1.80

TOXICITY
Duke's A, B, C and D Evaluable Pts.

Leukopenia (WBC $< 3.0 \times 10^9$ 1)	34/66	(52%)
Thrombocytopenia	1/66	(1.5%)
Alopecia (None required wigs)	6/66	(9%)
Nausea	0/66	(-)
Vomiting	0/66	(-)
Diarrhoea	0/66	(-)

The white cell count fell in all patients and this was indirect evidence that the drug was being absorbed.

The two patients who died with exacerbations of chronic bron-
chitis may have suffered from a functional impairment of neutrophil
activity, although there is no evidence on this point and neither
patient was neutropenic.

Alopecia and gastrointestinal disturbances were minimal and in
over 95% of all razoxane randomized patients the quality of life was
essentially unimpaired.

DISCUSSION

Razoxane had previously been shown to be active in CRC (5,6).
It had also been found to be well tolerated in high doses and even
better in the lower doses required for continuous treatment.

The number of patients in the present trial is small, but there
appears to be a statistically significant difference between control
and razoxane treated patients with Duke's stage B and C tumours
analysed as a single group.   It may also be significant that this
difference has remained steady and has shown no signs of disappearing
as the duration of the trial has increased.

The results stand in contrast to those with adjuvant 5-FU where
a merger of the non-significant results of five separate trials
(employing a number of different protocols) was required to obtain
a statistically significant difference.   This in itself speaks for
the fact that if there is any difference at all as a result of
adjuvant 5-FU it must be very small since it required large numbers
of patients to demonstrate it.

Our patients were well matched for age, sex, site of tumour and
Duke's stage, but there was a slight preponderance of poorly differentiated tumours amongst the controls in Duke's group C. Little
significance can be attached to this imbalance because not only is
Duke's stage the single most important prognostic criterion, but
Gill and Morris (4) have shown that differentiation had no
influence on prognosis. Furthermore all the control poorly differentiated cases were in Duke's stage C and a log rank analysis between

control and razoxane treated patients who fell into Duke's stage C showed that there was no difference between them.

REFERENCES

1. Moertel, C.G: Chemotherapy of gastrointestinal cancer. New England J. of Medicine. 299, 1049-1052, 1978.
2. Higgins Jr., G.A., Lee, L.E., Dwight, R.W. and Keehn, R.J. The case for adjuvant 5-fluorouracil in colorectal cancer. Cancer Clinical Trials, 1, 35-41. 1978
3. Davis, H.L. and Kisner, D.L. Analysis of adjuvant therapy in large bowel cancer. Cancer Clinical Trials 1, 273-287, 1978.
4. Gill, P.G. and Morris, P.J. The survival of patients with colorectal cancer treated in a regional hospital. British Journal of Surgery, 65, 17-20, 1978.
5. Marciniak, T.A., Moertel, C.G., Schutt, A.J., Hahn, R.G. and Reitemeier, R.J. Phase II study of ICRF-159 (NSC-129943) in advanced colorectal carcinoma. Cancer Chemotherapy Reports 59, 761, 1975
6. Bellet, R.E., Engstrom, P.F., Catalano, R.B., Creech, R.H. and Mastrangelo, M.J. Phase II study of ICRF-159 in patients with metastatic colorectal carcinoma previously exposed to systemic chemotherapy. Cancer Treatment Reports 60, 1395-1397 1976.

CHANGING ASPECTS IN THE SURGICAL APPROACH TO METASTATIC DISEASE; INFLUENCE OF CHEMOTHERAPY ON INDICATIONS FOR AND RESULTS OF METASTASECTOMIES

J.A. van Dongen

INTRODUCTION

Modesty is imperative in looking at the benefits of surgery in oncology. The surgeon is confronted with the metastatic problem by the mere fact that in many cases it is he who provokes the spread of the disease. In localised disease however surgery frequently is the only curative treatment. Even when metastases are already established surgical intervention can be of great importance and frequently the aim is cure.

In the surgical approach to metastatic disease, patterns are changing, not only in indications and option of intervention, but also in results to be expected.

The possibility of combining surgery with radiotherapy widens the indication for surgery of macroscopically involved nodes; the principles of pre- and post- operative radiotherapy are well known.

Elective radiotherapy can sometimes be as effective as elective surgery and it is less mutilating. Surgery is therefore becoming less attractive for some of the regions where elective treatment is indicated.

The possibilities of gaining information on the real extent of the disease (mainly serving as a base for further therapy) sometimes make surgery more attractive than other therapy modalities. This "staging" principle which is widely used in the lymphomas, is also used as an argument for surgery of the axilla in breast cancer.

By optimal treatment of regional node areas and elective treatment of "first hematogenous filters" (e.g. lung irradiation) eventually a number of cases with isolated and possible curable distant metastases may be seen with unusual "bizarre" localizations.

The influence on surgery of metastases caused by the introduction of chemotherapy is fascinating and merits special attention.

PULMONARY METASTASECTOMIES AFTER ADJUVANT CHEMOTHERAPY

The number of surgical interventions performed for distant, mainly pulmonary metastases is growing. Some 20-30 years ago a pulmonary metastasis was removed only by chance. The operation was thought to be done for an operable lung cancer and it was the pathologist who discovered that a solitary metastasis was removed of an almost forgotten tumor treated long ago. Now even multiple metastases are excised, sometimes at the same time as the removal of the primary tumor. The interval between treatment of the primary tumor and the appearance of metastases is considered to be of great prognostic significance. The longer the interval the better the prognosis of the metastasectomy. Also cases with solitary metastasis have a better prognosis after excision than those where several metastases are removed.

Looking at these prognostic factors we must realize that the present more aggressive attitude could be reflected by a worse final fate, with the risk of bringing metastasectomies into discredit.

The influence of previous adjuvant chemotherapy on the prognosis after metastasectomy is illustrated in the diagrams. Using a semilogarithmic presentation tumor growth can be (hypothetically) represented by a straight line. The most ideal situation for metastasectomy is given in the upper part of the diagram. The isolated metastasis, probably "born" just before extirpation of the primary tumor becomes apparent only after many years and is

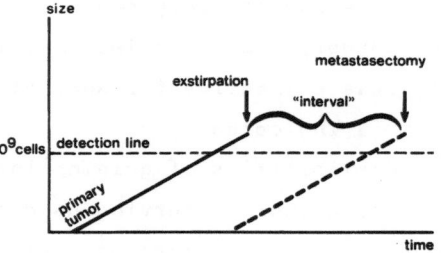

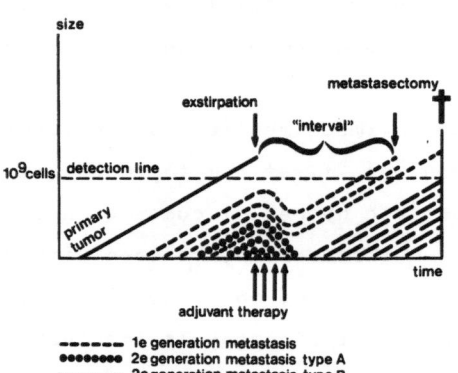

----- 1e generation metastasis
••••••• 2e generation metastasis type A
—— — 2e generation metastasis type B

removed in this hypothetical model prior to secondary spread from
the metastatic lesion and the patient is cured. Very seldom will
such cases be seen in this era of adjuvant therapy. The metastasis
shown in this diagram would probably have been killed by appropriate chemotherapy given at the time of the removal of the
primary tumor. The lower diagram represents the model of a
"modern" metastasectomy-case. The metastases "born" early are in
part killed by the adjuvant chemotherapy (or any other type of
adjuvant therapy if effective); the other ones, the oldest, are
not killed but do show an important retardation. They manifest
themselves late in the course of the disease. If the statement
is accepted that metastases have the same properties as the
primary tumor e.g. in this case to shed tumor emboli early, then
the metastases of the metastases will be numerous and the patient
will not be cured by the metastasectomy.

If we compare these hypothetical models we see that in both
cases the interval is just as long, but that it is no longer a
sign of good prognosis in the second case. The long interval is
a useful prognostic guideline only if consideration is given as
to whether or not adjuvant therapy has been given. These re-
flections and the fact that cases as represented in the first
model will be rare in these days of adjuvant therapy cause us to
re-evaluate our expectations after metastasectomies.

In the Netherlands Cancer Institute the number of pulmonary
metastasectomies has increased considerably. More patients with
multiple metastases have been operated on recently. The group of patients pretreated with adjuvant schemes is becoming larger and in all probability will increase further. More recently in some cases the interval was zero, but also patients with long intervals were seen (in part as effect of previous adjuvant therapy). In view of the

Netherlands Cancer Institute

Pulmonary metastasectomy

1960 - 1965	1975 - 1980
+ 2/year	+ 10/year
Only "solitary" metastases resected	+ 2 - 3 metastases/patient
interval: + 3 years	interval: + 3 years
No adjuvant therapy given	+ 30% of patients adjuvant therapy at time of therapy of primary tumor

pessimism already referred to the fate of the most recent patients should be worse than that of patients in the first group. It is remarkable that the early results in the recent past are quite superimposable on the curves of the first group in which a long term survival was seen in half of the cases. Probably the unexpectedly good preliminary results in the recent group are in part due to adjuvant chemotherapy used after metastasectomy.

CYTOREDUCTIVE SURGERY AS PART OF THE GENERAL TREATMENT OF WIDE SPREAD DISEASE

Cytoreductive surgery in wide spread disease is performed on those patients where modern chemotherapy schedules are effective but not so effective that "bulky" disease can be cured. At present "debulking" procedures are quite popular. However, from the technical point of view of a surgical oncologist these kinds of interventions are far from attractive. In many schedules debulking is proposed as the initial therapeutic step, prior to chemotherapy.

However, there are strong arguments for such interventions after having given the first courses of chemotherapy and not as initial treatment prior to chemotherapy. The risk of surgical propagation of metastases is reduced by debulking after starting chemotherapy. Furthermore chemotherapy is most active with an intact blood supply. The information gained during the first chemotherapy courses is of great importance. If no reaction is observed cure is not to be expected, not even after cytoreductive surgery; in that case a sound indication for a debulking procedure is absent. Another main point is that primary debulking can seriously delay the start of chemotherapy, a drawback which is of special importance in fast growing tumors.

In our opinion debulking procedures should not be started before chemotherapy. The "staging" information which is obtained by early debulking procedures should be collected by other means. Chemotherapy is more active on smaller tumor masses, which is an argument for early debulking, but from a theoretical point of view it does not greatly matter at what point during chemotherapy the

surgeon is of assistance.   The fact that small tumor masses are
difficult to find and hard to remove constitutes the major problem
in cytoreduction performed at a later point;   this may be an
argument for early debulking.

STAGING SURGERY AFTER INTENSIVE CHEMOTHERAPY

With the introduction of very active chemotherapy-schedules
patients with extensive disease who could not be cured in former
years, can now sometimes be treated successfully, as is seen e.g.
in testicular cancer.   At present more and more cancer centres
are faced with the conflicting situation of persisting tumor masses
on X-rays or by palpation, while the tumor markers are normalized.
It is then difficult to decide whether the aggressive chemotherapy
which is so hard to tolerate can be terminated and consolidated
therapy (if of any use), which is also far more attractive to the
patient, can be started.   Here it is not debulking which is the
aim, it is staging by collecting tumor material.

In the Netherlands Cancer Institute we recently acquired some
experience with 9 of such rare cases.   All were non-seminomatous
testicular malignancies with very extensive disease, palpable masses
in the abdomen with pulmonary and other distant metastases.   In
all cases the markers (βHCG 9 cases; α-foetoprotein 3 cases; LDH 3
cases) came down to normal levels after one or two cycles of the
very aggressive P.V.B. (Cisplatin, Vinblastine, Bleomycin) regimen
(Einhorn).   We expected the patients to be cured, but tumor masses
remained palpable or were still visible on the radiographs.
Despite repeated negative cytology we considered laparotomy or
thoracotomy indicated for removing tumor remnants (occasionally
large ones) or for taking several big biopsies out of the remaining
masses, to help decide what to do further.   Eight times necrosis
and fibrosis only was seen, but in one case active tumor was found.
In that case the P.V.B. regimen was continued.   In the other cases
consolidation chemotherapy only was given.   Maturation as was
described by Merrin and by Hong was not seen in the histology of
these 9 cases.   Only very recently in another patient we did
indeed find transformation from a malignant to a benign type of

teratoma after chemotherapy.   The X-ray appearances of the thorax
of one of the patients are given as an illustration. The patient
entered the hospital in a far advanced state (fig.1A).   The P.V.B.
regimen was quite effective but a large mediastinal mass persisted
after four cycles (fig.1B).   The markers decreased to normal levels
after the second course of chemotherapy and in biopsies only necrosis was found.   The aggressive chemotherapy was therefore discontinued. Now, almost two years later, the patient is in good
health with the same mass still persistent in the mediastinum
(fig.1C).

FIG.1A   FIG. 1B

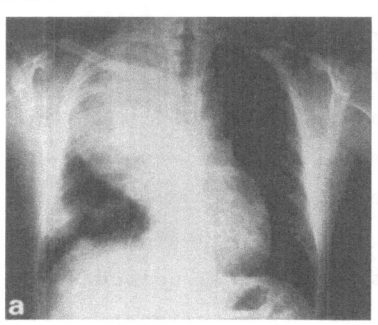   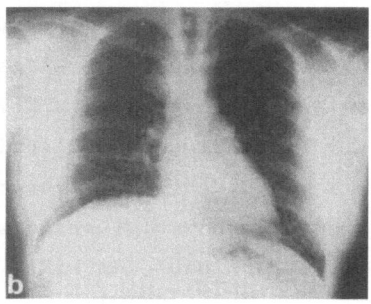

FIG.1C

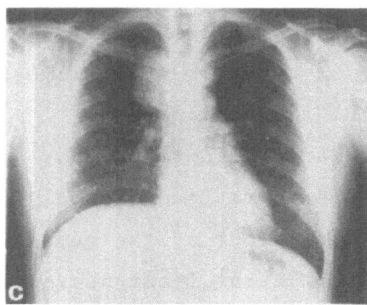

SUMMARY

The influence of chemotherapy on the surgical treatment of metastatic disease is considered. The prognosis after metastasectomy is greatly influenced by prior adjuvant therapy.

The timing of "cytoreductive" surgery is probably of great importance. Some chemotherapy courses should precede these debulking procedures.

The staging aspect of surgery of "metastasis" is of great help in deciding whether to discontinue aggressive chemotherapy in cases of testicular malignancies with normalized tumor markers, but with persistent tumor masses.

REFERENCES

Einhorn, L.H., Donohue, J.: Cis-diammunedichloroplatinum, Vinblastine and Bleomycin combination chemotherapy in disseminated testicular cancer. Ann.Intern. Med. 87:293-298, 1977.
Merrin, C., Takita, H., Weber,R. et al: Combination radical surgery and multiple sequential chemotherapy for the treatment of advanced carcinoma of the testis (stage III). Cancer, 37:20, 1976.
Hong, W.K., Wittes, R.E., Hajdu, S.T. et al: The evolution of mature teratoma from malignant testicular tumors. Cancer, 40: 2987-2992, 1977.

ACKNOWLEDGEMENTS
Thanks are expressed to the medical record department and to A.Linssen and W.W.ten Bokkel Huinink for the help in collecting the data of the discussed patients with testicular cancer and to E.R.D.Posthuma, who studied the pulmonary metastasectomy cases in the Netherlands Cancer Institute.

CLINICAL STUDY ON SELECTIVE ENHANCEMENT OF DRUG DELIVERY BY ANGIOTENSIN II IN CANCER CHEMOTHERAPY

H. Sato, K. Sato, Y. Sato, Y. Mimata, M. Asamura, R. Kanamuru,
A. Wakui, M. Suzuki and H. Sato

INTRODUCTION

In a series of experimental studies marked increase of blood flow was noted in tumor tissue with elevated blood pressure produced by angiotensin II, while no increase was detected in normal tissues (Suzuki et al., 1977a,1978,1979a,b). Thus, the functional difference between tumor and normal vessels could be applied selectively in cancer chemotherapy to enhance the delivery of drugs to tumor tissue (Suzuki et al., 1977b, 1980). This paper deals with the procedures and results obtained in clinical cancer chemotherapy studies (Sato et al., 1979b, c) which have used the concept based on the above experimental observations.

MATERIALS AND METHODS

Preparation of treatment

1. Angiotensin II (Hypertensin, CIBA-GEIGY Ltd., Basel, Switzerland, 2.5 mg/ampoule) was dissolved in 10ml physiological saline to a concentration of 250 μg/ml and was divided into about 10 sterile vials which were stored at $-20°C$ until use.

2. About 100ml of saline containing 3-10 μg/ml of angiotensin II was prepared just before treatment.

3. Instruments were set up as shown in Fig.1.

Clinical procedure of treatment

1. The blood pressure (BP) was measured to determine the mean BP before treatment ($\overline{BP}o$). $\overline{BP}o$ = diastolic BP + 1/3 pressure difference (PD).

2. The optimal elevation level of mean BP ($\overline{BP}e$) was estimated. $\overline{BP}e = 3/2 \ \overline{BP}o$.

3. Angiotensin II was infused continuously with great care until the mean BP was gradually elevated to the level of $\overline{BP}e$.

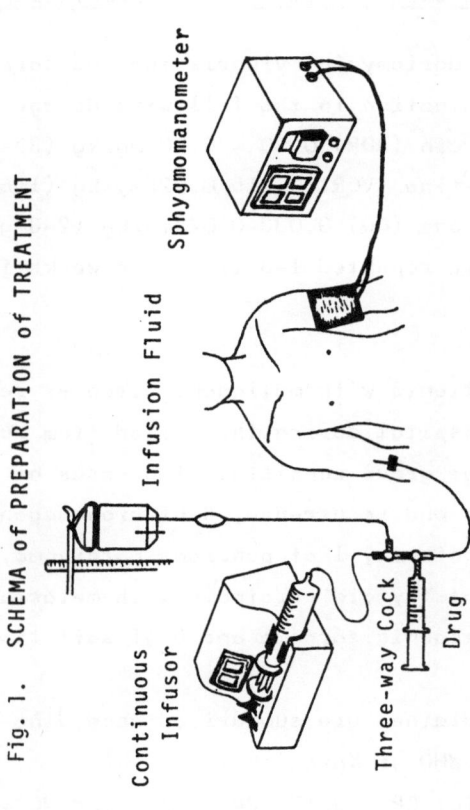

Fig. 1. SCHEMA of PREPARATION of TREATMENT

4.   The drug was administered intravenously with continuous
infusion of angiotensin II until the mean BP reached the mean BPe
level. $\overline{BP}e$ = diastolic BP + 1/2 PD.
5.   The $\overline{BP}e$ level was maintained for 10 minutes following
injection of drug.
6.   On stopping the infusion of angiotensin II the BP fell down
immediately to the pretreatment level.

Treatment schedules of combination chemotherapy (Sato et al., 1979a)

In this trial adriamycin, vincristine and carboquone were
mostly used in combination in the following dosage.

Day 1, adriamycin (ADR) 0.60 - 0.90 mg/kg (35-50mg)

Day 2, vincristine (VCR) 0.015-0.025mg/kg (1mg)

Day 3, carboquone (CQ) 0.033-0.075mg/kg (2-3mg)

VCR and CQ were repeated 1-3 times/3-4 weeks if toxicity
permitted.

Patients

Twenty-two patients with malignant diseases received this
treatment in our hospital during the period from July 1978 to
February 1980.   The group consisted of 3 cases of gastric carcinoma with metastasis and recurrence, 3 of bronchogenic carcinoma,
3 of esophageal carcinoma, 1 of pancreas carcinoma, 3 of head and
neck carcinoma, 3 of thyroid carcinoma with metastasis and recurrence, 1 of osteogenic sarcoma and 5 of soft tissue sarcoma.

RESULTS

The results obtained are summarized according to the evaluation
criteria of either WHO or Karnofsky:
1.   By WHO criteria; CR = 3/17, PR = 8/17 and NC + P = 6/17
2.   By Karnofsky's criteria; 1 - C = 1/17, 1 - B = 10/17,
1 - A = 1/17, 0 - C = 3/17 and 0 - 0 = 2/17.

The detailed data of the patients are shown in Table 1 and
the clinical course of 3 patients who showed complete response
to the treatment are given below.

Table 1.

Clinical Results of Angiotensin II Combination Chemotherapy*
in Cancer Patients evaluated according to the WHO criteria.

Tumor	NO. of cases	CR	PR	NC	PD
gastric carcinoma	2 (1)**	-	-	2	-
lung carcinoma	3	1	2	-	-
esophagus carcinoma	1 (2)	-	-	-	1
pancreas carcinoma	0 (1)	-	-	-	-
head & neck carcinoma	3	-	3	-	-
thyroid carcinoma	2 (1)	-	2	-	-
sarcoma	6	2	1	1	2
total	17 (5)	3	8	3	3

* *Drugs used, ADR,VCR,CQ,MMC,BLM,MTX,5-FU,NITROSOUREA etc.*
**The number in parentheses indicates the case not evaluable.*

Table 2.
Appearance of side effects and
frequency related to AVQ***

side effect	frequency
leucopenia 3000-2000	9/18 } 11/18
2000-1000	2/18
thrombopenia 10,000	2/18
nausea & vomiting*	11/18
alopecia*	13/18
change in ECG**	1/18
peripheral neuropathy	3/18

* *almost slight ones*
***reversible ST-depression*
****combination chemotherapy of adriamycin,*
 vincristine and carboquone

Table 3.
Time for appearance of initial response
and evaluation of the effects.

patient	initial response* (week)	effect evaluation (week)
1. K. S.	2	2
3. M. T.	1	3
4. H. I.	2	3
5. Y. W.	3	4
6. Y. O.	4	7
7. T. H.	2	3
11. Y. S.	0.4(3days)	3
12. T. C.	3	6
13. K. H.	2	4
14. K. C.	0.6(4day)	-
15. T. S.	1	6
16. T. M.	2	8
18. Y. M.	3	3
20. M. M.	8	8
21. U. M.	3	6

**Tumor regression and/or other sign of improvement*

Case 1: A 70 year old male with bronchogenic carcinoma (small cell
carcinoma), complained of productive cough, and anorexia for 3
months was admitted to hospital in August 1978. He had a fever and
a large shadow in the hilar region of the left lung. This disappeared completely after one course of combination chemotherapy of
AVQ with angiotensin II. The tumor recurred after 3 months and
the patient died in March 1979.

Case 2: A 51 year old male with a rhabdomyosarcoma (pleomorphic
type) in the left supraclavicular region, was admitted in March
1979. The painful and firm tumor extended rapidly into the left
cervical region before the treatment. A marked response was
observed within a few days after treatment and the tumor became in-
palpable after 3 weeks. The patient is still in complete remission
at present (1 year later), having received several repeated treatments intermittently.

Case 3: A 68 year old female with a leiomyosarcoma of the stomach,
was admitted complaining of epigastric discomfort in August 1979.
No response was obtained to chemotherapy over a few months, and
then AVQ combined with angiotensin II was administered in December
1979. Two months later the tumor had regressed completely.
The regression in the gastric mucosa was observed by means of
X-ray and endoscopic examination. No tumor was detected in the
biopsy specimen of the mucosa. She subsequently received surgery.

A variety of side effects were observed, although this was
not severe in most cases. The frequency is summarized in Table
2. Leucopenia was seen commonly as was alopecia in patients who
received adriamycin; however, the severity was slight in most
cases. Nausea and vomiting were experienced sometimes, particularly
after adriamycin. In general, the occurrence of these side
effects seemed to be no more frequent than that observed after
intravenous administration of adriamycin without angiotensin II
(Cortes et al., 1975, Hoogstraten, 1975).

DISCUSSION

Caution must be exercised in the method used to elevate blood pressure when carrying out this treatment. Careful attention must be paid not to elevate the blood pressure too rapidly. In animal experiments, it is known that the blood brain barrier was functionally destroyed when the mean pressure was elevated from 100 to 200 mmHg in rats (Häggendal and Johanssen, 1972., Suzuki et al., 1975, Suzuki et al., 1977a). Some patients complained of headache, shoulder dullness or breast discomfort when the pressure was elevated rapidly within one minute, while none had such symptoms if the BP was elevated carefully over 3 to 4 minutes.

The time of infusion of angiotensin II was 10 minutes, as it was known that the plasma half life of adriamycin, carboquone or mitomycin C are relatively short (Baucher, 1975, Fujita, 1971). However, further investigations should be carried out to determine adequate infusion times for the use of other anticancer drugs.

It was worth noting in our cases that the initial response appeared early and the effect evaluation time (the time required for evaluable effects) was relatively short as seen in Table 3. This seemed reasonable considering the experimental results obtained in animals (Suzuki et al., 1980). Based on these findings, it might be possible to estimate the sensitivity of a drug on the tumor of a patient in the early stages of treatment. Although some conditions are considered as a contraindication for our treatment, e.g. uncontrollable hypertension, active ischemic heart disease or severe bleeding lesion, the combination chemotherapy with angiotensin II based on the concept of enhanced drug delivery can be introduced safely into clinical trials without any technical difficulties.

REFERENCES

Baucher, N.R., 1975. Adriamycin pharmacology. Cancer Chemother. Rep. Part 3(6): 153-158.
Cortes, E.P., Holland, J.F., Wang, J.J. and Glidewell, O., 1975. Adriamycin in 87 patients with osteosarcoma. Cancer Chemother. Rep. Part 3(6): 305-313.
Fujita, H., 1971. The characteristics of tissue distribution, excretion and inactivation of anti-cancer drugs. Sogo-Rinsho 20: 1350-1359 (in Japanese).
Hoogstraten, B., 1975. Adriamycin in the treatment of advanced brest cancer. Studies by the Southwest Oncology Group. Cancer Chemother. Rep. Part 3(6): 329-334.
Häggendal, E. and Johansson, B., 1972. On the pathophysiology of the increased cerebrovascular permeability in acute arterial hypertension in cats. Acta Neurol. Scand., 48: 265-270.
Suzuki, T., Tominaga, S., Standgaad, S. and Nakamura, T., 1975. Fluorescein cineangiography of the pial microcirculation in the rat in acute angio-tensin-induced hypertension. Blood Flow and Metabolism in the Brain. Harper, A.M. et al. (Editors) Churchill Livingstone, Edinburgh, London and New York. pp. 5.8-5.9.
Suzuki, M. and Sato, H., 1977a. Experimental studies on local penetration of anticancer drug in tumor tissue. Cancer and Chemotherapy, 4(Suppl.): 97-102.
Suzuki, M., Hori, K., Abe, I., Saito, S. and Sato, H., 1977b. Characteristic blood circulation in tumor tissue, with reference to local permeation of drug in cancer chemotherapy. Proc. Jap. Cancer Assoc., The 36th Ann. Meeting. P.149.
Suzuki, M., Hori, K., Abe, I., Saito, S. and Sato, H., 1978. Characteristic blood circulation in tumor tissue, with reference to cancer chemotherapy. Cancer and Chemotherapy, 5(Suppl. 1): 77-80.
Suzuki, M., Hori, K., Abe, I., Saito, S. and Sato, H., 1979a. Characteristics of microcirculation in tumor. Cancer and Chemotherapy, 6(Suppl. II): 287-291.
Suzuki, M., Hori, K., Abe, I., Saito, S. and Sato, H., 1979b. Characteristic microcirculation of tumor. J. Jap. Coll. Angiol., 19: 233-236.
Suzuki, M., Hori, K., Abe, I., Saito, S. and Sato, H., 1980. Experimental study on characteristics of microcirculation in tumor tissue, with reference to cancer chemotherapy. Proceedings of the E.O.R.T.C. Metastasis Group Conference on clinical and Experimental Aspects of Metastasis, Hague, in print.
Sato, H., Asamura, M., Kanamaru, R. and Wakui, A., 1979a. Sequential designing of combination modalities based on the analysis of cell population kinetics in cancer chemotherapy. Proc. Jap. Cancer Assoc. The 38th Ann. Meeting. p.174.
Sato, H., Asamura, M., Kobayashi, Y., Kanamaru, R., Sato, K., Wakui, A., Suzuki, M., Hori, K., Abe, I. and Saito, S., 1979b. Clinical cancer chemotherapy based on the concepts of enhanced drug delivery in tumor tissue by angiotensin II. Proc. Jap. Cancer Assoc. The 38th Ann. Meeting. p. 180.
Sato, H., Asamura, M., Kanamaru, R., Sato, K., Wakui, A., Suzuki, M. and Sato, H., 1979c, (Abstract) Clinical cancer chemotherapy based on a concept of enhanced drug delivery to tumor by angiotensin II. J. Jap. Soc. for Cancer Therapy, (in print).

DIFFERENCES AND SIMILARITIES IN ADJUVANT CHEMOTHERAPY IN MOUSE AND MAN

L.M. van Putten and A.F.C. Gerritsen

The effectiveness of adjuvant chemotherapy is easily demonstrated in many mouse models, whereas in man the response is good but far less spectacular. With the aid of a mathematical model the following variables in which differences may exist between mouse and man were tested:

1. Uniformity of tumour load in population

2. Cell kinetic factors in drug sensitivity

3. Variation of drug sensitivity among tumours

4. Drug penetration into tumour

5. Tumour antigenicity

6. Variation in growth rate among tumours

It is concluded that factors. 1. and 3. are responsible for the difference. Mouse models are more sensitive by selection of an effective drug and an optimal tumour load. Other factors seem not to affect the results.

(The full paper is accepted for publication in 'Cell and Tissue Kinetics')

Studies were supported by the Queen Wilhelmina Fund for Cancer Research.

DRUG RESPONSE OF TWO DIFFERENT IN VITRO TUMOUR LINES DERIVED FROM LUNG METASTASES OF 3LL

M. Caputo, A. Corsi, A. Sacchi and G. Zupi

INTRODUCTION

The selection of cell lines derived from the same tumour and with different metastatic potential has been claimed to be a suitable approach to the problem of cancer metastasis (Fidler, 1978). In our laboratory,two cell lines were isolated from the lung metastases of a Lewis lung carcinoma. They were characterized and found different. This study was designed to verify whether such a difference in malignant properties would also correspond to a different sensitivity to various antineoplastic drugs.

MATERIALS AND METHODS

The cell lines used in these experiments were derived from lung nodules of a Lewis lung carcinoma. The procedure followed,to isolate and select the lines was described in detail in a previous paper (Sacchi,et al.,1979).The cells were grown as monolayers adherent to the plastic surface of a culture flask.The optimal growth conditions were achieved using a Waymouth's medium supplemented with 15% Calf serum in 10% CO_2 + 7% O_2 + 90% N_2.

Cell lines properties. The two lines (labelled BC215 and C108 respectively) are quite similar as regards the growth curve and plating efficiency in vitro (P.E. values : 35% for BC215 vs 40% for C108). Moreover the kinetic parameters have been studied using the Flow cytometry analysis (FCM) and measuring the DNA content of the cells stained with propidium iodide. Fig.1 shows the cell cycle distribution during the log and the log to plateau transition phase of growth.As it is possible to see, the G1 - S - G2/M distribution of the BC215 cells is closely similar to that of C108 cells.

Their tumorigenic ability was tested by the TD50 assay. Graded inocula of viable cells (without addition of H.R. cells) were implanted i.m. in C57Bl/6 mice in a range of concentrations differing by a factor of two.TD50 values were calculated 60 days after tumour implant by the method of Spearmann-Karber (Finney,1964). In both the cases the values were identical:800 cells (95%C.L.: 641 - 1167).

The lung colony forming ability was then studied by injecting 0.5 ml of a cell suspension in the tail vein of syngeneic mice without addition of heavily irradiated (H.R.) cells or microspheres (Suzuki et al.,1978).Fig.2 shows that the CIO8 line has a far greater colony forming ability than the BC215 line.It is interesting to point out here that the C108 line,when reinjected i.m. in the mice, gave rise to an in vivo subline (M1087) whose spontaneous metastatic ability is greater than that of both the parent line and the other derivative subline.

(%) OF CELL IN DIFFERENT PHASES OF THE CYCLE ACCORDING TO DNA CONTENT MONITORED BY FLOW CYTOMETRY

	C108 LINE		BC215 LINE	
	LOG. PHASE	LOG. to PLATEAU TRANSITION	LOG. PHASE	LOG. to PLATEAU TRANSITION
	(3rd day of growth)	(4th day of growth)	(4th day of growth)	(5th day of growth)
G_1/G_0	27	56	22	40
S	57	24	63	41
G_2/M	16	20	15	19

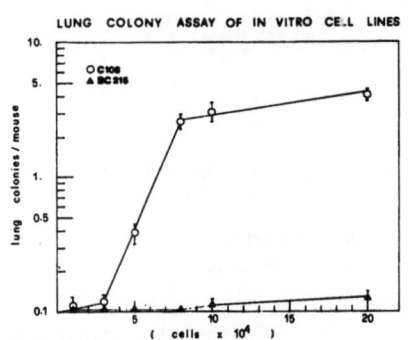

LUNG COLONY ASSAY OF IN VITRO CELL LINES

Fig.1 FCM analysis of the
two lines.

Fig.2 Lung colony forming ability of the two lines.

Cell survival studies.All the experiments were carried out using cells in the exponential phase of growth.After each treatment the medium containing the drug was removed,the cells growing as monolayer in 6 cm Petri dishes were washed with Earle's BSS,trypsinized (0.3% trypsin x 4' at 37°C) counted in a Coulter counter (mod. ZB1) and replated in appropiate dilutions.After 7 - 8 days the dishes were stained with methylene blue and colonies of more than 50 cells were scored. Drugs.Adriamycin (Adriblastina, Farmitalia - ADM),Hydroxyurea (Squibb - HOU) and Bleomycin (Roger Bellon - BLM) were diluted in the medium up to 10 times the final concentration. ICRF159 (Razoxane,kindly supplied by Dr. Hellmann) was dissolved in 0.4 N HCl before diluting in the medium.

RESULTS AND DISCUSSION

398

In fig.3,the effects of HOU (10 mM) on both the lines are represented .

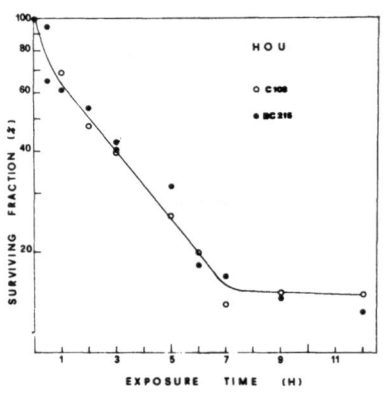

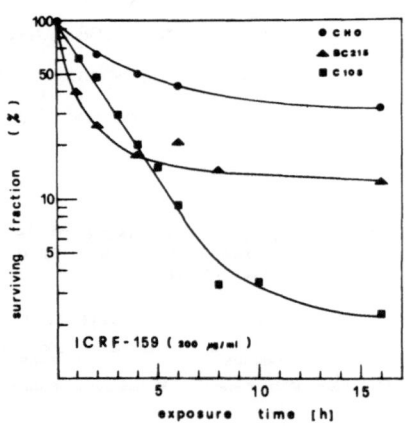

Fig.3 HOU effects on BC215
      and C108 lines.

Fig.4 Response of the two
      lines to ICRF159.

As can be seen,the time dependent survival curve follows an identical trend
for C108 line as well as for the BC215 line and reaches the same plateau value of
15-16% after a time exposure of 7 hours.This particular case is the only exception
to the different behaviour of the two lines to the agents tested throughout our
study.This could probably be explained on the basis of the strict similarity in
their main kinetic parameters,as indicated by the FCM analysis.

Fig.4 represents the effects of ICRF159 as a function of the exposure time on
the cell lines.In sharp contrast with the previous results,the C108 line is the
most sensitive to this agent As is widely known,Razoxane is considered as a specific
antimetastatic agent and its peculiar activity was first   evaluated just on lung
metastases of the Lewis lung carcinoma (Salsbury,et al.,1973).It is worth mentio-
ning that the C108 line cells have the higest (spontaneous and artificial) metastatic ability when reinjected either intravenously or intramuscularly in syngeneic
C57Bl/6 mice.

The data presented here are consistent with the hypothesis mentioned above.As a matter of fact,different cell lines derived from the same tumour
are also different in regard to their chemosensitivity to various antineoplastic
drugs.In our opinion,the use of cell variants with different metastatic potential

can be of valuable help in planning strategies for developing optimum treatment regimens,either in the **choice** of drug and dose and in the effort to overcome the phenomenon of drug resistance.

Table I summarizes the response of the two lines to ADM,evaluated as a function of the dose.

TABLE I

SURVIVING FRACTION (S.F.) AFTER TWO HOURS EXPOSURE TO ADRIAMYCIN

DOSES	CELL LINES	
	BC215	C108
(g/ml)	% S.F.	% S.F.
1×10^{-7}	65.	65.
1×10^{-6}	10.	55.
2×10^{-6}	4.5	20.
5×10^{-6}	0.55	13.
1×10^{-5}	0.02	4.
5×10^{-5}	0.02	1.2

The dose dependent response to ADM is completely different in the two lines:the C108 line exhibits a significant resistance to this agent,in sharp contrast with the other line.Furthermore,using doses higher than 2×10^{-6} g/ml the linear dose effect relation is missed and an increase in the dose does not correspond to a li-near increase of the C108 cell killing.This finding could be interesting for its clinical implications,particularly as concerns the overdose problem.

TABLE II

SURVIVING FRACTION (S.F.) AFTER BLEOMYCIN TREATMENT

DOSES	EXPOSURE TIME	CELL LINES	
		BC215	C108
(g/ml)	(hours)	% S.F.	% S.F.
1×10^{-6}	4	10.	14.
1×10^{-6}	16	2.	6.
1×10^{-5}	4	1.5	3.
1×10^{-5}	16	0.15	1.5

Similar results were found when BLM was tested as a function of both the expo-sure time and the doses employed.Also in this case,as shown in Table II,the C108 line was affected to a lesser extent,whereby the BC215 line elicited a greater sensitivity.

Supported by CNR grant: PFCCN – n° 790069096.

REFERENCES

Fidler, I.J.,1978.Tumor heterogeneity and the biology of Cancer invasion and me-
    tastasis. Cancer Res., 38: 2651 – 2660.

Finney, D.J.,1964.Statistical methods in Biological Assay.525 – 529, 2nd ed.
    Griffin and Co. London.

Sacchi, A.,Corsi, A., Caputo, M.,Zupi, G.,1979.In vitro and in vivo selection of
    two Lewis lung carcinoma cell lines.Tumori, 65: 657 – 664.

Salsbury, A.J.,Burrage, K. and Hellmann, K.,1973.Inibition of metastatic spread
    by ICRF159: selective **deletion** of a **malignant** characteristic.Brit. Med. J.,
    4: 344 – 346.

Suzuki, N. and Withers, H.R.,1978.Isolation from a murine fibrosarcoma of cell
    lines with enhanced plating efficiency in vitro.J. Natl. Cancer Inst. ,60 :
    179 – 183.

ACKNOWLEDGMENTS

We thank Dr. F. Mauro and Dr. G. Starace for collaboration with the Flow cytometry experiments.

THERAPEUTIC IMPLICATIONS OF HETEROGENEOUS TUMOR CELL POPULATIONS

J. Lundy, P. Roberts, E.J. Lovett III, S. Elgebaly and J. Varani

Heterogeneous subpopulations of tumor cells with varying biologic properties have been demonstrated in animal and human tumors (Fidler, 1978; Dexter, 1979; Barranco, 1973).

We have isolated from a 3-methylcholanthrene induced syngeneic murine fibrosarcoma several clones which vary greatly in malignant potential (Varani, 1979a; Varani, 1979b). No differences were observed in in-vitro growth kinetics between the parent tumor (P), high malignant (Ll) or low malignant (NP) clones. However, in-vivo growth kinetics were significantly different with Ll growing most rapidly, P intermediate, and NP the slowest. Both Ll and P primary tumors can be established in 100% of mice with doses of 1×10^4 - 1×10^5 cells. However, the antigenic NP clone requires an inoculum of at least 3×10^6 cells to produce a similar effect. This data suggests that not only tumor properties but also host factors are significant determinants of tumor growth in-vivo.

Since we knew that P and Ll have the capacity to spontaneously metastasize and kill, we developed a protocol using chemotherapy and immunotherapy directed at the specific clones in order to obtain optimal tumor kill.

METHODS

<u>Mice</u> - Six to eight-week-old C57Bl/6 J female mice were obtained from Jackson Laboratory, Bar Harbor, Maine. Mice were fed and watered ad libitum.
<u>Tumor</u> - A 3-methylcholanthrene induced syngeneic murine fibrosarcoma was serially passed in-vivo and maintained in tissue culture in-vitro. Ll and NP clones were maintained in a similar fashion. The method by which these clones were initially obtained has been described previously (Varani, 1979a).

For all in-vivo experiments, single cell suspensions were injected intradermally in the flank and tumor diameters measured three times per week. Tumor volumes were determined according to the method of Sparks, et al (Sparks, 1974). The correlation of tumor weight to the calculated volume was .974.

For in-vitro experiments, tumor cells were grown in 35 mm culture dishes. On days 1,3 and 5 following the addition of chemotherapeutic agents, dishes were harvested and the number of viable cells determined.

In both in-vitro and in-vivo experiments, growth inhibition was determined
by the following formula:

$$\% \text{ Inhibition} = \left[1 - \frac{\text{Experimental (Treated)}}{\text{Control (Untreated)}} \right] \times 100$$

Drugs - 1,3-bis (2-chlorethyl)-1-nitrosourea (BCNU), Bristol Laboratories,
was administered at the optimal in-vivo dose of 30 mg/kgm on day 2 post tumor
transplantation.

Fluorouracil (5FU), Adria Laboratories, Inc., was given intraperitoneally
at a dose of 20 mg/kgm on day 2 when used as a single agent. When combined
with BCNU, it was given on the same day at a dose of 20 mg/kgm.

Corynebacterium parvum (C. parvum), Burroughs Wellcome Co., when used
alone was given at a dose of 350 ugm intratumorally on day 2. When combined
with chemotherapy, the drug was given on day 5 (3 days after BCNU).
Statistical Analysis - Arc sin transformation of percent inhibition of tumor
growth was compared in a one-way analysis of variants and Duncan's procedure.

RESULTS

Both 5FU and BCNU were tested against P, L1 and NP in-vitro (Figure 1).
5FU was most effective against L1 ($>$70% inhibition). BCNU showed the
greatest tumor inhibition against L1 and P, but also demonstrated activity
at the highest concentration against NP.

The in-vivo drug activity did not correlate well with in-vitro results
(Figure 2). After establishing dose/response curves for all chemotherapeutic
and immunotherapeutic drugs in-vivo, the optimal dose of BCNU, 5FU, or C.
parvum as single agents was employed as described in the methods section.
BCNU was most effective in inhibiting growth of L1 (87% inhibition), but less
effective against P or NP. 5FU demonstrated no in-vivo efficacy against P
or L1. When BCNU and 5FU were used in combination, the observed effect on P
or L1 was no greater than the effect of BCNU alone.

A single intratumoral dose of C. parvum demonstrated maximum activity
against NP (65% inhibition) with limited efficacy against P or L1.

Since BCNU inhibited L1 and C. parvum inhibited NP, it was logical that
the combination should have the optimal efficacy against parent tumor.
Figure 3 demonstrates the combination inhibited parent tumor growth by 85%.
The only short term cures (less than 4 weeks) of mice bearing parent tumor
were observed in this group (50%).

For detailed explanation of Figures, see text.

FIGURE 1.

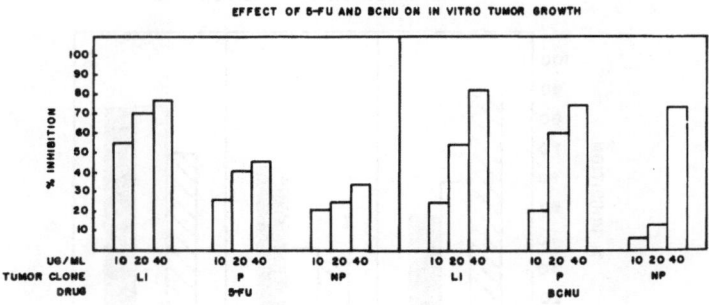

EFFECT OF 5-FU AND BCNU ON IN VITRO TUMOR GROWTH

FIGURE 2.

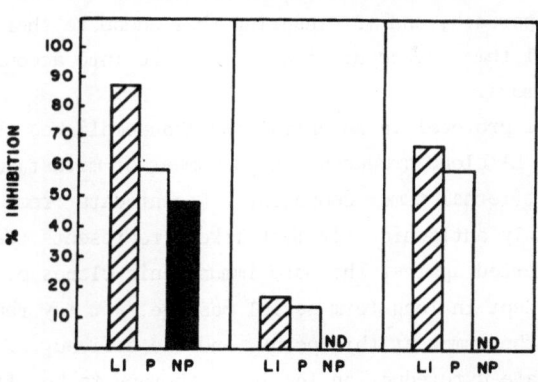

% INHIBITION OF TUMOR GROWTH

FIGURE 3.

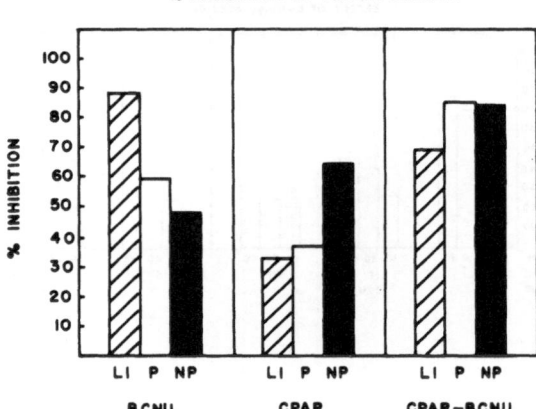

DISCUSSION

A multimodal approach to therapy of solid tumors that metastasize should take into account several basic principles including (1) reducing tumor bulk to allow host defenses to be effective, (2) appropriate timing of drugs in a combined modality approach, and (3) insuring that adequate therapy has been directed against all tumor subpopulations, i.e. take into account the heterogeneity of tumors.

Our experimental protocol in an animal model accomplishes the above. The rapidly growing L1 clone produces a high number of metastases and probably is the most lethal tumor component. Recent data from our laboratory indicates it is weakly antigenic. It most likely represents the result of immune selection exerted against the more immunogenic clones of a methyl-cholanthrene tumor kept in long-term serial passage. It may represent the major component of the tumor at this point, and the efficacy of BCNU against L1 allows for adequate cytoreduction for immunotherapy to be effective.

NP is antigenic and slowly growing. C. parvum's efficacy may be on the basis of an augmentation of tumor-specific immune reactivity in the host or a local effect involving the macrophage. The possibility of an innocent bystander effect has also been suggested (Kreider, 1978). Our timing for using C. parvum with BCNU was arbitrary and based in part upon drug schedules used by Fisher in combination chemoimmunotherapy protocols with C. parvum

(Fisher, 1978). Clearly, our combination therapy met criteria (c), i.e. it was directed effectively against both clones. Olsson and Ebbesen's work with AKR mouse thymomas is another example of the necessity to attack, at least immunologically, all components of a polyclonal tumor (Olsson, 1979).

In summary, solid tumors with the capacity to metastasize and kill can be most effectively treated in part by better understanding the biology of tumor cell subpopulations.

REFERENCES

Barranco, S.C., Drewinko, B., and Humphrey, R.M. 1973. Differential response by human melanoma cells to 1,3-(bis) - (2-chloramethyl)-1-nitrosurea and bleomycin. Mutation Res. 19:277-280.

Dexter, D.L., Kowalski, H.M., Blazar, B.A., Fligiel, Z., Vogel, R., and Heppner, G. 1978. Heterogeneity of tumor cells from a single mouse mammary tumor. Cancer Res. 38:3174-3181.

Fidler, I. 1978. Tumor heterogeneity and the biology of cancer invasion and metastasis. Cancer Res. 38:2651-2660.

Fisher, B., Gebhardt, M., Linta, J. and Saffer, E. 1978. Comparison of the inhibition of tumor growth following local or systemic administration of corynebacterium parvum of other immunostimulating agents with or without cyclophosphamide. Cancer Res. 38:2679-2687.

Kreider, J.W., Bartlett, G.L., Purnell, D.M. and Webb, S. 1978. Immunotherapy of an established rat mammary adenocarcinoma (13762A) with intratumor injection of corynebacterium parvum. Cancer Res. 38:689-692.

Olsson, L. and Ebbesen, P. 1979. Natural polyclonality of spontaneous AKR leukemia and its consequences for so-called specific immunotherapy. J. Natl. Cancer Inst. 62:623-627.

Sparks, F.C. and Breeding, J.H. 1974. Tumor regression and enhancement resulting from immunotherapy with bacillus calmetter-guerin and neuraminidase. Cancer Res. 34:3262-3269.

Varani, J., Orr W., Ward, P.A. 1979a. Comparison of subpopulations of tumor cells with altered migratory activity, attachment characteristics, enzyme levels and in-vivo behavior. Eur. J. Cancer 15:582-592.

Varani, J., Orr, W., Ward, P.A. 1979b. Hydrolytic enzyme activities, migratory activity and in-vivo growth and metastatic potential of recent tumor isolates. Cancer Res. 39:2376-2380.

EFFECT OF BLEOMYCIN SCHEDULING ON LUNG METASTASES OF 3LL AND A SUBLINE OF DIFFERENT METASTATIC POTENTIAL

C. Greco, F. Calabresi, M. Caputo, A. Sacchi, G. Zupi

INTRODUCTION

In the past ten years several reports have shown the hetero-geneous nature of both the human and experimental neoplasm.   In fact, many authors demonstrated the existence of distinct cell subpopulations in the tumours differing in various characteristics like number of chromosomes, DNA content, antigenic properties, metastatic potential (Fidler, 1978).   Moreover, it has been pointed out that the employment of such tumour sublines selected within the same tumour represents a useful tool for experimental chemo-therapy studies (Lotan et al., 1979).

As previously reported (Zupi et al., 1980) in our own laboratory, several lines were isolated either in vitro and in vivo from the Lewis lung carcinoma (3LL), differing in some bio-logical characteristics from the parent tumour.   In particular, the subline named M1087 markedly differs from the original line in that it elicits a more exponential trend of tumour growth, a higher oncogenicity, an early spreading of the metastatic cells, a higher number of both spontaneous and artificial lung nodules.

The aim of the present study was : (i) to investigate if the differences observed between both the original line and the M1087 subline, mainly in oncogenicity and in metastatic potential, would correspond to a different response with a known antineo-plastic agent, Bleomycin, at the level of secondary tumours, (ii) to verify whether a variation of scheduling-either as function of the dose or of the interval of administration - could influence the response of lung metastases of both tumour lines to Bleomycin.

MATERIALS AND METHODS

3LL tumour lines.   The original line is maintained in our laboratory biweekly i.m. transplanted into C57BL/6 mice, its strain of origin.   During the experiments, each animal was injected with 0.1 ml of a suspension containing 2.5×10^5

viable cells (0.02% Trypan blue). The tumour cell suspension was mechanically prepared as previously reported (Sacchi et al., 1979).The M1087 subline was obtained after two in vitro selections of cells derived from a biopsy of lung nodules of the original 3LL line (Zupi et al., 1980). When these experiments were performed the M1087 subline was in the 54th animal passage . Tumour cell suspension and transplantation of this subline were performed as for the original line.

TD50 determination . Graded inocula of viable tumour cells (without the addition of H.R. cells) were implanted i.m. within a range of concentrations differing by a factor of 2. Tumour takes were periodically detected and 60 days after tumour cells implantation the TD50 values were calculated by the method of Spearman and Karber

Lung colony assay . The tumour suspensions containing the appropriate concentration of viable cells in 0.5 ml were injected into tail veins of C57BL/6 mice (15 animals/group), without the addition of H.R. cells or microspheres. Eighteen days after inoculation the mice were killed, lungs removed and fixed in a Bouin's solution to score the colonies .

Drug and scheduling . Bleomycin (BLM)(Roger Bellon)was dissolved in sterile 0.9% NaCl. The appropriate concentrations of the drug were injected i.m. in a volume of 0.01ml/g body weight.For every treatment, groups of at least 20 animals were used. Throughout this study, the following treatments were performed : schedule (a)-single dose of BLM(80mg/Kg or 40mg/Kg)on day 1st or 3rd after tumour implantation; schedules b (b_1)- five times injections of 4mg/Kg/dose (24 hr interval) from the 1st to the 5th day after tumour implantation ;(b_2)- ten times injections of 8mg/Kg/dose or 4mg/Kg/dose (12 hr interval) from the 1st to the 5th day after tumour implantation ;(b_3)- 1,6mg/Kg/dose every 3 hr for 12 hr, followed by a 12 hr interval,from the 1st to the 5th day after tumour implantation.

RESULTS

The oncogenicity of both tumour lines was assessed by determining the number of cells required to produce 50% takes in syngeneic recipient animals. In our experimental conditions, the TD50 value was 730 cells(95% c.1.=949-561)for the original line and 225 cells(95% c.1.= 330-154) for the M1087 subline .

As regards the differences in metastatic potential elicited by the two lines, they are shown in Tables 1 and 2. As is evident a higher metastatic ability is exhibited by the M1087 subline respect to the parent line, either as production of

spontaneous pulmonary metastases or as cloning efficiency in the
lung following i.v. injection of the tumour cells.

TABLE 1
Spontaneous pulmonary metastases of the original 3LL line and of the M1087 subline after i.m. tumour implantation

Days after 3LL implant	N° Metastases (mean ± S.E.)	
(2.5 x 10^5 viable cells)	Original line	M1087 subline
13 th	2.25 ± 0.25	14.5 ± 4.5
15 th	19.0 ± 4	32.0 ± 10
17 th	20.2 ± 5	34.0 ± 10
21 st	38.0 ± 2	69.0 ± 9

TABLE 2
Artificial lung colonies/mouse after i.v. injection of viable tumour cells from
both the original 3LL line and the M1087 subline

Size of inoculum	N° Colonies (mean ± S.E.)	
	Original line	M1087 subline
1 x 10^4	0.55 ± 0.15	1.8 ± 0.2
3 x 10^4	1.1 ± 0.5	3.0 ± 0.8
5 x 10^4	2.2 ± 0.6	6.0 ± 1.0
1 x 10^5	8.0 ± 1.5	20.0 ± 2.0
2 x 10^5	19.0 ± 2.0	50.0 ± 8.0

Previous experiments in our laboratory have shown that the M1087
subline exhibits an earlier dissemination of the metastatic cells from
the primary tumour, in comparison to the original parent line (Greco
et al., 1980).

The antimetastatic effect produced with both tumour lines by
different treatment schedules of BLM is reported in Table 3. As
can be observed, no significantly different responses are elicited in
either tumour line after 40 mg/kg or 80 mg/kg BLM given in single
doses. Conversely, after fractionated administration of the drug,

a different antimetastatic effect is produced. In particular, while
the fractionated schedules induce a marked improvement on metastases
reduction of the original line, no similar decrease in the metastases
number is observed on the M1087 derivative subline.

TABLE 3

Effects of Bleomycin dose schedule on metastases reduction of the original 3LL
line and of the M1087 subline

Treatment schedule	% Metastases Reduction [*]	
	Original line	M1087 subline
BLM 80mg/Kg, day 1st	38.8	33.3
80mg/Kg, day 3rd	57.5	43.1
8mg/Kg/dose (q12h x 10)[**]	100.0	56.3
BLM 40mg/Kg, day 1st	n.e.	24.0
40mg/Kg, day 3rd	61.1	36.0
4mg/Kg/dose (q12h x 10)[**]	92.7	48.0

[*] % M.R. $= (\dfrac{n^\circ \text{ Metastases T} - n^\circ \text{ Metastases C}}{n^\circ \text{ Metastases C}}) - 1 \times 100$

[**] BLM was given beginning on day 1st after tumour implantation

Successively, other kinds of fractional schedules were tested on the original
3LL line, using the total lower dose of BLM (40mg/Kg). Data relative to the effect on the metastases reduction are reported in Table 4.

TABLE 4

Effect of Bleomycin scheduling (total dose 40mg/Kg) on lung metastases of the
original 3LL line

Treatment schedule	% Metastases Reduction
	Original Line
BLM 8mg/Kg/dose (q24h x 5)	90.8
1.6mg/Kg/dose(q3h x 4; 12 h interval)	99.4

As shown, by reducing the interval of BLM administration we obtained a remarkable effect on the secondary tumour outgrowth, quite similar to that observed after the higher dose of BLM (80mg/Kg).

In conclusion, the findings of our preliminary study indicate that:

(i) the M1087 subline of the 3LL tumour elicits a resistance to BLM

(ii)it is possible to reduce drastically the BLM dose without reducing the antimetastatic effect on the 3LL tumour

(iii) it is possible to improve the therapeutic effectiveness of BLM on lung metastases using a fractionation scheduling with a very low dose of drug (40mg/Kg).

Supported by C.N.R. grant PFCCN N° 790.0690.96

REFERENCES

Fidler,I.J.,1978. Tumor heterogeneity and the biology of cancer invasion and metastasis. Cancer Res.,38: 2651-2660

Greco,C.,Calabresi,F.,Caputo,M., Corsi,A.,Sacchi,A.,Zupi,G.,1980. Adriamycin effect on the Lewis lung carcinoma : comparison between the original line and its derivative subline . Europ.J.Cancer, in press

Lotan,R. and Nicolson,G.L.,1979. Heterogeneity in growth inhibition by β transretinoic acid of metastatic B16 melanoma clones and in vivo-selected cell variant lines. Cancer Res., 39: 4767-4771

Sacchi,A., Corsi,A., Caputo,M., Zupi,G., 1979. In vitro and in vivo selection of two Lewis lung carcinoma cell lines . Tumori, 65: 657-664

Zupi,G., Mauro,F., Sacchi,A.,1980 . Cloning in vitro and in vivo of Lewis lung carcinoma : properties and characteristics . Brit.J.Cancer, 41: Suppl.IV

METASTASIS OF LEWIS LUNG CARCINOMA (LL) REGROWING AFTER CYTOTOXIC TREATMENTS

T.C. Stephens, K. Adams and J.H. Peacock

INTRODUCTION

The cytotoxic effects of drugs and radiation on primary tumours and their metastases have been extensively studied and small metastases are often found to be more sensitive to cytotoxic treatments than larger primary tumours (Shipley, Stanley and Steel, 1975; Steel, Adams and Stanley, 1976; Hill and Stanley, 1977). The implications are that treatment that fails to control a bulky primary tumour might control systemic metastases and under these circumstances the primary tumour will regrow and may re-metastasize.

We have examined the metastatic behaviour of untreated LL tumours and tumours regrowing after irradiation or treatment with cyclophosphamide (CY). Since it is well established that pretreatment of mice with CY or thoracic irradiation can enhance the production of artificial lung metastases resulting from i.v. injected tumour cells (Brown, 1973; van Putten et al, 1975; Carmel and Brown, 1977; Steel and Adams, 1977) we have also attempted to establish whether there is similar enhancement of naturally produced lung metastases by thoracic irradiation.

The relationship between the initiation of metastases and the size, age and clonogenic tumour cell content of untreated tumours

Intramuscular LL tumours were produced by implanting between 10^2 and 10^5 tumour cells and their volume growth curves were measured (Fig. 1A). The metastatic behaviour of these tumours was also examined, by sterilizing the implants at various times by local exposure to 50 Gy of γ-radiation and counting the number of macroscopic metastases present in the lungs when the animals were killed 14 days later. The patterns of metastasis for each implant size are shown in Fig. 1B.

Metastasis is clearly dependent on tumour size rather than age, and begins when tumours reach about 0.15g. By using an excision assay involving trypsinization to produce a cell suspension and clonal growth of the tumour cells in soft agar (Stephens, Currie and Peacock, 1978), tumours of 0.15g were found to contain about 2 to 3 x 10^6 clonogenic tumour cells.

The metastatic behaviour of LL tumours regrowing after cytotoxic treatments

Intramuscular tumours were allowed to grow until they had just begun to metastasize. They were then given a test treatment of 15 Gy local γ-radiation, or 75 mg/kg CY.

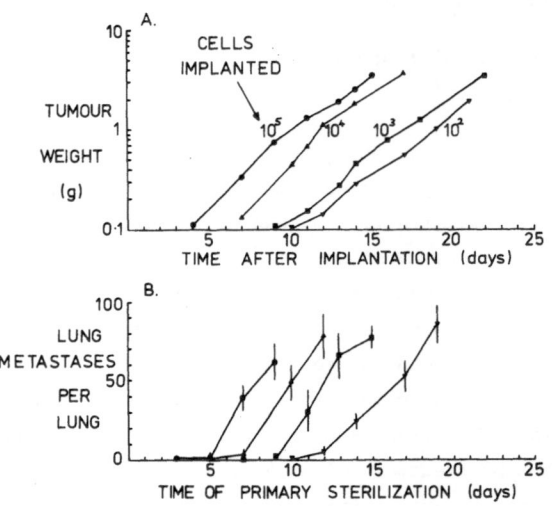

Fig. 1 Panel A shows the volume growth curves of untreated LL tumours derived from different sized cell implants and Panel B indicates the incidence of lung metastases observed by sterilizing the primary implant at various times after implantation.

The volume responses of the treated primary implants are shown in Fig. 2A and 3A. Each treatment produced a small growth delay, followed by regrowth at a rate similar to the untreated control.

The metastatic behaviour of the regrowing tumours was determined by the sterilization procedure outlined above. Any lung metastases produced prior to primary treatment were eradicated by 15 Gy thoracic irradiation 3 h after primary treatment. The extent of re-metastasis of regrowing tumours is shown in Figs. 2B and 3B. After both treatments regrowing tumours started to re-metastasize when they reached about 0.4 to 0.5g.

Cell survival measurements showed that the initial effect of each treatment was to reduce the number of clonogenic cells per tumour from about 3×10^6 to about 5×10^4. However by the time the tumours began to re-metastasize, some repopulation had occurred and there were about 2 to 3×10^5 clonogenic tumour cells per tumour.

Thus, after treatment tumours began to re-metastasize with about 1 decade fewer clonogenic cells than were present in untreated tumours when they began to metastasize.

There are several possible reasons why treated tumours may begin to re-metastasize with fewer clonogenic tumour cells present than in untreated tumours. It may simply reflect the presence of a pre-existing vascular system in regrowing tumours. Metastasis may be more rapid especially if the vascular bed has been

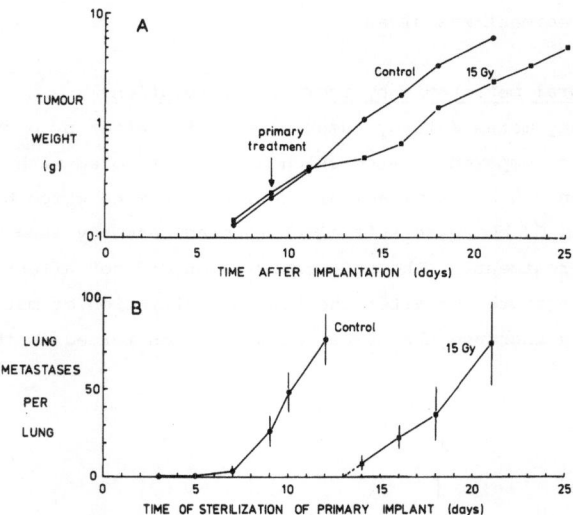

Fig. 2. Panel A shows the growth delay induced when primary LL tumours were treated locally with 15 Gy γ-radiation and panel B shows the incidence of lung metastases from the regrowing tumours.

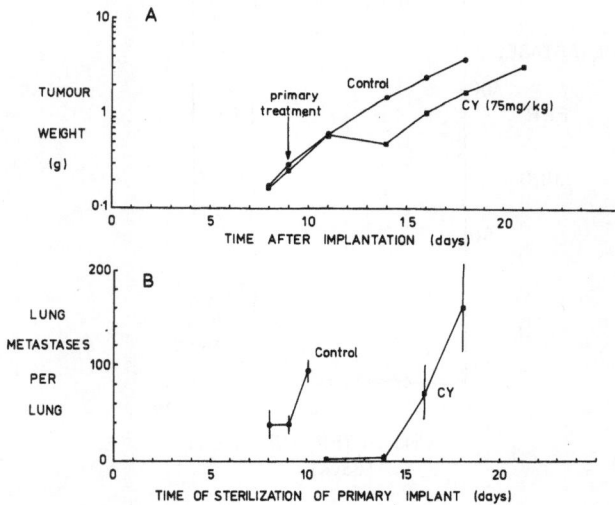

Fig. 3. Panel A shows the growth delay induced when primary LL tumours were treated with 75 mg/kg cyclophosphamide and panel B shows the incidence of lung metastases from the regrowing tumours.

damaged by treatment.   Alternatively, there may be enhancement of natural metastasis by the thoracic irradiation given to eradicate lung metastses seeded before the primary treatment was given.

Enhancement of natural metastasis by thoracic irradiation
    The extent of lung metastasis by tumours regrowing after primary treatment
with 75 mg/kg CY was compared in mice which had been treated with 15 Gy local
thoracic irradiation 3 h after CY administration, and mice which had received CY
only (Fig. 4).   The CY dose was sufficient to eradicate any lung metastases
present before CY treatment.   Thoracic irradiation did not affect the pattern
of primary tumour regrowth, or alter the time of initiation of metastasis, but
it did significantly increase the number of metastases formed as the tumours re-
grew.

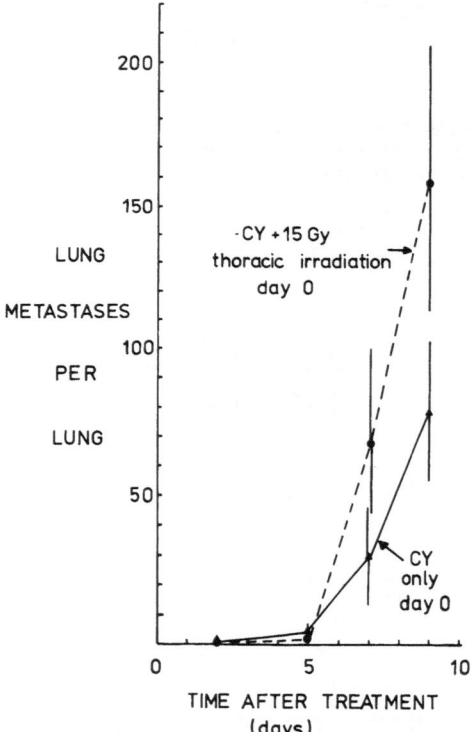

Fig. 4.   Shows the influence of thoracic irradiation on the incidence of lung
metastases from tumours regrowing after primary treatment with 75 mg/kg
cyclophosphamide.

SUMMARY AND CONCLUSIONS

We have found that pulmonary metastasis of untreated LL tumours is directly related to tumour size and to clonogenic tumour cell content. After cytotoxic treatment of primary tumours with γ-irradiation or CY, the relationship is changed and metastasis takes place when fewer clonogenic cells are present. Local thoracic irradiation leads to increased metastasis of tumours regrowing after CY treatment.

If a similar pattern of metastatic behaviour after treatment occurred in man, the implications are considerable. A cytotoxic treatment may fail to control a primary tumour which may then re-metastasize more quickly and more widely as it regrows.

REFERENCES

Brown, J.M., 1973. The effect of lung irradiation on the incidence of pulmonary metastases in mice. Br. J. Radiol., 46: 613-618.
Carmel, R.J. and Brown, J.M., 1977. The effect of cyclophosphamide and other drugs on the incidence of pulmonary metastases in mice. Cancer Res. 37: 145-151.
Hill, R.P. and Stanley, J.A., 1977. Pulmonary metastasis of the Lewis lung tumor-cell kinetics and response to cyclophosphamide at different sizes. Cancer Treatment Rep. 61: 29-36.
Shipley, W.U., Stanley, J.A. and Steel, G.G., 1975. Tumour size dependency in the radiation response of the Lewis lung carcinoma. Cancer Res. 35: 2488-2493.
Steel, G.G. and Adams, K., 1977. Enhancement by cytotoxic agents of artificial pulmonary metastasis. Br. J. Cancer 36: 653-658.
Steel, G.G., Adams, K. and Stanley, J.A., 1976. Size dependence of the response of Lewis lung tumours to BCNU. Cancer Treatment Rep. 60: 1743-1748.
Stephens, T.C., Currie, G.A. and Peacock, J.H., 1978. Repopulation of γ-irradiated Lewis lung carcinoma by malignant cells and host macrophage progenitors. Br. J. Cancer 38: 573-582.
van Putten, L.M., Kram, L.K.J., van Dierendonck, H.H.C., Smink, T. and Fuzy, M., 1975. Enhancement by drugs of metastatic lung nodule formation after intravenous tumour cell injection. Int. J. Cancer 15: 588-595.

ADJUVANT CHEMOTHERAPY FOLLOWING SURGERY FOR SMALL-CELL CARCINOMA OF THE LUNG

K. Karrer, N. Pridun and H. Denck

In spite of the fact that cancer of the lung is usually a
lethal disease increasing numbers of reports are generating
important information which can lead to further improvement of
therapeutic results in this disease. If adequately used, currently
available chemotherapy combined with surgery can produce prolongation of survival time and increasing experience warrants some
degree of optimism. Surgery is the therapy by which cure might
be obtained if preoperative assessment has unequivocally established
the presence of limited primary disease, but progress in preventing
or controlling carcinoma of the bronchus is contingent upon finding
methods that will either supplement or enhance the therapeutic
effectiveness of surgery.

It is generally accepted that, at the time of diagnosis, the
majority of bronchogenic carcinomas are systemic diseases. Any
material or really meaningful improvement in survival will therefore only be obtained if effective adjunctive treatment is
employed.

Amongst the various types of bronchogenic carcinomas, small,
or 'oat-cell' carcinoma of the lung has a particularly poor
prognosis. Because of the early spread of this type of tumour
it is not considered as operable. These patients are therefore
not resected, but receive intensive chemotherapy from the time of
diagnosis.

Impressive results with different chemotherapeutic regimes
in prolonging the survival time of oat cell carcinoma patients
have been obtained. However, no cures have been achieved, but
this might be possible by using surgery as an adjuvant to chemotherapy (Karrer 1978, 1979). There is evidence from clinical
research that the effectiveness of chemotherapy is closely related
to the degree of tumour body burden (Humphreys 1970, Friedl 1971).

From these results the following can also be concluded: the more advanced the tumour, the less is the probability that effective chemotherapeutic schedules can be given. On the other hand, the earlier and smaller the tumour appears to be the more effective chemotherapeutic schedules may be. A third point is that the more advanced the tumour is, the more unfavourable is the relation of therapeutic effectiveness of chemotherapy and its side effects (Karrer 1965). Patients with early stages of malignant disease can tolerate doses of chemotherapy closer to optimal than patients with advanced tumours. The host's defence mechanisms may also become exhausted during the advance of the disease.

For these reasons, surgical removal of the primary tumour may increase the chances of chemotherapy. For the small cell bronchial carcinomas there is no need to make an exception. The risk of surgery and the contraindications are identical for patients with small cell carcinomas and patients with other bronchial carcinomas.

As long as the primary small cell bronchial carcinoma can be removed by surgery without particular difficulty this should be performed in combination with effective chemotherapy. This seems to be in line with the usual surgical procedures for metastases and palliative tumour reduction. Recent results from our co-operative clinical trial support this point of view (Karrer 1979).

A co-operative randomized study of patients receiving surgery for cure of bronchial carcinomas of all histological types has been carried out in Vienna since 1969. High dose intermittent polychemotherapy consisting of 13 courses of three infusions separated by intervals of a week was administered over 3 years. Each infusion contained 12 mg/kg cyclophosphamide, 12 mg/kg 5-Fluorouracil (5-FU), 0.5 mg/kg methotrexate and 0.1 mg/kg vinblastine.

The evaluation of this study as of 1st March, 1980 is based on a total of 639 patients. They are classified into 3 groups by histology as 369 squamous-cell, 140 adeno-, 51 small-cell and 79 with all other types of carcinomas. In all, 2,762 such infusions were given to 246 patients who had undergone radical surgery. This treatment was generally well tolerated; and the incidence of leucopenia was within acceptable limits.

Comparisons of survival rates of the sub-divided treatment groups and control groups, calculated by the life-table method, show differences in the prognoses, as well as in the effectiveness of the chemotherapeutic used regime. These differences also existed with regard to tumour size (TNM-staging (Harmer 1978)) to clinical symptoms FEINSTEIN-classification (Feinstein 1969) and to histology.

For patients receiving chemotherapy and belonging to Feinstein class 3 or 5 (fast growing tumours), their survival curves show (in comparison to the controls) a slight beneficial effect in increased survival time, lasting for 1-2.5 years after operation, which disappeared thereafter. Five years after operation, the survival rate of the treated group was about 25%. which is similar to the controls.

The survival rate of patients receiving chemotherapy and belonging to Feinstein classes 2 or 4 (slow growing tumours) at the five year point was only about 10%, while the comparable figure of the controls was about 45% indicating the unfavourable effect of chemotherapy in this particular group of patients.

The subdivision of patients, according to the main histo-logically different groups without regard to TNM-staging or to the Feinstein categories, demonstrates a further differential effectiveness of this adjuvant chemotherapy.

While patients with squamous- and adenocarcinomas did not benefit from the chemotherapy there was an increased survival of patients with small-cell tumours in comparison with controls.

Thirty-one patients were randomized to the chemotherapy group, 23 of them have been observed for more than 3 years and 4 of them are surviving at this point. In contrast 19 randomized control patients died within 2 years as expected from general experience.

The 51 patients with small-cell carcinomas are from a total of 815 patients operated for bronchial carcinomas (6.2%).

Figure 1 compares the survival of patients operated on for small-cell bronchial carcinoma and either receiving or not receiving adjuvant chemotherapy after radical surgery.

The comparison of the life-tables of patients operated for bronchial carcinoma of the other histological types, non small-cell, i.e. adeno- or squamous cell, also indicated a prolongation of survival time in the group receiving the adjuvant chemotherapy.

According to the results mentioned above, these groups of patients should also be subdivided according to Feinstein- and TNM classifications, but this would only be meaningful if the numbers of patients treated is increased by further co-operative trials within larger international study groups.

We concluded from our results that there was a strong indication for further clinical trials of such combined modality treatment. Therefore we started a new randomized co-operative trial in patients who were radically operated for small-cell bronchial carcinoma, one group received the same polychemotherapy as given in the trial referred to above. The other group of this two-armed randomized trial receives a newly designed, intermittent polychemotherapy and radiation. In the new protocol the chemotherapy regimen uses the following 3 different schemata:

A: Cytoxan $1.500mg/m^2$	B: Cytoxan $1.000mg/m^2$	C: Ifosfamid $40mg/kg$
CCNU $100mg/m^2$	Adriamycin $40mg/m^2$	VP-16 $200mg$
MTX $15mg/m^2$	Vincristin $1mg/m^2$	for 5 days

The chemotherapy starts in all patients one week after radical surgery. Half of them receive the combination by infusions as before, consisting of 12mg/kg Cytoxan, 12mg/kg 5-FU, 0.5mg/kg MTX and 0.1mg/kg Velbe. 5 x 3 such infusions are given intermittently within 1 year.

The other half of the patients receive scheme A twice with 4 week intervals, thereafter twice scheme B and then twice scheme C.   Thereafter local radiation (3000 rad) to the mediastinal area and to the area of the bronchial stump, fractionated over 4 weeks is given 25-29 weeks after surgery.   Following a 5 week interval 2 further courses of schemes A,B,C each at 4 week intervals are given.   In this way each scheme is administered intermittently 4 times within the first postoperative year.

Fig. 1

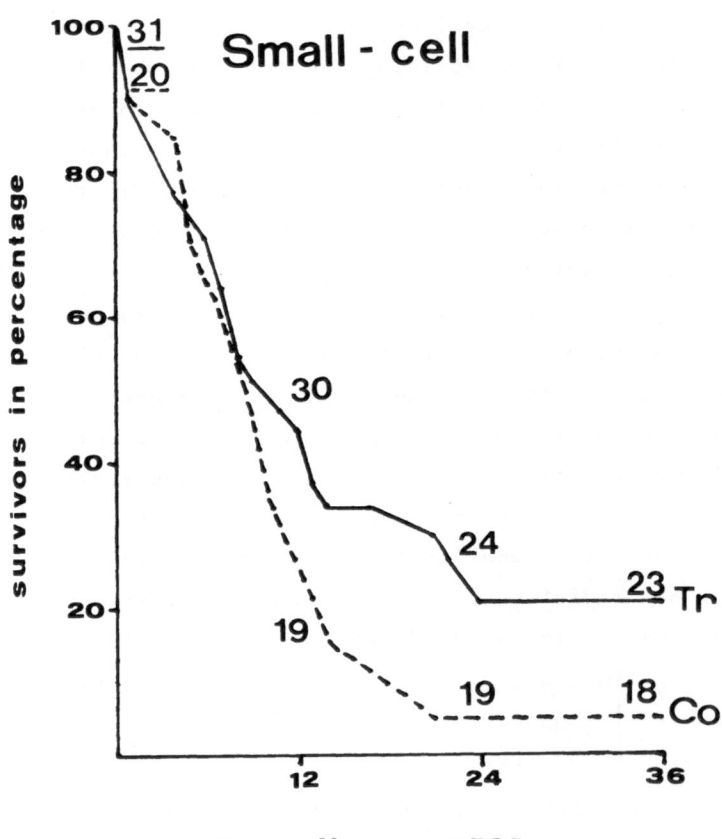

REFERENCES

Feinstein, A. R., (1964). Symptomatic patterns, biologic behavior and prognosis in cancer of the lung. Ann. Intern. Med. 61: 27.

Friedl, H. P., Karrer, K. and Kühböck, J., (1971). The relation of tumor size to the results of chemotherapy in malignant tumors. Europ. J. Clin. Biol. Res., 16: 268 - 272.

Harmer, M. H. (Editor), (1978). TNM-classification of malignant tumors, Third edition. UICC, Geneve 1978.

Humphreys, S. R., Karrer, K., (1970). Relationship of dose schedules to the effectiveness of adjuvant chemotherapy. Cancer Chemother. Report 54: 379 - 392.

Karrer, K., Humphreys, S. R. and Goldin, A., (1965). Relationship of drug toxicity to chemotherapeutic effectiveness. Antimicrob. Agents Chemother. 539 - 543.

Karrer, K., Pridun, N. and Denck, H., (1978). Chemotherapy as an adjuvant to Surgery in Lung Cancer, Cancer Chemother. Pharmaccl. Cancer Chemother. Pharmacol., 1: 145 - 159.

Karrer, K., (1979). Adjuvant Chemotherapy of Post-Surgical Minimal Residual Bronchial Carcinomas in G. Bonadonna, G. Mathé and S. E. Salmon (Editors) Recent Results in Cancer Research 68:
Springer-Verlag Berlin-Heidelberg-New York: 246-259

CELL SURFACE SIALYLATION OF METASTATIC VARIANT MURINE TUMOR CELL LINES

G. Yogeeswaran and P.L. Salk

Much attention has recently been focused on understanding the factors responsible for determining the metastatic behavior of tumor cells. A number of parameters have been suggested to contribute to the metastatic potential of tumor cells, including their adhesiveness, motility, and their ability to evade destruction by host immune mechanisms (1). Because cell surface sialic acid has been directly or indirectly associated with these aspects of cell behavior, we have examined the sialic acid content and cell surface expression of sialic acid in a number of rat and mouse tumor cell lines of diverse types which vary in their spontaneous metastatic properties.

The cultured cell lines used in these experiments are described in the legend to Figure 1. The metastatic properties of the cell lines were determined by injecting syngeneic animals subcutaneously in the midback with tumorigenic doses of cultured cells and excising the resulting tumors when they reached a size corresponding to approximately 2-6 grams in the rat systems and 1-3 grams in the mouse systems. Animals were sacrificed when external lymph node or visceral metastases were clinically apparent, or after a prolonged period of observation, if the animals remained tumor-free. The percent of animals developing macroscopic metastases to any site was then determined. Eleven of the cell lines were classified as low-metastatic (0-38% incidence of metastasis) and 21 as highly-metastatic (57-100% incidence of metastasis). Three of the lines examined were nontumorigenic.

The total sialic acid content of the cultured cells, determined colorimetrically as previously described (3), is shown in Figure 1A. The mean total sialic acid content of cells from the high-metastatic lines was 1.4-fold greater than that of cells from the low-metastatic lines (p<.03), while the sialic acid content of the low-metastatic cells was comparable to that of the cells from the nontumorigenic cell lines.

423

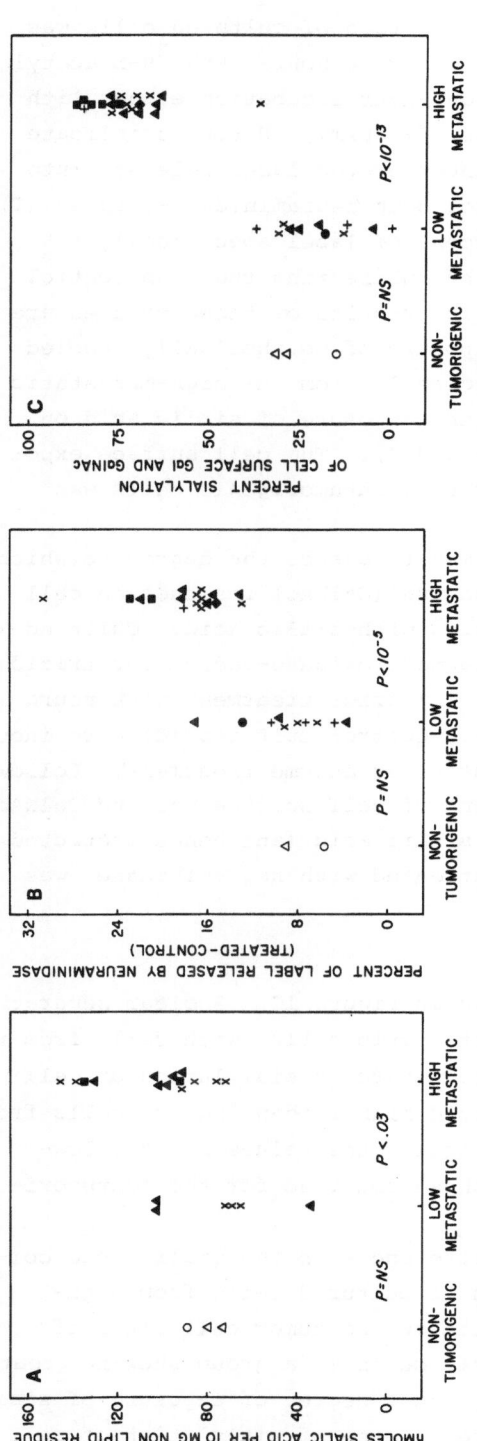

FIGURE 1. A) Total sialic acid content of cultured cells. B) Cell surface exposure of metabolically-labeled sialic acid. C) Sialylation of cell surface glycoconjugates. Methods are described in the text. Cell lines and symbols: ten derivatives of the polyoma-virus induced PW20 Wistar-Furth rat renal sarcoma (X) (2), two derivatives of the methylcholanthrene-induced MT/W9A Wistar-Furth rat mammary adenocarcinoma (+), the dimethylbenzathracene-induced DMBA #8 and the spontaneous R3230AC Fischer rat mammary adenocarcinomas (+), twelve SV40-transformed (●) and Moloney and Kirsten sarcoma virus-transformed (▲) (3, 4) BALB/3T3 mouse embryo cells, two nontumorigenic flat revertants of the K234 Kirsten sarcoma virus-transformed BALB/3T3 cell line (△) (3), the nontumorigenic parental BALB/3T3 A31 cell line (o) (5), the F1 and F10 derivatives of the B16 C57Bl/6 mouse melanoma cell line (6) and three further derivative lines (■), and a cell line established from the spontaneous C57Bl/6 mouse Lewis lung carcinoma (◆). The percent incidence of metastasis was determined in 1-5 experiments involving a total of 5-64 animals per cell line. Total sialic acid levels (A) represent the mean of 2-3 independent determinations, and values for percent sialylation (C) the mean of 2-7 independent determinations.

The exposure of sialic acid on the surface of cultured cells was studied by metabolically labeling cells for 48 hours with ^{3}H-N-acetyl mannosamine (1 μCi/ml) followed by a one-hour incubation either with or without Vibrio cholera neuraminidase (25 U/ml, pH 6.0, triplicate samples). The percent of the total incorporated label released into the supernatant was then calculated for both neuraminidase-treated (T) and control (C) cultures, and the percent of label specifically released by neuraminidase calculated by subtracting the mean control from the mean treated values (T-C). The results of these studies are shown in Figure 1B. The degree of exposure of metabolically-labeled sialic acid on the surface of cultured cells from the high-metastatic lines averaged 2.0-fold greater than the exposure of sialic acid on cells from the low-metastatic lines ($p < 10^{-5}$). The cell surface exposure of sialic acid on low-metastatic and nontumorigenic cells was similar.

A third set of studies was performed to assess the degree to which galactose (Gal) and N-acetyl galactosamine (GalNAc) residues on cell surface glycoconjugates were substituted with sialic acid. Cultured cells were surface-labeled by the galactose oxidase-sodium borotritide technique either with (NG) or without (G) prior treatment with neuraminidase, as previously described (3). Control cultures (C) were incubated with sodium borotritide, without prior enzyme treatment. Following scintillation counting, the percent of cell surface Gal and GalNAc residues terminally substituted with sialic acid (and hence protected from labeling in the cultures not pretreated with neuraminidase) was then calculated by the formula:

$$\% \text{ sialylation} = \frac{(NG-G)}{(NG-C)} \times 100\%$$

The results of these studies are shown in Figure 1C. A clear separation was observed between high- and low-metastatic cells, with cells from the high-metastatic lines showing an average percent sialylation of cell surface Gal and GalNAc residues 3.6-fold higher than that of cells from the low-metastatic lines ($p < 10^{-13}$). Again, the values for the low-metastatic cells were comparable to those obtained for the nontumorigenic cells.

These studies thus demonstrate differences in the sialic acid composition and cell surface sialylation of cultured cells from high-metastatic as compared to low-metastatic murine tumor cell lines of diverse types, with the high-metastatic cells as a group showing greater levels of total cell sialic acid, a greater degree of exposure of sialic acid on the cell surface, and a greater degree of sialylation of cell

surface Gal and GalNAc residues. Of these parameters the degree of
sialylation of cell surface Gal and GalNAc was most strongly associated
with the metastatic properties of the cells. Low-metastatic cells
were similar to nontumorigenic cells with respect to each of the
parameters tested.

The mechanisms responsible for producing the differences in sialylation of the low- and high-metastatic cells have not been determined.
Nor is it understood whether the high degree of sialylation of cell
surface glycoconjugates in the high-metastatic cells is causally
related to their enhanced ability to metastasize, or is secondarily
associated with some other aspect of cellular physiology which is more
directly responsible for producing the observed differences in the
metastatic properties of the cells. However, since removal of sialic
acid from cells has previously been observed to alter their adhesive
properties (7-9), change their patterns of invasiveness in organ culture (10), alter the organ distribution of intravenously injected cells
(11, 12), and increase the treated cells' immunogenicity (13), it is
tempting to speculate that cell surface sialylation may play a role in
determining the metastatic properties of tumor cells through effects
on one or more of these processes.

ACKNOWLEDGMENTS

We thank Henry Sebastian, Eric Hoffer, Barry Stein, Elsie Ward,
Francis Yurochko and Chon Garcia for their technical help and Dr. Jonas
Salk for his continued support. The studies were funded by PHS
research grant CA 19312-01 from the National Cancer Institute, and
grants from the National Foundation-March of Dimes, the Dorothy Grannis
Sullivan Foundation, and the Mildred and Leonard A. Javer Medical
Research Fund

REFERENCES

1. Roos E, Dingemans KP: Biochim. Biophys. Acta 560, 135, 1979.
2. Salk P, Yogeeswaran G: Fed. Proc. 37, 1760, 1978.
3. Yogeeswaran G, Sebastian H, Stein BS: Int. J. Cancer 24, 193, 1979.
4. Yogeeswaran G, Stein BS, Sebastian H: J. Natl. Cancer Inst. 64,
   951, 1980.
5. Aaronson SA, Todaro GJ: Science 162, 1024, 1968.
6. Fidler IJ: Nature New Biol. 242, 148, 1973.
7. Berwick L, Coman DR: Cancer Res. 22, 982, 1962.
8. Weiss L: Exp. Cell Res. 30, 509, 1963.

9. Kemp RB: J. Cell Sci. 6, 751, 1970.

10. Yarnell MM, Ambrose EJ: Eur. J. Cancer 5, 265, 1969.

11. Weiss L, Glaves D, Waite DA: Int. J. Cancer 13, 850, 1974.

12. Sinha BK, Goldenberg GJ: Cancer 34, 1956, 1974.

13. Ray PK: Adv. Appl. Microbiol. 21, 227, 1977.

POTENTIAL FOR SELECTIVE INHIBITION OF METASTASIS

A. Goldin

In antitumor screening programs the target in the test models has generally been early disease rather than advanced disseminated disease or the metastatic process (Goldin et al, 1975; Goldin et al, 1979). These models clearly do not reflect the clinical setting since when cancer is first detected there may already be the presence of metastatic disease (DeVita et al, 1975). Although with drugs discovered primarily through screening against early disease there has been successful treatment of a number of types of advanced clinical cancers (DeVita et al, 1979), there is nevertheless a great need for the discovery of new and more effective drugs for the treatment of metastatic neoplasia.

Important obstacles must be overcome in order to increase the specificity of therapy against metastatic disease. 1) As the body burden of tumor cells is increased, the drugs must meet an increasing demand. When the inoculum level is increased (Goldin et al, 1956; Skipper et al, 1957) or with increasing delay in the initiation of therapy, there is in general a loss in drug effectiveness (Goldin, 1969; Goldin, 1973; Laster, 1975; Karrer et al, 1967). 2) There is an increased requirement for generalized drug distribution and tumor cell exposure and the need to treat effectively the largest and most resistant metastases. 3) The drugs must reach relatively sequestered tumor sites such as the brain (Chirigos et al, 1962). 4) There may be an increase in incidence of spontaneous or drug induced resistant mutants. 5) There may be a decrease in host tolerance to drug toxicity. 6) Decrease in immune capacity of the host may occur resulting in an increase in tumor growth and dissemination and further reduced tolerance to drug.

Procedures that may be employed in efforts to overcome the difficulties in treating advanced disseminated metastatic tumors may be outlined as follows:

1. Search for drugs with greater specificity of antitumor action and optimization of their usage, taking into account the host-tumor-drug inter-relationship. In this regard, a number of compounds of interest are active in the new NCI screen involving human tumors growing in athymic mice.

2. Testing of drugs for their capability of reaching sequestered and metastatic sites and means for increasing selective delivery. Systems such as advanced leukemia L1210, where the disease is systemic and death is expected within a few days, may provide useful models for this type of study (Goldin et al, 1959).

3. Drug action to prevent metastasis. There is a need for the development of models for the testing of drugs against various steps in the process
of metastasis. This includes detachment of cells from the primary tumor,
invasion at the local site and penetration into capillaries, transport in the
blood and lymph, re-entry into normal tissue, and establishment of metastatic
foci at the new site followed by proliferation (Spreafico and Garattini, 1974;
Fidler, 1978). For example, treatment of Lewis lung carcinoma with the drug
ICRF-159, by normalization of the capillary structure in association with the
tumor markedly reduced metastasis even at doses that did not appreciably retard
the growth at the primary tumor site (Hellmann and Burrage, 1969).

4. Combination Chemotherapy with drugs having differing mechanisms of
action. Advantages that may accrue include a) reduction of limiting toxicity;
b) ability to use higher effective doses; c) delay in origin and treatment of
resistant tumor cells (Skipper et al, 1978); d) action at differing host sites;
e) a second drug may improve distribution, prevent detoxification and maintain
tissue levels of a primary active drug; f) priming dose therapy with a tumor
cytotoxic drug may reduce tumor mass, leading to more effective therapy with a
second drug; g) opportunity to manipulate host-tumor relationship with drug
combinations resulting in reduction of host toxicity without concomitant loss
of antitumor effectiveness. This may be accomplished through appropriate drug
scheduling, the administration of a metabolite in conjunction with an anti-
metabolite (Goldin et al, 1955), and by supportive measures for the host that
may increase tolerance to drugs. There are a variety of mechanisms of multiple
biochemical blockade and cooperative biochemical interactions that may result
in improved antitumor activity (Mihich and Grindey, 1977).

5. Surgery plus chemotherapy. Surgical adjuvant chemotherapy, by reduction of tumor mass, may permit more effective chemotherapy of advanced disseminated disease (Karrer et al, 1967; Schabel, 1977; Goldin, 1978; DeVita, 1977).
Advantages of surgical adjuvant chemotherapy include: a) surgery by reduction
of tumor mass may increase life duration sufficiently to permit further drug
therapy; b) surgery may lead to improved host tolerance so that higher dosage
can be employed; c) surgery may reduce the immunosuppressive effect of drug
treatment; d) surgery by retardation of the metabolic depletion of the host
may diminish immunosuppressant action resulting from progressive tumor growth;
e) surgery may reduce the absolute number of spontaneous and drug induced
resistant mutants and the degree of metastatic spread and attendant tumor cell
sequestration; f) surgery may be followed by an increase in the proliferative
fraction of tumor cells and thereby result in increased drug sensitivity;

g) the reduction in tumor challenge by surgery may result in sufficient increase in drug effectiveness against metastatic disease so that total tumor cell eradication can become a more attainable objective.

6. Radiation plus chemotherapy. This modality may contribute in the same manner as surgery plus chemotherapy and awaits development of its full potential in preclinical studies. The current interest in the employment of radiopotentiators and radioprotectants in preclinical test systems is undoubtedly contributing in an important manner to therapy of metastatic disease.

7. Biological response modifiers. Utilization of agents or approaches that will modify the host's biological response to tumor cells may contribute to improved therapy of metastatic disease. It is the subject of a broad program in process of development at the Division of Cancer Treatment, NCI. Antecedent to this program is a broad base of programs involving as general approaches (a) the employment of non-specific immunological stimulants (b) adoptive immunological procedures including the utilization of allogeneic or syngeneic immune cells (c) active or passive immunization.

8. Immunotherapy plus chemotherapy. Approaches that may be employed include (a) prevention of immunosuppression by treatment with a chemotherapeutic agent or by other means; (b) the use of non-specific immunostimulants plus chemotherapy; (c) chemotherapy plus adoptive immunotherapy; (d) passive immunization plus chemotherapy; (e) active immunization plus chemotherapy; (f) alteration of tumor cell antigenicity and collateral sensitivity.

9. Additional approaches may be investigated for the improvement of therapeutic effectiveness against metastatic disease such as (a) approaches to prevention of tumor cell adhesiveness; (b) hyperthermia; (c) manipulation of tumor cell kinetics.

Thus, the potential for selective inhibition of disseminated metastatic tumor encompasses a broad array of approaches. There is an important reed for further emphasis on model development and fundamental investigations for improved selective inhibition of metastasis.

REFERENCES

Chirigos, M.A., Humphreys, S.R., and Goldin, A., 1962. Effectiveness of cytoxan against intracerebrally and subcutaneously inoculated lymphoid leukemia L1210. Cancer Research 22: 187-195.

DeVita, V.T., Jr., 1977. Adjuvant therapy - An overview. In: S.E. Salmon and S.E. Jones (Editors), Adjuvant therapy of Cancer, Elsevier, North Holland Publishing Company, Amsterdam, pp. 613-641.

DeVita, V.T., Oliverio, V.T., Muggia, F.M., Wiernik, P.W., Ziegler, J., Goldin, A., Rubin, D., Henney, J. and Schepartz, S., 1979. The drug development and clinical trials programs of the Division of Cancer Treatment, National Cancer Institute, Cancer Clin. Trials 2: 195-216.

DeVita, V.T., Young, R.C. and Canellos, G.P., 1975. Combination versus single agent chemotherapy. Review of basis for selection of drug treatment of cancer. Cancer 35: 98-110.

Fidler, I. J., 1978. Tumor heterogeneity and the biology of cancer invasion and metastasis. Cancer Research 38: 2651-2660.

Goldin, A., 1969. Factors pertaining to complete drug-induced remission of tumor in animals and man. Cancer Res. 29: 2285-2291.

Goldin, A., 1973. Effects of drugs on disseminated tumor. In: S. Garattini and G. Franchi (Editors), Chemotherapy of Cancer Dissemination and Metastasis, Raven Press, New York, pp. 341-354.

Goldin, A., 1978. Rationale of chemotherapeutic adjuvant treatment. Arch. Geschwulstforsch 48/7: 627-635.

Goldin, A., Humphreys, S.R., Venditti, J.M. and Mantel, N., 1959. Prolongation of the lifespan of mice with advanced leukemia (L1210) by treatment with halogenated derivatives of amethopterin. J. Natl Cancer Inst. 22: 811-823.

Goldin, A., Johnson, R.K., and Venditti, J.M., 1975. Preclinical characterization of candidate antitumor drugs. Cancer Chemotherapy Reports, Part 2: 5, No. 1, pp. 21-81.

Goldin, A., Schepartz, S.A., Venditti, J.M. and DeVita, V.T., Jr., 1979. Historical development and current strategy of the National Cancer Institute Drug Development Program. In: V.T. DeVita, Jr. and H. Busch (Editors), Methods in Cancer Research, Vol. XVI, Academic Press, New York, pp. 165-245.

Goldin, A., Venditti, J.M., Humphreys, S.R., Dennis, D. and Mantel, N., 1955. Studies on the management of mouse leukemia (L1210) with antagonists of folic acid. Cancer Res. 15: 742-747.

Goldin, A., Venditti, J.M., Humphreys, S.R. and Mantel, N., 1956. Influence of the concentration of leukemic inoculum on the effectiveness of treatment. Science, 128: 840.

Hellmann, K. and Burrage, K., 1969. Control of malignant metastases by ICRF 159. Nature, 224: 273-275.

Karrer, K., Humphreys, S.R. and Goldin, A., 1967. An experimental model for studying factors which influence metastasis of malignant tumors. Int. J. Cancer 2: 213-223.

Laster, W.R., Jr., 1975. Ridgway osteogenic sarcoma - A promising model for special therapeutic trials against an advanced-staged, drug-sensitive animal tumor system. Cancer Chemother Rep (Part II) 5(1): 151-168.

Mihich, E. and Grindey, G.B., 1977. Multiple basis of combination chemotherapy Cancer 40: 534-543.

Schabel, F.M., Jr., 1977. Surgical adjuvant chemotherapy of metastatic murine tumors. Cancer 40: 558-568.

Skipper, H.E., Schabel, F.M., Jr., Bell, M., Thompson, J.R. and Johnston, S., 1957. On the curability of experimental neoplasms I. Amethopterin and mouse leukemia. Cancer Res. 17: 717-726.

Skipper, H.E., Schabel, F.M., Jr. and Lloyd, H.H., 1978. Experimental therapeutics and kinetics: Selection and overgrowth of specifically and permanently drug-resistant tumor cells. Semin. Hematol. 15: 207-219.

Spreafico, F. and Garattini, S., 1974. Selective antimetastatic treatment - current status and future prospects. Cancer Treatment Reviews, 1: 239-250.

TUMOUR LOAD DEPENDENT EFFECTIVENESS OF CYCLOPHOSPHAMIDE IN LEWIS LUNG CARCINOMA

J.H. Mulder, C. Bignell and L.M. van Putten

The concept of adjuvant chemotherapy is attractive: when the residual tumour load is minimal, a given treatment will be more effective than in the advanced stage of the disease. In the design of a treatment protocol, the chemotherapist must take at least two basic problems into account: 1) which drugs should be applied in the adjuvant format? and 2) which group of patients should be selected for the adjuvant treatment?

The choice of drugs in the adjuvant format generally depends on results obtained in advanced disease. As 5-Fluorouracil is the most effective drug in advance colorectal tumours, the same agent is applied in almost all adjuvant protocols for this type of disease. Although this policy of extrapolation of results obtained in the late stage of the disease to the early stages seems very sensible, it was decided to investigate whether this policy was indeed valid. For this purpose, the effect of Cyclophosphamide (Cyclo) was evaluated in the metastasizing Lewis lung tumour model. A comparison was made between the volume response of the "primary" tumour and the response in small lung metastases determined by the increase in lifespan of the animals. The results of pre-operative Cyclo treatment are given in Table 1.

TABLE 1.

Pre-operative Cyclophosphamide treatment: the discrepancy between "primary" tumour response and the effect on lung metastases.

	Primary tumour response growth delay (days) Mean $\pm$ S.E.	Micrometastases response	
		MdSt (range)	cure rate
no Cyclo pre-operative, amputated (n = 27)		33 (24 -61)	41%
Cyclo pre-operative, amputated (n = 28)	0 $\pm$ 0.6	41 (18 - 63)	79%

Lewis lung tumour cells (10^5.0.01 ml^{-1}) were implanted into the foot pad of C57BL/Ka mice on day 0. Cyclo (100 mg.kg^{-1} i.p.) was given on day 29; tumour volume at that time was approximately 120 mm^3. After the volume of the "primary" tumour was determined to establish the growth delay, the tumour bearing leg was amputated on day 36. Death was caused by the outgrowth of lung metastases. Mice with no evidence of disease on day 120 were assumed to be cured. The median survival time (MdST) of the non-survivors was calculated from the day of amputation.

The effect of Cyclo treatment on the volume of the foot pad tumour was negligible. Seven days after drug administration, control and Cyclo treated mice were amputated and their survival time was determined. Although pre-operative Cyclo treatment resulted in no tumour volume reduction in the "primary" tumour, the effect of Cyclo on the micro-metastases in the lungs was clearly measurable. The percentage of animals without evidence of disease on day 120 increased from 41 to 79% as a result of Cyclo treatment.

From "primary" tumour characteristics such as tumour volume (T-classification), the risk of dying from metastatic disease can be calculated. As a rule, the more advanced locally (T3), the larger the residual metastatic tumour load. In experiments, described in this report, Cyclo adjuvant chemotherapy was applied in carefully staged groups of Lewis lung disease mice with low, medium and high risks of lung metastasis. The aim was to establish a correlation between "primary" tumour volume at the time of surgical intervention (T-classification) and the increase in lifespan after adjuvant therapy.

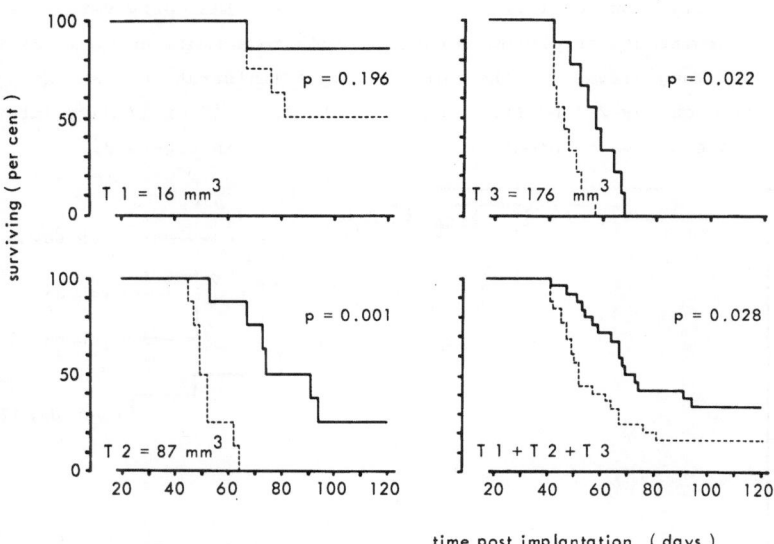

Fig. 1. Tumour stage dependent effectiveness of Cyclophosphamide adjuvant chemotherapy. Lewis lung tumour cells (10^5.0.01 ml^{-1}) were implanted into the foot pad of C57BL/Ka mice on day 0. On day 29, immediately before amputation, mice were separated on the basis of their tumour volume into 3 groups of at least 8 animals each. The mean tumour volume per tumour stage group is presented. Three days after amputation, Cyclo (100 mg.kg^{-1} i.p.) was administered. Mice with no evidence of disease on day 120 were assumed to be cured. The log rank test was used to compare the survival curves of treated (solid lines) to that of control mice (dashed lines).

434

In Figure 1, survival curves for mice amputated after staging according to the volume of their foot pad tumour are presented. All amputated control animals with originally large tumours (T3) died of lung metastases, in contrast to 50% of control mice with small "primary" tumours (T1). Adjuvant chemotherapy with Cyclo in T3-staged mice resulted in death delay (delay curve). However, an increase in cure rate was observed in T2 and T1 staged animals (cure curves). When the data of all stages are grouped together, a combined delay and cure curve can be constructed. What is clear from the various survival curves is a tumour stage and residual tumour load dependent effectiveness of the adjuvant chemotherapy. If the aim of adjuvant therapy is to increase the cure rate, then low stage tumours (T1-T2) should preferably be submitted to adjuvant chemotherapy post-operatively. In more advanced stages (T3), only a delay in time of tumour related death can be anticipated. The appreciation of increase in survival-versus-increased cure rate depends on a cost-benefit analysis which is beyond the scope of this report.

In the third type of experiment, mice were submitted to adjuvant therapy either immediately after amputation of the tumour bearing leg or at a later time in the post-operative course of the disease. This so-called early-versus-late treatment of micrometastases presumably corresponds to a small and a large tumour load of residual lung disease at the time of drug administration. Data for groups of mice amputated on day 29 and treated with Cyclo 2, 7, 12 or 17 days later (early-versus-late adjuvant chemotherapy) are presented in Figure 2.

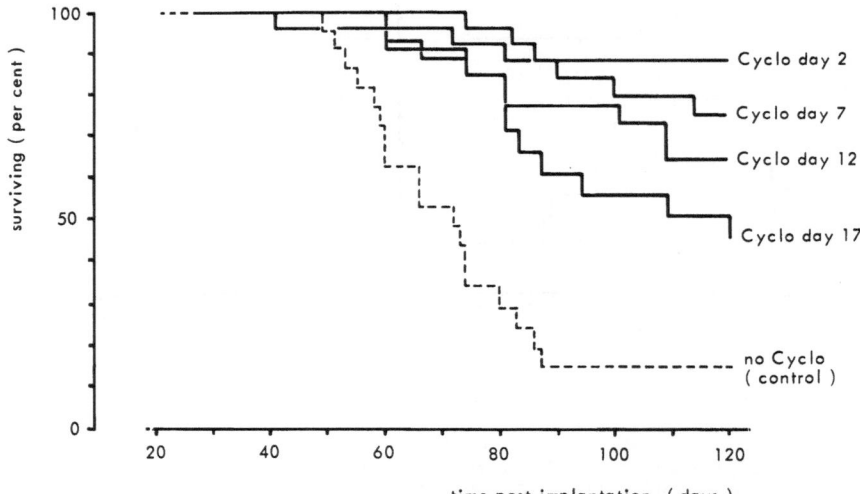

Fig. 2. Adjuvant chemotherapy applied at various time intervals after amputation: the residual tumour load dependent effectiveness of Cyclophosphamide treatment. Lewis lung tumour cells ($10^5.0.01$ ml^{-1}) were implanted into the foot pad of C57BL/Ka mice on day 0. After amputation on day 29, each group of a minimum of 20 mice was treated with Cyclo (100 mg.kg^{-1}i.p.) at the time interval indicated in the figure. The animals died of lung metastases.

An increase in the time interval between primary operation and adjuvant chemotherapy resulted in a dramatic decline in efficacy of Cyclo treatment. Presumably, the efficacy of chemotherapy depends on the size of the residual tumour load in the lungs at the time of Cyclo administration.

In conclusion, negative results of cytostatic treatment derived from volume measurements in advanced disease do not necessarily indicate ineffectiveness of treatment in early, microscopic disease. If the aim of the study of adjuvant therapy is to achieve an increase in cure rate, it may be preferable to treat individuals with a low risk of tumour relapse. Although a non-tumour bearing subpopulation in the low risk group will be overtreated in this way, the chance of being cured as a result of the chemotherapy in the low staged tumour groups is considerably greater than in a high staged or high risk population. Adjuvant chemotherapy should start as soon as possible after local treatment of a metastasizing tumour.

PROPHYLACTIC ANTIMETASTATIC AGENTS: DIMETHYLTRIAZENES, N-DIAZOACETYLGLICINE DERIVATIVES AND OTHER NEUTRAL PROTEINASE INHIBITORS

T. Giraldi, G. Sava, R. Cuman, C. Nisi and L. Lassiani

The differential effects of several substances on the growth of subcutaneous Lewis lung carcinoma and on the formation of spontaneous lung metastases, have been investigated in our laboratory. All of the agents examined have in common the property of inhibiting "in vitro", at "in vivo" attainable concentrations, the activity of neutral proteinases (Table 1). At the same time, these drugs resulted in selective antimetastatic effects in the experimetal system employed, consisting of a depression of the formation of spontaneous lung metastases with no significant inhibition of subcutaneous primary tumor growth (Table 1). These findings are in agreement with the proposed role of a high level of neutral proteinases present in the primary tumor for the early phases of the process of metastasis formation, namely tumor cell detachement and vascular invasion leading to tumor cell entrance into the blood stream.(Easty, 1975; Kleinerman and Liotta, 1977).

The three nitrosoureas derivatives examined do not appear to act as selective antimetastatic drugs, since they depress also primary tumor growth. However, it is interesting to note that the compound which does not appreciably produce the proteinase inhibiting metabolite (isocianate), is the least active.

TABLE 1.

Selective antimetastatic effects in mice bearing Lewis lung carcinoma and proteinase inhibition of the tested agents.

Agent	Activity	Reference	Enzymes inhibited
Aurintricarboxylic acid	High	T. Giraldi et al., 1980b	Broad spectrum non-specific inhibitor (Bina-Stein and Tritton, 1976).
Chloroquine	Moderate	T. Giraldi et al., 1980b	Cathepsin B and collagenase (Poole et al., 1977; Cowey and Whitehouse, 1966).
Indomethacin	Moderate	T. Giraldi et al., 1980b	Collagenase (Wojtecka-Lukasik and Dancewicz, 1974; Wirl, 1977).
Phenylbutazone	High	T. Giraldi et al., 1980b	Collagenase (Wojtecka-Lukasik and Dancewicz, 1974; Wirl, 1977).
Aprotinin (Trasylol[R])	Moderate	T. Giraldi et al., 1977a	Broad spectrum inhibitor (Trautschold et al., 1967), active on trypsin, chymotrypsin, kallikrein, plasmin elastase and cathepsin G (Starkey,

		1977).	
N-diazoacetylglycin-amide	Very high	T. Giraldi et al., 1977c, 1979	Elastase, chymotrypsin-like neutral proteinase (histonase) (Kopitar et al., 1977a).
p-carboxamidophenyl-3,3-dimethyltriazene	Very high	T. Giraldi et al., 1978, 1980a	Elastase, chymotrypsin-like neutral proteinase (histonase) (Kopitar et al., 1977b).
p-(3,3-dimethyl-1-triazeno)benzoic acid potassium salt (DM-COOK)	Very high	G. Sava et al., 1979	
(+)1,2-di(3,5-dioxo-piperazin-1-yl)propane (ICRF 159, Razoxane)	Very high	Bakowski, 1976 T. Giraldi et al., 1980c	Inhibits collagen peptidase activity (assayed using p-phenylazo-benzyloxycarbonyl-L-prolyl-L-leucyl-L-prolyl-D-arginine as substrate) of human tumor homogenates (Boggust and Mc Gauley, 1978).
Leucocyte intracellular inhibitor of neutral proteinases (LNPI)	Moderate	T. Giraldi et al., 1977b	Elastase, chymotrypsin-like neutral proteinase (histonase) (Kopitar and Lebez, 1975; Kopitar et al., 1977a).
Spleen intracellular inhibitor of neutral proteinases (SNPI-1)	Moderate	T. Giraldi et al., 1980b	Trypsin, chymotrypsin-like neutral proteinase (histonase), cathepsin B and H (Brzin et al., 1977; Kopitar et al., 1978).
Spleen intracellular inhibitor of neutral proteinases (SNPI-2)	Moderate	T. Giraldi et al., 1980b	Trypsin, α-chymotrypsin, chymotrypsin-like neutral proteinase (histonase), elastase (Brzin et al., 1977; Kopitar et al., 1978).
BCNU, CCNU	Very high (also on primary tumor)	(unpublished results)	Elastase and chymotrypsin (by production of isocianates (Babson et al., 1977).
Chlorozotocin	Moderate (also on primary tumor)	(unpublished results)	Do not produce appreciably isocianates (Kann, 1978).

Moderate: weight of spontaneous lung metastases significantly reduced to about 30-50%.
High: weight of spontaneous metastases significantly reduced to 20%; some animals free of metastases.
Very high: weight of spontaneous metastases significantly reduced to less than 5%; some animals free of metastases.
The growth of subcutaneous tumor is not reduced significantly.

The most active compound in the series examined, in terms of the magnitude of effects caused at maximum tolerated dosages, is DM-COOK: the mechanism of its action has therefore been investigated in more detail. This dimethyltriazene sharply depresses the formation of spontaneous lung metastases. It appears that the mechanism of its antimetastatic action is different from cytotoxicity, since DM-COOK is devoid of effects on subcutaneous tumor growth and on the development of artificial lung colonies obtained by i.v. injection of tumor cells (G. Sava et al., 1979). Furthermore, the fractional incorporation of ^{3}H-thymidine in pulmonary and subcutaneous tumor is unaffected (T. Giraldi et al., 1980c). The i.v. injection

438

of tumor cells in pretreated hosts has the same efficiency in lung colony formation
as compared with non-pretreated controls, showing that DM-COOK does not affect the
lodgement in the lungs of tumor cells present in the blood stream. This agent,
thus, appear to act preventing tumor cell entrance into the blood stream.

DM-COOK has been consequently used as a prophylactic adjuvant to the surgical
removal of primary tumor in mice bearing Lewis lung carcinoma. C57BL mice were
implanted i.m. in the calf of the hindleg with 5×10^5 viable tumor cells (trypan
blue excluding) prepared by mechanical dissociation. Amputation was performed 9
days later, when the tumor weight was about 2 g. The daily dosage employed is the
maximum tolerated for 8 days: the treatment schedules employed are daily administrations on days 1-8, on days 7-9 and one hour before amputation only (day 9).
The results, illustrated in Figure 1 show that in controls treated by surgery only, the average survival time is about 26 days, all of the animals dying within
42 days. The treatment with DM-COOK on days 1-8 and 7-9 causes 36.7 and 34.6% survivors at four months respectively: the average survival time of uncured mice is
significantly increased by 30.5 and 13.5%. The preoperative treatment (day 9 only)
is markedly less effective, causing 10% long term survivors and no significant
increase of the life span of uncured animals.

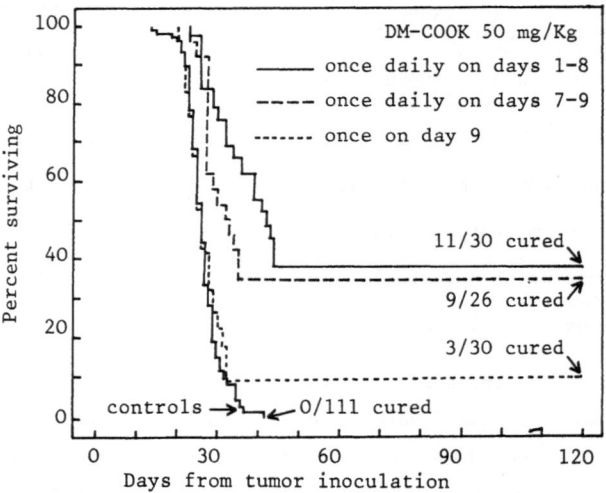

Fig. 1. Survival of mice bearing Lewis lung carcinoma treated with DM-COOK or
DM-CH$_3$ and surgical removal of primary tumor. Animals having local tumor regrowth
at surgical site have been excluded from the plot: all of the animals considered
died because of metastases, as evidenced by necroscopic examination.

These data indicate that a selective antimetastatic drug, acting with a mechanism different from cytotoxicity for tumor cells, can be usefully employed as an
adjuvant to the surgical treatment of a solid metastasizing tumor, also when the
treatment is started in advanced phases of tumor growth. Further investigation is
in progress in order to ascertain whether an inhibition of tumor proteinases is
involved in the action of DM-COOK, and also to examine whether its antimetastatic
action is independent from the type of tumor treated.

This work was supported by Italian National Research Council - Special Project
"Control of Neoplastic Growth", Contract n°79.00635.96.

REFERENCES

Babson, J.R., Reed, D.J. and Sinkey M.A., 1977. Active site specific inactivation
of chymotrypsin by cycloexyl isocianate formed during degradation of the car-
cinostatic 1-(2-chloroethyl)-3-cyclohexyl-1-nitrosourea. Biochemistry, 16:
1584-1589.
Bakowski, M.T., 1976. ICRF 159 (+)1,2-di-(3,5-dioxopiperazin-1-yl)propane NSC
129,943; Razoxane. Cancer Treat. Rev., 3: 95-107
Bina-Stein M. and Tritton T.R., 1976. Aurintricarboxylic acid is a non specific
enzyme inhibitor. Mol. Pharmacol., 12: 191-193.
Boggust W.A. and Gauley H., 1978. Inhibition of collagen peptidase in HeLa cells
and human tumors by compounds including drugs used in cancer therapy. Br. J.
Cancer, 38: 329-334.
Brzin, J., Kopitar, M. and Turk, V., 1977. Isolation and characterization of inhibitors of neutral proteinases from spleen. Acta Biol. Med. Ger., 36: 1883-1886.
Cowey, F.K. and Whitehouse, M.W., 1966. Biochemical properties of antiinflammato-
ry drugs VII. Biochem. Pharmacol., 15: 1071-1084.
Easty, G.C., 1975. Invasion by cancer cells. In: E.J. Ambrose and F.J.C. Roe (Editors), The biology of cancer. Ellis Horwood, London, pp. 58-73.
Giraldi, T., Nisi, C. and Sava, G.,1977a. Lysosomal enzyme inhibitors and antimetastatic activity in the mouse. Europ. J. Cancer, 13: 1321-1323.
Giraldi, T., Kopitar, M. and Sava, G., 1977b. Antimetastatic effects of a leukocy-
te intracellular inhibition of neutral proteases. Cancer Res., 37: 3834-3835.
Giraldi, T., Nisi, C. and Sava, G., 1977c. Antimetastatic effects of N-diazoacetyl-
glycine derivatives in C57BL mice. J. Natl. Cancer Inst., 58: 1129-1130.
Giraldi, T., Houghton, P.J., Taylor, D.M. and Nisi, C., 1978. Antimetastatic action
of some triazene derivatives against the Lewis lung carcinoma in mice. Cancer
Treat. Rep., 62: 721-725.
Giraldi, T., Guarino, A.M., Nisi, C. and Baldini, L., 1979. Selective antimetastatic effects of N-diazoacetylglicinamide derivatives in mice. Europ. J. Cancer,
15: 603-607.
Giraldi, T., Guarino, A.M., Nisi, C. and Sava, G., 1980a. Antitumor and antimetastatic effects of benzenoid triazenes in mice bearing Lewis lung carcinoma. Pharmacol. Res. Commun., 12: 1-11.
Giraldi, T., Sava, G., Kopitar, M., Brzin, J. and Turk, V., 1980b. Neutral proteinase inhibitors and antimetastatic effects in mice. Europ. J. Cancer in the press.
Giraldi, T., Sava, G., Cuman, R., Nisi, C. and Lassiani, L., 1980c. Selectivity of the
antimetastatic and cytotoxic effects of 1-p-(3,3-dimethyl-1-triazeno)benzoic
acid potassium salt (DM-COOK), (+)1,2-di(3,5-dioxopiperazin-1-yl)propane (ICRF
159) and cyclophosphamide in mice bearing Lewis lung carcinoma. Manuscript submitted to Cancer Res.
Kann, H.E. Jr., 1978. Comparison of biochemical and biological effects of four nitrosoureas with differing carbamoyllating activities. Cancer Res., 38: 2363-2366.

Kleinerman, J. and Liotta, L., 1977. Release of tumor cells. In: S.B. Day, W.P.L. Meyers, P. Stansly and S. Garattini (Editors), Cancer invasion and metastasis: biological mechanism and therapy. Raven Press, New York, pp. 135–143.

Kopitar, M. and Lebez, D., 1975. Intracellular distribution of neutral proteinases and inhibitors in pig leucocytes. Isolation of two inhibitors of neutral proteinases. Europ. J. Biochem., 56: 571–581.

Kopitar, M., Babnik, J., Kregar, I. and Suhar A., 1977a. Neutral proteinase and inhibitors of leucocyte cells. In: F. Rossi, P. Patriarca and D. Romeo (Editors), Movement, metabolism and Bactericidal mechanism of phagocytes. Piccin, Padova, pp. 117–127.

Kopitar, M., Suhar, A., Giraldi, T. and Turk, V., 1977b. Biochemical and biological properties of cell and tissue neutral proteinases and inhibitors. Acta Biol. Med. Germ., 36: 1863–1871.

Kopitar, M., Brzin, J., Zvonar, T., Locnikar, Kregar, I. and Turk, V., 1978. Inhibition studies of an intracellular inhibitor on thiol proteinases. FEBS Letters, 91: 355–359.

Poole, B., Ohkuma, S. and Warburton, M.J., 1977. The accumulation of weakly basic substances in lisosomes and the inhibition of intracellular protein degradation. Acta Biol. Med. Germ., 36: 1777–1788.

Sava, G., Giraldi, T., Lassiani, L. and Nisi, C., 1979. Mechanism of the antimetastatic action of dimethyltriazenes. Cancer Treat. Rep., 63: 93–98.

Starkey, P.M. and Barret, A.J., 1976. Human cathepsin G. Catalytic and immunological properties. Biochem. J., 155: 273–278.

Starkey, P.M., 1977. Elastase and cathepsin G; the serine proteinaes of human neutrophil leucocytes and spleen. In: A.J. Barret (Editor), Proteinases in mammalian cells and tissues. North Holland Publishing Company, Amsterdam, pp. 57–89.

Trautschold, I., Werle, E. and Zickgraf-Rudel, G., 1967. Trasylol. Biochem. Pharmacol., 16: 59–72.

Wirl, G., 1977. Croton oil induced collagenolytic activity in the mouse skin. In: V. Turk and N. Marks (Editors), Intracellular protein catabolism II. Plenum Press, New York, pp. 154–162.

Wojtecka-Lukasik, E. and Dancewicz, A.M., 1974. Inhibition of human leukocyte collagenase by some drugs used in the therapy of rheumatic diseases. Biochem. Pharmacol., 23: 2077–2081.

SELECTIVE CHEMOTHERAPY OF METASTASIS BY DRUG CARRYING FAT EMULSION OR TUMOR SPECIFIC ANTIBODY

T. Takahashi, T. Yamaguchi and K. Kohno

To ensure a sufficiently high concentration of anticancer agents to metastases with minimal side effects, we have used drug carrying fat emulsions or tumor specific antibody. We previously reported experimental work on fat emulsion (Takahashi, 1973, 1977), this paper reports mainly on clinical trials of the emulsion and experimental study of chemotherapy by a drug carrying tumor specific antibody.

CHEMOTHERAPY OF LYMPH NODE METASTASIS BY DRUG CARRYING FAT EMULSION

A fat emulsion injected into tissues is taken up by lymphatic capillaries and conveyed to regional lymph nodes. Utilizing this property, we used fat emulsion as a drug carrier to regional lymph nodes. Various types of emulsions containing anticancer agents were prepared by ultrasonification technique. The detailed procedures for preparation of the emulsion have already been described (Takahashi, 1973). Water soluble drugs (Mitomycin-C (MMC), bleomycin, adriamycin, etc) were encapsulated by fat in the inner-most phase as water in oil (W/O) or water in oil in water (W/O/W) type emulsion. The lipid soluble drug methyl-CCNU was dissolved in sesame oil and oil in water (O/W) emulsion was made up. The O/W emulsion in which the drug is contained in the oil phase was the most stable one.

To know whether the emulsions can carry anticancer drugs to the lymphatic system, the drug concentrations in thoracic lymph was measured. Rabbits were used in this experimental series.

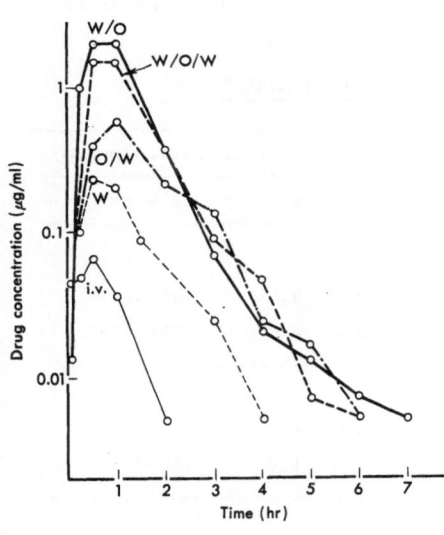

Fig. 1

The drugs were injected into the subserosa of the stomach and the thoracic lymph was collected at various intervals. Fig. 1 shows the drug concentration in the thoracic lymph after injection of 2mg of MMC in various forms. In W/O and W/O/W emulsions, the maximum values were 3 times as high as the maximum value after subserosal injection of normal MMC. The drug concentration in lymph of the emulsion groups persisted at a higher level when compared with intravenous injection.

We conducted clinical trials of the emulsion in patients with stomach, skin and breast cancer. The results of this trial have been reported in part previously (Takahashi, 1976). In later cases receiving the emulsion the results were as favourable as those reported earlier.

In stomach cancer which has the highest incidence in Japan, we tried oral application of the emulsion. For this purpose we prepared oil in water emulsion attached to 5-fluorouracil (5-FU).

Table 1 illustrates 5-FU concentrations in the regional lymph nodes in 13 stomach cancer patients 2 hours after administration of 5-FU emulsion or 5-FU solution. The mean 5-FU levels both in the paragastric nodes and in the retroperitoneal nodes were higher after the administration of 5-FU emulsion, compared with those given 5-FU in solution form.

TABLE 1. 5-FU CONCENTRATION IN REGIONAL LYMPH NODES

	No. of cases	No. of lymph nodes	5-FU concentration (mcg/g)	
			range	m $\pm$ SE
Emulsion group	8			
paragastric nodes		23	trace-9.0	1.55$\pm$0.42
retroperitoneal nodes		13	trace-4.0	1.79$\pm$0.34
Solution group	5			
paragastric nodes		14	trace-1.9	0.54$\pm$0.16
retroperitoneal nodes		8	trace-1.0	0.18$\pm$0.11

A total of 231 patients with stomach cancer were given oral 5-FU emulsion preoperatively. The dose of 5-FU was 500mg every day in three divided doses for 7-30 days and total dose of 5-FU was 3,500mg to 15,000mg. After this treatment, patients had a gastrectomy with lymph node dissection. Cancer changed in shape following this treatment. We examined macroscopical changes of the stomach cancer before and after treatment by means of x-rays and endoscopy. Borrmann type II was most changeable to shallow ulcers.

To evaluate the effect of this treatment on metastatic lesions of the regional lymph nodes, histological examinations of the specimen were carried out. Of the 700 lymph nodes removed from 69 stomach cancer patients, 242 were histologically proven to have metastasis. Various changes of metastatic foci were seen, but the changes were not uniform, showing a mosaic of cell nests consisting of various damaged cells. Therefore we graded the histological changes into four categories (Majima, 1978). Grade I: no remarkable changes, Grade II: showing slight changes in most portions, Grade III: showing moderate changes in most portions, Grade IV: exhibiting extensive necrosis or marked degeneration of cancer cells.

Table 2 shows the grade of histological changes in metastatic lesions. One hundred and fifty of 242 (62%) metastatic nodes (Grade II & III) were markedly damaged. The histological changes were seen not only in the paragastric nodes, but also in the retroperitoneal lymph nodes remote from the stomach.

TABLE 2. GRADE OF HISTOLOGICAL CHANGES OF METASTATIC LESION

	Grade			
	0	I	II	III
Paragastric nodes	32(20.3%)	28(17.7%)	66(41.8%)	32(20.2%)
Retroperitoneal nodes	11(13.1%)	21(25.0%)	41(48.8%)	11(13.1%)
Total	43(17.8%)	49(20.2%)	107(44.2%)	43(17.8%)

Since 1976 we have given oral 5-FU emulsion for patients
with stomach cancer as adjuvant chemotherapy for surgery (in Akita
University). Three-year survival rate of patients given the
emulsion seems to indicate better outcome than that of patients
without the emulsion at all stages:

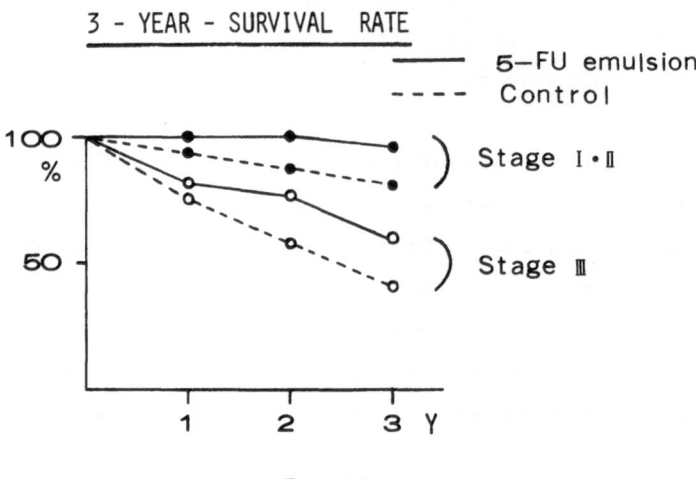

Fig.II

SELECTIVE CANCER CHEMOTHERAPY WITH ANTIBODY CARRYING CYTOTOXIC DRUGS

One possible approach to tumor specific chemotherapy is to
use tumor specific antibodies as carriers of cytotoxic drugs.
However tumor specific antibodies against human tumor are not
available yet and we therefore used antibodies against α-feto-
protein (AFP) which was produced by rat ascites hepatoma AH66.

Rabbits were used to obtain the antibody against AFP, four
weeks after injection of purified AFP with Freund's complete
adjuvant.   Anti-AFP IgG was purified by the affinity chromatography
technique. The cytotoxic drug Mitomycin-C (MMC) was successfully
coupled with anti-AFP IgG by a 2-step method using glutaraldehyde
as indicated in Table 3.   The optimum concentration of glutaraldehyde was 0.01 to 0.02% and the reaction time 2 hours. The anti-
AFP IgG - MMC conjugate produced by the affinity chromatography
technique was used to obtain the complex with antibody activity.
The conjugates retained their cytotoxic activity, as assessed by

Binding of MMC to anti AFP by
glutaraldehyde—— two·step method

MMC 1mg

  ├──── PBS 600 μl

  ├──── 1% glutaraldehyde 10 μl

12hrs at room temp

  ├──── anti AFP 1mg in 500 lμPBS

2hrs at room temp

 affinity chromatography

    (AFP bind Sepharose 4B)

elute with 8M urea

dialyze in saline at 4°C

    ⌠ gel—filtration on Sepharose 4B
    ⌡ bioassay with subtilis ATCC

bioassay, and were also found to have retained antibody activity, as tested by immuno-electrophoresis in agar. _In vitro_ study suggests the possibility of tumor specific chemotherapy with antibody carrying drug.

There are however _in vivo_ problems to overcome and we are now engaged in the experiments to elucidate these problems.

TABLE 3

REFERENCES

Majima, S., Watanabe, S., Nakao, E., Ueda, T., Morisawa, K., Cho, K., Nishioka, B., Fujita, Y. and Takahashi, T., 1978. Histological evaluation of the effect of 5-FU emulsion on lymph node metastasis of stomach cancer. Jap. J. Surg., 8: 111-118.

Takahashi, T., Mizuno, M., Fujita, Y., Ueda, S., Nishioka, B. and Majima, S., 1973. Increased concentration of anticancer agents in regional lymph nodes by fat emulsion, with special reference to chemotherapy of metastasis. Gann, 64: 345-350.

Takahashi, T., Ueda, S., Kohno, K. and Majima, S., 1976. Attempt at local administration of anticancer agents in the form of fat emulsion. Cancer, 38: 1507-1514.

Takahashi, T., Kono, K. and Yamaguchi, T., 1977. Enhancement of the Cancer Chemotherapeutic Effect by Anticancer Agents in the Form of Fat Emulsion. Tohoku J. exp. Med., 123: 235-246.

TREATMENT OF METASTASES IN LONG BONES

O Bertermann, T. Mischkowsky and H. Krebs

Pathological fractures of a bone are fractures under physiological strain. The causes may be benign or malignant. About one third of all carcinomas give rise to metastases in bones. During this process the local osseus tissue is eliminated and substituted by tumor tissue, especially in long bones. Consequently, the weight-transmitting and supporting function of these bones is impaired. It is therefore the primary aim of treatment to obtain pain-free movement of the affected bone as rapidly as possible.

RESULTS

The data on 56 patients with pathological fractures were analyzed during a retrospective study. Table 1 shows the aetiology of these pathological fractures.

TABLE 1   Aetiology in 56 pathological fractures of the extremities

Ca.	
Breast	32
Hypernephroma	5
Solid or tubular unknown primary tumor	5
Lung	3
Prostate	3
Melanoma	1
Plasmocytoma	1
Hepatoma	1
Reticulo Sarcoma	1
Haemangiopericytoma	1
Malignant giant cell tumor	1
Radionecrosis after Ca.Uterus	1
Colon	1
	56

Table 2 shows the localisation of the 56 pathological fractures.

TABLE 2   Localisation of 56 pathological fractures of the
          extremities

Femur	28
Femur neck	18
Humerus	9
Tibia	1
	56

Table 3 shows the therapy received by our pathological fractures.

TABLE 3   Therapy in 56 pathological fractures of the extremities

Nail	14
130° plate	16
Arthroplasty	11
Condylar plate	9
Straight plate	4
Excochleation and	
bone cement	1
Exarticulation	1
	56

Figures la and lc show an example of the treatment of a
pathological fracture

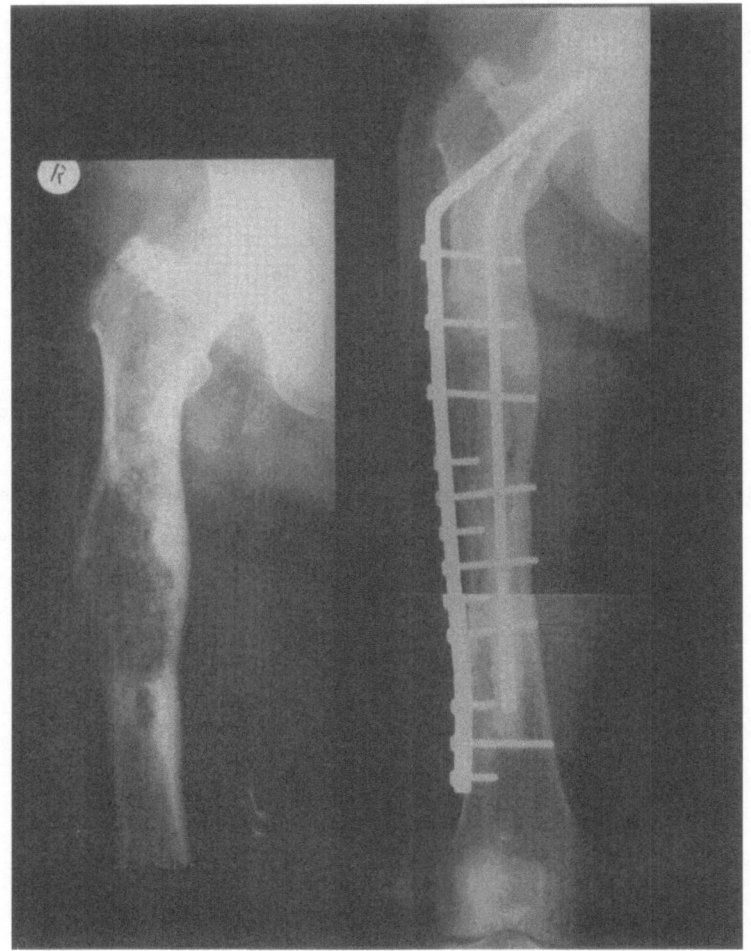

Relief of pain was observed in over 70% and satisfactory
healing and functional results in about 80%.

The median survival time was 18 months.

Most authors agree that radiation therapy plays an integral
role in the management of these patients.   Two points however
should be stressed: 1.   irradiation of the entire length of
the involved bone is important because of the propensity of the
tumor to spread along the medullary cavity;   2.   the use of
relatively high doses of radiation thereapy in a short period of

time produces better tumor control for prolonged periods of time.
The use of prophylactic internal fixation and radiation therapy
for the treatment of an impending fracture particularly in
weight-bearing bones of large osteolytic lesions has received
increasing publicity in recent years.   The primary
 indication for this method of treatment is as follows:
1.   the existence of a definite danger of fracture;   2.   relatively
isolated lesion;   3.   relatively localized disease and 4. satisfactory condition of the patient who should in general be fully
ambulatory and pursuing a normal life.

It is thus possible to achieve an immediate rehabilitation
of a cancer patient with pathological fracture by means of an
osteosynthesis which can tolerate maximum stress.

IMMUNOTHERAPY AS ADJUVANT TREATMENT FOR RESIDUAL TUMORS

J. Stjernswärd

The relevance of tumor immunology depends partly on the demonstration that malignant transformation is associated with specific immunogenic changes which provoke tumor-retarding immune reactions in the primary host.   In the cancer patient, postulated immunological surveillance mechanisms have been out-flanked, which makes the interpretation of immunological investigations difficult.

Positive results on immunotherapy in animal models are usually not reproducible in humans.   The irrelevance of many of these animal models for therapy in man must be recognized.

More than 400 ongoing controlled clinical studies are registered exploring immunotherapy but it is questionable how many of these will give conclusive answers, negative or positive due to e.g. prevalent deficiencies in the clinical trial design. The relevance of existing positive results on 'immunotherapy' in strictly controlled studies may still be questioned due to e.g. sample size.   Unknown prognostic factors disbalancing the randomized arms in the clinical trials cannot be excluded as an explanation for false positive answers, although statistically significant.

To date the medical community has not been convinced by existing data, and rightly so, that adjuvant 'immunotherapy' for residual disease works as judged from routine treatments applied. Adjuvant immunotherapy is still at the experimental stage with more promises and hopes than positive results in the clinic.

INDEX

INDEX

INDEX